Reaching *for* Health

The Australian women's health movement and public policy

Reaching *for* Health

The Australian women's health movement and public policy

Gwendolyn Gray Jamieson

Australian
National
University

E PRESS

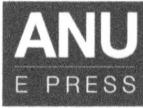

ANU E PRESS

Published by ANU E Press
The Australian National University
Canberra ACT 0200, Australia
Email: anuepress@anu.edu.au
This title is also available online at http://epress.anu.edu.au

National Library of Australia Cataloguing-in-Publication entry

Author: Gray Jamieson, Gwendolyn.

Title: Reaching for health [electronic resource] : the Australian women's health
               movement and public policy / Gwendolyn Gray Jamieson.

ISBN: 9781921862687 (ebook) 9781921862670 (pbk.)

Notes: Includes bibliographical references.

Subjects: Birth control--Australia--History.
               Contraception--Australia--History.
               Sex discrimination against women--Australia--History.
               Women's health services--Australia--History.
               Women--Health and hygiene--Australia--History.
               Women--Social conditions--History.

Dewey Number: 362.1982

Cover design and layout by ANU E Press

Contents

Preface

In sifting through boxes and filing cabinets of material collected for this book, I am struck by how much attitudes towards women, and attitudes of women themselves, have changed since the 1970s. The argument that women are not genetically equipped to participate in public-sector life is not often heard today, for example. Where possible, therefore, I attempt to create a sense of the atmosphere in which the women's health movement emerged by including selected anecdotes and quotations. The passion and commitment of early Australian women's health movement activists and the extraordinary efforts they made to improve the circumstances of women's lives and to fill gaps in service provision can only be understood, I believe, in the context of the times. The intensity of the critiques they developed was a product of their inferior position, the scarcity of health information, the insensitivity of some health professionals and the gaps in available health services, leaving many needs unmet.

It is impossible within the pages of a single volume to document more than a fraction of the work done by members of the movement. Similarly, only a brief outline can be given of the influence of the movement on public policy in nine jurisdictions over 40 years. Moreover, although I have interviewed scores of women and collected mountains of documents, there is a wealth of experience that I have been unable to record and there are parts of the story about which little is now known.

Space also prevents me from naming the women and the handful of men who have played important roles. The text necessarily contains reference to a few women who carried out crucial work or held key positions. Such a mention should not, however, suggest a more important role or a greater contribution than women not mentioned at all. Indeed, so many women have been involved in so many arenas that it would be impossible to calculate individual contribution. All the women who were interviewed for this book either formally or informally are listed in Appendix 2. Where no reference is provided, the information presented derives from interviews or from personal involvement in the events described.

One of the difficult decisions I have had to make in writing is whether to use the past or the present tense when discussing the movement's ideas and the criticisms that developed. None of the problems that feminists identified in the early 1970s has disappeared, although some are less pressing than they were. For example, information about women's bodies and women's health is far more readily available now and medical attitudes are less patronising. Serious concerns remain, however, and the social health perspective that the movement has promoted since the early days is not yet central in mainstream debate. The past tense, therefore, is often inappropriate. Mixed time frames are therefore used but, try as I might to achieve stylistic elegance, even the casual reader will notice an ungainly 'wobbling' between tenses.

At the outset, my involvement in the Australian women's health movement must be declared. Since the mid-1980s, I have been an active member, first, of the ACT Women's Health Network and then of the Australian Women's Health Network (AWHN). I represented the ACT Women's Health Network on the Australian Capital Territory's Women's Health Advisory Committee (WHAC) from 1989 until 1996. From the early 1990s until 2008, I was a member of the Board and sometime President of Sexual Health and Family Planning ACT and represented the Australian Capital Territory on the Board of Sexual Health and Family Planning Australia (SH&FPA) from 2002 until 2008. I was a member of the interim management committee of AWHN in the early 1990s when the constitution was written and the organisation was incorporated, Convenor from 1995 to 1998, Deputy Convenor from 1998 until 2008 and Convenor again from 2008 onwards.

Acknowledgments

There are many people to thank for their assistance, support and encouragement during the production of this book—so many that I am afraid some will be overlooked. First and foremost, I thank the scores of women in the Australian women's health movement and in political parties, trade unions and bureaucracies who so generously gave their time to talk with me, formally and informally. Those interviewed are listed in Appendix 2. Women supported my research in many other ways as well. They provided me with contacts, made appointments for me with key policymakers and activists in their regions, gathered local women together to facilitate group discussion and, in some cases, even offered me a bed for the night. As well as agreeing to be interviewed, women gave me access to written materials and pointed me in the direction of relevant sources. Many have been willing to talk to me on the telephone, and answer follow-up questions sent by email. These women include Esther Alvares, Morven Andrews, Moira Carmody, Karin Cheyne, Cathy Crawford, Denele Crozier, Glynis Flower, Vig Geddes, Robyn Gregory, Jocelyn Hanson, Maree Hawken, Lekkie Hopkins, Judith Ion, Libby Lloyd, Toni Makkai, Lynnley McGrath, Roxanne McMurray, Heather Nancarrow, Cathy North, Anne O'Byrne, Andrea Shoebridge, Mandy Stringer, Tammy Vu, Veronica Wensing, Karen Willis and Faye Worner. Researching the history of the movement has been a socially rewarding experience. I have been privileged to meet many wonderful women and make new friends.

Dorothy Broom, Helen Keleher and Marian Sawer read the full draft manuscript and I thank all three for their invaluable comments and suggestions and for their friendship and support. Marian Sawer has been a wellspring of ideas, support and encouragement throughout the writing process. People who gave me excellent feedback on parts of the manuscript include Morven Andrews, Marilyn Beaumont, Justine Cairns, Denele Crozier, David Denham, Carolyn Frohmader, Peter Howe, Lynnley McGrath, Adele Murdolo, Anne O'Byrne and Kerreen Reiger. Kerreen Reiger gave me great assistance with the first half of Chapter 6, including providing documents, some of which were still in press at the time of writing. Marilyn Beaumont generously gave me a copy of her extensive notes on the four-year process through which abortion was decriminalised in Victoria.

My thanks go to those who helped me with photographs, including Tony Adams, Dorothy Broom, Peter Howe, Gail Radford and Romaine Rutnam. Tracey Wing, photographer extraordinaire, combed through her files, freely sharing her women's health collection with me. Ann Pettigrew, Genevieve Ebeck and Bridget Gilmour-Walsh volunteered to edit the manuscript—acts of generosity well beyond the bounds of friendship and filial duty. Peter Howe fixed leaky taps, regained control of errant formatting and supplied me with relevant press clippings.

Staff at the Australian National Library cheerfully and efficiently helped me find sources and locate obscure references. I thank Duncan Beard and the staff of ANU E Press for their assistance and cooperation and the ANU Publications Subsidy Committee for its grant. The book was written during my time as an Adjunct Fellow in the School of Politics and International Relations, Research School of Social Sciences, College of Arts and Social Sciences, at The Australian National University. I thank the University for supporting my work and providing congenial surroundings in which to write.

Abbreviations

ABS	Australian Bureau of Statistics
ABSP	Alternative Birthing Services Program
ACCHS	Aboriginal Community Controlled Health Service
ACM	Australian College of Midwives
ACON	AIDS Council of New South Wales
ACSSA	Australian Centre for the Study of Sexual Assault
ACT	Australian Capital Territory
ACTU	Australian Council of Trade Unions
ACTWHN	ACT Women's Health Network
AD	Australian Democrats
AHMAC	Australian Health Ministers Advisory Council
AH&MRC	Aboriginal Health and Medical Research Council of New South Wales
AIHW	Australian Institute of Health and Welfare
ALMA	Australian Lesbian Medical Association
ALP	Australian Labor Party
ALRA	Association for the Legal Right to Abortion
AMA	Australian Medical Association
AMS	Aboriginal Medical Service
ANF	Australian Nursing Federation
ARHA	Australian Reproductive Health Alliance
ATSIC	Aboriginal and Torres Strait Islander Commission
AVO	apprehended violence order
AWHN	Australian Women's Health Network
BCNA	Breast Cancer Network Australia

C by C	Children by Choice
CAAC	Central Australian Aboriginal Congress
CASA	Centres Against Sexual Assault
CEDAW	Convention on the Elimination of All Forms of Discrimination against Women
CEP	Community Employment Program
COAG	Council of Australian Governments
COAL	Coalition of Activist Lesbians
COCAITH	Coalition on Criminal Assault in the Home
CR	consciousness raising
CWA	Country Women's Association
DES	diethylstilboestrol
DOHA	Department of Health and Ageing
DPIA	Disabled Peoples International Australia
DVCS	Domestic Violence Crisis Service
DVRCV	Domestic Violence Resource Centre Victoria
FaHCSIA	Department of Families, Housing, Community Services and Indigenous Affairs
FORWAARD	Foundation of Rehabilitation with Aboriginal Alcohol Related Difficulties
FVIP	Family Violence Intervention Program
FVPLS	Family Violence Prevention Legal Service
FVPP	Family Violence Partnership Program
FVRAP	Family Violence Regional Activities Program
EMSN	Extended Medicare Safety Net
GLBT	gay, lesbian, bisexual and transgender
GLBTIQ	gay, lesbian, bisexual, transgender, intersex and queer

HCC	Hospitals and Charities Commission
HHSC	Health and Hospitals Services Commission
HRT	hormone replacement therapy
HRWWC	Hunter Region Women's Working Centre
IUD	intrauterine device
IWD	International Women's Day
IWDVS	Immigrant Women's Domestic Violence Service
IWHS	Immigrant Women's Health Service
IWOT	Independent Women's Organisations of Tasmania
LPA	Liberal Party of Australia
LWCHC	Leichhardt Women's Community Health Centre
MC	Maternity Coalition
MCWH	Multicultural Centre for Women's Health
MGPs	Midwifery Group Practices
MWSAS	Migrant Women's Support and Accommodation Service
NACCHO	National Aboriginal Community Controlled Health Organisation
NAIHO	National Aboriginal and Islander Health Organisation
NASASV	National Association of Services against Sexual Violence
NECB	non-English cultural background
NESB	non-English-speaking background
NESBWHS	Non-English Speaking Background Women's Health Strategy
NGO	non-governmental organisation
NHHRC	National Health and Hospitals Reform Commission
NHMRC	National Health and Medical Research Council
NHS	National Health Service

NWH Program	National Women's Health Program
NWHP	National Women's Health Policy
NIFVGP	National Indigenous Family Violence Grants Program
NMA	Nursing Mothers Association
NOHSC	National Occupational Health and Safety Commission
NPY	Ngaanyatjarra Pitjantjatjara Yankunytjatjara
NQDVRS	North Queensland Domestic Violence Resource Service
NT	Northern Territory
OATSIH	Office of Aboriginal and Torres Strait Islander Health
OECD	Organisation for Economic Cooperation and Development
OHS	occupational health and safety
OSW	Office of the Status of Women
OWN	Older Women's Network
PADV	Partnerships Against Domestic Violence
PANDA	Post and Antenatal Depression Association
PANDSI	Post and Antenatal Depression Support and Information
PCP	Primary Care Partnership
PGPD	Parliamentary Group on Population and Development
PHOFA	Public Health Outcomes Funding Agreement
PND	postnatal depression
PNDSA	Postnatal Depression Support Association
PTSD	post-traumatic stress disorder
QWHN	Queensland Women's Health Network
RACOG	Royal Australian College of Obstetricians and Gynaecologists
RANZCOG	Royal Australian and New Zealand College of Gynaecologists

RCA	Reproductive Choice Australia
REWP	Refuge Ethnic Workers Program
RHS	Reproductive Health Service
RSI	repetitive strain injury
SA	South Australia
SAAP	Supported Accommodation Assistance Program
SACS	Social and Community Services
SANDS	Stillbirth and Neonatal Death Support
SARC	Sexual Assault Resource Centre
SASS	Sexual Assault Support Service
SH&FPA	Sexual Health and Family Planning Australia
SHFPACT	Sexual Health and Family Planning ACT
SIDS	sudden infant death syndrome
TGA	Therapeutic Goods Administration
TUTA	Trade Union Training Authority
UN	United Nations
VAW Strategy	Violence Against Women Strategy
VicHealth	Victorian Health Promotion Foundation
VLRC	Victorian Law Reform Commission
WA	Western Australia
WAAC	Women's Abortion Action Campaign
WARS	Women's Addiction and Recovery Service
WAWHO	Western Australian Women's Health Organisation
WCAG	Women's Centre Action Group
WEL	Women's Electoral Lobby
WESNET	Women's Emergency Services Network

WESP	Women's Emergency Services Program
WHAC	Women's Health Advisory Committee
WHAM	Women in Health around Melbourne
WHAV	Women's Health Association of Victoria
WHIRCCA	Women's Health and Information Resource and Crisis Centres Association
WHO	World Health Organisation
WHSU	Women's Health Strategy Unit
WHV	Women's Health Victoria
WICH	Women in Industry Contraception and Health
WISN	Women's Incest and Survivors Network
WL	women's liberation
WODEB	Women of Different Ethnic Backgrounds
WWDA	Women with Disabilities Australia
WWDACT	Women with Disabilities ACT

Introduction

> Once upon a time, before the feminists carried their banners emblazoned with the women's sign and the inscription 'Women's Liberation', there was a luxury tax on the contraceptive pill. (Stevens 1995:13)

When the women's health movement burst onto the Australian political scene as part of the resurgent women's movement, resentment about social arrangements was intense. Women knew how it felt to be trivialised, disbelieved and dismissed. They had experienced frustration, indignity and stigmatisation in their daily lives. For many, encounters with the health system were unsatisfactory and often humiliating and traumatising. In the early 1970s, the gatherings organised by mobilising feminists provided an opportunity for women to ventilate their concerns, often for the first time. The gender order would never be quite the same again.

At a packed public 'speak-out' organised by Melbourne feminists in early 1973, poor health care and lack of relevant information emerged as the dominant concerns. Women told stories that shocked those listening, stories that were confirmed by the doctors, nurses and healthcare workers who were present. Women's health care was condemned as too often 'demeaning, discriminatory, judgemental and of poor quality' (Hull 1986:14). Sydney women reached a similar verdict at another gathering a few weeks later. Unmarried women told of lectures that implied immorality and promiscuity when they requested contraceptives, which were often denied them, and married women talked about the difficulties and the humiliation of requesting an abortion. Older women reported being unable to get information about menopause and of being summarily dismissed or referred to a psychiatrist. All women shared the distress they felt at being made to feel 'dirty, shameful, unbalanced, neurotic, stupid and guilty'. Out of these meetings, the first dedicated women's health groups were formed. The intention was to set up centres where skilled medical care would be available, where women could speak openly about their lives and share their experiences 'in an atmosphere of warmth, acceptance and understanding' (Cooper and Spencer 1978:149).

Feminists, as well as feeling anger about their encounters with the health system, objected strongly to the entrenched gender order. From the 'best' clubs to local pubs, women were frequently excluded from sporting and social venues. The bar obliging married women to resign from permanent jobs in the Public Service had been lifted in 1966 but women were still largely absent from public-sector life. Domestic violence, rape and child sexual abuse were not discussed openly. A feminist-produced sex education pamphlet for young women was branded 'obscene' by major newspapers in 1971 and abortion-squad detectives carried out investigations at Sydney girls' schools, even though the brochure had been approved by parents' and citizens' associations (Stevens 1995:14–15). Sanitary pads were wrapped in brown paper and hidden under pharmacy counters and women's sexuality was still depicted in Australian obstetrical and gynaecological textbooks from a heterosexual perspective with women's natural aspirations portrayed as marriage and mothering (Koutroulis 1990).

There were few publicly funded support services for women or anyone else who needed them. After more than 20 years of conservative national government, the Australian welfare system was in a primordial state, having missed out on most of the expansion that had taken place in comparable countries after World War II (Gray 2003; Jones 1990:29–48). The hospital and medical system was sorely in need of reform; financial barriers to access were high and the range of services was narrow (Gray 1984, 1991; Sax 1984). Aboriginal communities and Aboriginal health were ravaged by the combined impacts of colonisation, racism and government policies. Despite high immigration rates in the 1950s and 1960s, services for newly arrived people were scarce. It was extremely difficult to find an interpreter, for example, even in the largest hospitals in the country. There was no public income support for single parents, and about 80 per cent of court orders for family maintenance were never honoured. Only the wealthy could afford child care. Some lone mothers, who needed paid work to survive, took small children with them to early morning cleaning jobs. Others left them at home to take themselves to school, sometimes hours before the starting bell.

It was in this context that the embryonic women's health movement made its first faltering efforts to respond to the calls for help that were being made. As one participant remembers the early situation: 'the phone calls and letters were coming in from women everywhere…They desperately needed information on abortion, contraception, and many other things that were affecting their health so badly. And we didn't know the answers!' (Zelda D'Aprano, quoted in Robertson n.d.:Ch. 16).

With few resources and, in many cases, very little knowledge about politics or medical care, small groups of women set out not only to provide health services but also to achieve fundamental social change and public policy transformation. From the beginning, they knew that many of the circumstances of women's lives, not least their second-class status, had a detrimental impact on their health and needed to be changed. They articulated the problems arising from gender roles, identified domestic violence as a serious women's health issue and broke the silence surrounding sexual assault. Where they found glaring gaps in the services available they tried to fill them by establishing services themselves: health centres, sexual assault services and refuges for women and children who had nowhere to go were set up on precarious foundations. They set up telephone help lines to provide information and support. They took to the streets to fight for a woman's right to choose a safe abortion and they campaigned on factory floors and within the union movement to modernise occupational health and safety regimes. Mothers' groups agitated for women's control of childbirth and to achieve maternity-care reform. Feminist-inspired training modules for the police, the judiciary and other relevant professions were developed, so that sexual assault and violence services might be delivered more appropriately. Healthcare providers were trained and educated about feminist health perspectives. The underlying philosophy was to provide services and support 'by women, for women'. Critiques of the social, political and economic organisation of society were developed, along with strategies for how to promote change. In carrying out this work, women faced huge obstacles, particularly a shortage of resources of all kinds.

As time went on, it became increasingly clear that the structural forces supporting the existing system were not going to be dislodged easily. In health, the power of organised medicine was brought to bear against every reform proposal, while pharmaceutical giants continued to peddle their wares. Bureaucracies—not accustomed to being challenged and comfortable with longstanding structures and practices—resisted new ideas, especially the notion that there should be separate women's services. In the cultural sphere, ideas proved to be durable, especially discourses around domestic violence and rape. And when women suggested changes that would improve their economic position, the power of business and its acolytes mobilised against them. Whether it was community-based child care, national superannuation or paid maternity leave, the arguments against were that markets do a better job and are cheaper for the public purse. The political environment of the very early years was, however, a rare moment—one that was unusually favourable for the articulation of radical change proposals.

Radical Reform on the Radar: The context of the early women's health movement

In public policy terms, the context in which proposals are developed has a strong impact on outcomes. Some political contexts facilitate change while others retard it. The environment in which the Australian women's health movement emerged presented perhaps a 'once in a lifetime' policy opportunity. Internationally, change was in the air as radical challenges to the status quo were mounted in all Organisation for Economic Cooperation and Development (OECD) countries. Equality-seeking social movements—interested in such issues as civil rights, peace, sexuality, the environment, self-help, and consumer, student, worker and women's issues—were generating proposals for root-and-branch reform of existing power relations.

In Australia, the health system was highly controversial. The publicly subsidised private health insurance system was inequitable, unpopular, complicated and expensive. Approximately 20 per cent of Australians had no health insurance coverage and hundreds of thousands had inadequate coverage. Frustration was widespread because the Liberal Coalition Government[1]—in power for more than 20 years—had failed to countenance reform except within the parameters of a private insurance regime. Competition between the major parties was intense as the Australian Labor Party (ALP), in opposition, developed a series of reform proposals that generated fierce public debates. Inside the ALP, opinions were divided between those who supported traditional Labor approaches to health, including a national, community-based medical service, staffed by salaried doctors, and those who supported the newer idea of universal health insurance. The former group opposed the entrenchment of the private fee-for-service medical practice that would come with national insurance because they thought it inimical to good health care. Many within the party, therefore, viewed health insurance as a transitional measure, a step along the way to a comprehensive public health service, which would have strong primary health care as its foundation (Gray 2003:274–5). Meanwhile, as well as women and other low-income groups, Aboriginal people found that the existing system failed to meet their needs for many reasons, not least of which was widely experienced racism. An Aboriginal health movement developed that led the way in establishing community-controlled primary healthcare centres, based on a social view of health. A social health perspective recognises the impact of political, social, economic, environmental and cultural factors on health outcomes. It points out that the full circumstances of people's lives need to be taken into account when considering healthcare options. Because life circumstances can be altered, strategies to achieve that change need to be developed. Income security, housing security, physical security and the like are essential components of improved population health. Moreover, disease-prevention strategies are fundamental elements of a health system, alongside treatment services. A social view of health is part of the cultural heritage of Aboriginal people. The women's health movement and the 'new' public health movement had to develop and articulate this perspective for themselves in the 1960s and 1970s.

---

1   While several parties are usually represented in the national Parliament, in practice, Australia has a two-party system. The Liberal Party of Australia (LPA) is the major party of the 'right' and, when in office nationally, it forms a coalition with the small, rural-based party, The Nationals. The ALP is the major party on the 'left'. The historical distance between the two parties on health and social policy has, however, gradually narrowed. Indeed, in 2011, analysts point to the centrism of both. There are two significant minor parties: the Australian Democrats (AD) and the Australian Greens. After 30 years of success, however, the electoral fortunes of the AD are presently in decline.

The Limits to Medicine

Internationally, health reform and healthy public policy movements were developing. Analyses of the limitations of modern, scientific medicine had been developing since the 1950s and provided a theoretical underpinning for structural change proposals. Twentieth-century advances in medical science, such as improvements in anaesthetics and blood transfusion, had helped to legitimise a focus on scientific medicine; however, epidemiological research suggested the need for a broader approach. Health experts began to argue that hospital and medical systems placed too much emphasis on treatment and high-tech cures and too little emphasis on prevention and support services. An individual explanation of the causes of health and illness was challenged by a social determinants approach, grounded in social, economic and political structures.

On the basis of work done in the United States, René Dubos drew early attention to the now well-known idea that medical science was not responsible for the nineteenth-century decline in mortality from infectious diseases. Rather, improvements came about as a result of public health measures, including improvements in water, air and sewage disposal (cited in Conrad 2004:6). This work was followed by that of McKeown and colleagues, who, in the 1950s, 1960s and 1970s, showed that declines in mortality in England and Wales in the nineteenth century were the result of social determinants: rising standards of living, including a healthier diet, improvements in housing and water quality and better sewerage and waste-disposal systems, accompanied by favourable trends in the relationship between some micro-organisms and human beings. Biomedical interventions had made little contribution (McKeown et al. 1975:391). Other work produced similar findings for Sweden, France, Ireland, Hungary and the United States (McKinlay and McKinlay 2004:8). Victor Fuchs' (1974) well-known work in the United States found that the very different health outcomes in the neighbouring States of Nevada and Utah were attributable to social determinants and lifestyle factors, rather than biomedical causes or health system differences.[2] The twentieth century probably presents a more mixed picture in that lifestyle factors, such as smoking cessation, and medical interventions have helped to improve population health.

The body of evidence about the importance of the social determinants has not been well accepted in scientific medical circles. As McKinlay and McKinlay (2004) report, the notion that modern medical care is not responsible for improvements in population health (as distinct from improving the outcomes

---

2   Thirty years later, major differences remain between health outcomes in the two States (Rodwin and Croce-Galis 2004).

of individual episodes of disease), is seen as 'heresy'. Lack of acceptance by the most powerful political group in the health landscape is the main reason that public investment in health services—beyond those produced in hospitals and doctors' offices—is low.

Community Health Movements and the 'New' Public Health

On the basis of emerging evidence, proposals to change health system structures were gradually developed. It is often argued that the internationally influential *Lalonde Report*, released in Canada in 1974, marks the birth of what is loosely called the 'new' public health. As in public policy generally, however, radical proposals are invariably built upon previous experience and action. From the early 1960s onwards, Canadian health experts developed a critique that was sceptical of excessive reliance on hospital and medical services. They argued for the establishment of community-based, community-controlled health centres where care would be provided by teams of health professionals, including allied health professionals. A full range of preventive and support programs would be delivered alongside treatment services.

The community-health movement in western Canada has its foundation in the strong cooperative movement that emerged in the Prairie Provinces about the beginning of the twentieth century. A municipal doctor scheme was instituted in the town of Sarnia, Saskatchewan, in 1914. The scheme expanded steadily, operating in hundreds of towns and villages by 1948 with some services established in neighbouring Provinces. A network of between 30 and 40 community health centres was set up in Saskatchewan by the early 1960s, where doctors who wished to accept a salary could practice (Taylor 1979:319). In terms of the ideas of the day, Canadian health system thinking was radical. The benefits of community participation in health decision making were endorsed by the Minister for National Health and Welfare, the Honourable John Monro, in 1969. In a statement that the Australian women's health movement would endorse, Munro argued that 'the key is contact, the place is the community, the concept is preventative...group practice, community health centres, mobile outpatient clinics, increased case findings through home visitation, greater availability of local alternative institutions, better home care, increased teamwork with community social agencies' (Munro 1969, quoted in Donner and Pederson 2004:5).

The Province of Quebec put many of these ideas into action. On the basis of recommendations in the *Castonguay Report*, released in 1967, a Province-wide network of community-controlled health centres was established from

1971 onwards (Government of Quebec 1970). The best centres provided comprehensive, holistic care and worked on an outreach model, making contact with the individuals for whom they were responsible in their catchment areas. In the same year, the health ministers of Canada set up an inquiry into community health centres, which reported in 1972 and recommended adoption by provincial governments (Health and Welfare Canada 1972). Community participation was stressed in the Manitoba Government's *White Paper on Health Policy*, released in 1972. The *Foulkes Report* (1973) in British Columbia recommended that health and social services be integrated, that investment be made in preventive services and that care be coordinated, with patients assisted to traverse their way through the system. The Ontario Health Planning Task Force in its 1974 report argued that primary health care should be the centre of the health system and that services should be comprehensive, continuous and delivered by teams of health professionals.

Thus, when the *Lalonde Report*, *A New Perspective on the Health of Canadians*, was published, it built upon Saskatchewan tradition, Quebec innovations and a decade and a half of discussion about how to achieve a more comprehensive health system. It argued for broad reforms, including the establishment of networks of community health centres.

By the late 1960s, community health and new public health movements began to appear outside Canada. A resurgent community health centre movement emerged in the United States[3] as the healthcare arm of the civil rights movement. An Aboriginal health movement and a community health movement developed alongside the women's health movement in Australia. In turn, by the time the World Health Organisation (WHO) produced the Alma Ata declaration in 1978, there was Canadian and Australian experience on which to draw. A social view of health, preventive primary health care, and improved environments for health, community participation and inter-sectoral action were all central to the WHO strategy of 'Health for All' by the year 2000.

The Aboriginal Health Movement

The Australian Aboriginal health movement arose in part from intense dissatisfaction with mainstream hospital and medical care, where a 'cultural chasm' separated Aboriginal people and mainstream service providers (Palmer and Short 1989:235; Saggers and Gray 1991:144, 147). In addition to discrimination and racism, user charges prevented low-income earners from accessing services. Recent research shows that health spaces need to be

---

3   There was a previous mobilisation in the 1920s.

'Aboriginal friendly', especially Aboriginal-women friendly, to allow people to feel welcome and comfortable. Where everything in the space pertains to the dominant culture, colonial stereotypes are 'reinscribed' (Fredericks 2009:41). In order to provide culturally appropriate and accessible services, the Aboriginal Medical Service (AMS) was set up in 1971 at Redfern, Sydney, by a community group that included Shirley Smith and Gordon Briscoe. Within a year, the Aboriginal population of Sydney had increased from a couple of thousand to 32 000 people as a result of freedom from confinement on reserves and subsequent congregation in cities in search of a means of survival (Foley 1984:112). Like early women's health centres, Redfern AMS opened in extremely humble premises and relied on donations and volunteer staff. Also as in women's health, it gradually secured precarious funding after extensive lobbying and submissions and, over the years, was able to expand. By 1974, Redfern was 'a free first-class medical service, created by Aborigines for Aborigines in the Redfern area, with similar facilities at the La Perouse settlement and with medical teams, headed by Aborigines, visiting country settlements' (Briscoe 1974:169).

Redfern AMS, the first community-controlled health service in Australia, was ahead of its time (Palmer and Short 1989:235) and it inspired Aboriginal communities across the country to set up their own health services. The Central Australian Aboriginal Congress Health Centre in Alice Springs, the Fitzroy Aboriginal Health Service in Melbourne and Derbarl Yerrigan Health Service in Perth were all established in 1973. In 1974, at a national AMS meeting in Albury, New South Wales, it was proposed that a national health organisation be established. The National Aboriginal and Islander Health Organisation (NAIHO) came into being in 1976—its first meeting funded by Redfern AMS. An office was established in Melbourne and the organisation survived on donations for nine years until it received its first government funds in 1985. In 1992, its name was changed to the National Aboriginal Community Controlled Health Organisation (NACCHO), and in 1997 it was funded to establish a secretariat in Canberra—a location that facilitates access to policymakers. Similar peak organisations have been established at the State and Territory levels (NACCHO web site).

The Aboriginal health movement takes a social health perspective, focusing on support, empowerment and community control through elected boards of management, local participation, disease prevention and provision of care by multidisciplinary teams. Aboriginal health is defined by NACCHO as

> not just the physical wellbeing of an individual but the social, emotional and cultural wellbeing of the whole community in which each individual is able to achieve their full potential, thereby bringing about the total wellbeing of their community. It is a whole-of-life view and includes the cyclical concept of life-death-life. (NACCHO web site)

From the beginning, Aboriginal Community Controlled Health Services (ACCHSs) aimed to deliver holistic, comprehensive and culturally appropriate care, with a preventive and health education focus. The Central Australian Aboriginal Congress (CAAC), in a submission applying for Commonwealth funding in 1974, argued that the new centre being proposed should have 'both a preventive and [a] curative approach', should be oriented towards the community and should provide appropriate training for Aboriginal health workers (Perkins 1975:32). The emphasis on community participation and community control was partly based on awareness that such structures can readily respond to changing needs—a bottom-up rather than a top-down approach (Bartlett and Boffa 2001). In the view of the congress, health cannot be considered separately from people's access to other resources, such as housing, education, employment, land rights, food, recreation facilities and community development (Rosewarne et al. 2007:10). The new centre was to have a good relationship with secondary and tertiary services to provide what, in present-day language, is called 'continuity of care'.

The origins of a holistic health perspective among Aboriginal people appear to be embedded in the importance placed on each member of the community. When Grace Kong, an Aboriginal women's health nurse practitioner in New South Wales, was asked whether her family was proud of her achievements, she replied: 'I think that with Koories our outlook on life is very different from yours. Every single person that belongs to a Koori community is important, regardless of what their role is, so that the fact of what I have achieved is nice but so what?' (Kong quoted in Smith 1992:27).

Moreover, it appears that there is no word meaning 'health' in Aboriginal languages. Words that might mean something like the English word suggest an approach to wellbeing that encompasses all aspects of life, including food, housing and family—a truly social perspective. The Redfern AMS founders thought that a health service should be able to meet the day-to-day needs of consumers (Briscoe 1974:170). A CAAC submission in 1974 recognised that the curative services provided by European medical systems 'did not and could not' meet Aboriginal needs. By 1976, it was being argued that 'healthy living cannot be developed without total community development under total community control' (Rosewarne et al. 2007:10).[4]

The Aboriginal concept of community health is exemplified in the rationale for women's stress-free days organised by Aboriginal health workers in La Perouse, New South Wales, in 2001. The primary concern in this case was not for women

4   This conclusion was reached by Aboriginal people in Australia prior to and independently of the WHO's adoption of a social view of health at the end of the 1970s. The WHO's own revision of thinking was strongly influenced by the failure to improve population health in developing countries through the provision of conventional medical services (Cueto 2004).

but for local youth. The reasoning is that the best way to empower young people is to empower their mothers, who benefit from the support networks formed as they come together (Aboriginal and Islander Health Worker Journal 2001a:14).

About the same time that Aboriginal people were setting up their first community-controlled health services, health system restructuring plans were being developed in the States, particularly in New South Wales. Community-based services were being proposed, including aged care and mental health services. A few limited-scale community health centres were set up in New South Wales, providing child health services, dental and mental health care and rehabilitation, domiciliary nursing and home-care services. Health education outreach teams worked from some centres. In 1972, the *Health Commission Act* was passed, which was informed by social health principles and provided for the representation of consumer interests. Ideas from New South Wales spread to other States through a body of Commonwealth and State officials known as the Hospitals and Allied Services Advisory Council, set up to advise Australian health ministers (Sax 1980; Shea 1970). Other States gradually enacted similar legislation but the capacity of Australia's sub-national jurisdictions to advance policy reform was severely constrained by the financial centralisation of the Australian federation. In other words, spare cash was, and still is, in short supply in State and Territory coffers.

The reforms being developed in the Australian States were in line with historical ALP support for locally based medical services. The new ideas found their way into ALP policy partly through the office of the leader, Gough Whitlam, who was keenly interested in the problems of the rapidly expanding, under-serviced, outer-metropolitan areas of Sydney and Melbourne. Members of Whitlam's electoral office were in regular contact with officials in the Health Department of New South Wales. They were supplied with research papers and detailed policy proposals.[5] By 1971, the ALP had developed plans for comprehensive health system reform, including regionalised, community-based services, community health centres, refurbished hospitals and national health insurance. 'Preventive, occupational and rehabilitation services' were to be 'key elements' of the health system (Sax 1984:100–3).

The women's health movement in Australia, then, emerged at a time when ideas about the social causes of ill health were beginning to run hot. The movement drew upon these ideas, endorsed them and contributed to their development and expansion. Together with the Aboriginal and community health movements, it played a pioneering role in taking health and health care out of the personal

---

5 Information about health policy developments in New South Wales and other Australian States and about contact between the New South Wales Health Department and Whitlam's office was provided by the late Dr Sidney Sax, Director of Health Research and Planning in New South Wales in the 1960s and early 1970s and Chairman of the Hospitals and Health Services Commission, 1973–78.

sphere and into the public domain, understanding that good health for all is impossible without social and economic changes (Donner and Pederson 2004:2). As commentators have argued, the principles underpinning women's health services are 'almost identical' to those of the new public health and community health (Auer et al 1987:2; Dwyer 1992a:212). In Table 1, the similarities between approaches are readily apparent.

Table 1

OLD PUBLIC HEALTH	NEW PUBLIC HEALTH	FEMINIST HEALTH	ABORIGINAL HEALTH
Focus on improving physical infrastructure to provide adequate housing, clean water and sanitation.	Focus on physical infrastructure, but also on social support, behaviour and lifestyle.	Focus on physical infrastructure, but also on social support and empowerment, especially through information provision and respectful interactions.	Focus on improving physical infrastructure to provide adequate housing, clean water, sanitation and so on, but equally on social support and empowerment through community development.
Legislation the key policy mechanism especially in the nineteenth century.	Legislation and policy rediscovered as crucial tools for public health.	Legislation and policy seen as crucial tools for women's health, especially in relation to the social determinants of health.	Not much expected from legislation and policy in view of past experiences. Some emphasis on lobbying to change the shape of healthcare delivery system.
Medical profession has a central place.	Recognition of inter-sectoral action as crucial. Medicine only one of the many professions contributing.	Recognition of inter-sectoral action as crucial. Medicine only one of many professions and service providers contributing.	Recognition of inter-sectoral action as crucial. Medicine, including traditional medicine, only one of many professions and service providers contributing.
In nineteenth century, public health was one of a series of social movements that worked to improve living conditions. Primarily expert driven but some legitimation of community movement. Progressively more expert dominated in twentieth century.	Philosophy places strong emphasis on community participation, but, in practice, this is not often achieved, despite some real successes.	Philosophy places strong emphasis on women's participation and community participation. Often achieved at the local level. Consumers and professionals considered to be equals.	Philosophy places strong emphasis on community control and community participation the sine qua non. Consumers and professionals considered to be equals.

OLD PUBLIC HEALTH	NEW PUBLIC HEALTH	FEMINIST HEALTH	ABORIGINAL HEALTH
Epidemiology legitimate research method.	Many methodologies recognised as legitimate.	Many methodologies legitimate. Validation of women's experiences.	Many methodologies recognised as legitimate. Validation of people's own experiences.
Focus on disease prevention. Health is seen as absence of illness.	Focus on disease prevention, health promotion and a positive definition of health.	Focus on disease prevention and health promotion, with emphasis on group sessions, support and education services and community development. A positive definition of health.	Focus on disease prevention, with strong emphasis on culturally appropriate, integrated, holistic care. A positive, holistic definition of health.
Primary concern was the prevention of infectious and contagious threats to human health.	Concern with all threats to health (including chronic disease and mental health issues) but also growing concern with sustainability and viability of the physical environment.	Concern with all threats to health, including neglected issues, such as mental health. Concern with avoidable health inequalities. Focus on the social determinants of health, especially economic, social, political and cultural threats to health. Concern with sustainability and viability of the physical environment.	Concern with all threats to health, including seriously neglected issues. Concern with avoidable health inequalities. Focus on the social determinants of health especially racist, economic, social and political threats. Concern with preservation of the physical environment and access to land.

In Table 1, feminist and Aboriginal health principles have been added to Fran Baum's (2007) comparison of the main elements of the old public health and the new public health. The parallels are clear, especially between the Aboriginal health movement and the women's health movement, as Jenny Baker (1998) has noted. In her view, non-Aboriginal women's struggles for control over their bodies are similar to Aboriginal struggles for the rights of freedom and control over their own lives against *Aborigines Protection Acts* and other acts of 'confinement and segregation'. She points out that collectives were set up and celebrated in both movements. Moreover, both movements, she argues, 'fundamentally challenge the Australian health system to pursue primary health care and community development, based on community management, input and ownership' (Baker 1998:92).

The harmony between the principles of the three movements was an important factor facilitating policy implementation in the early 1970s. Policymakers at the Hospitals and Health Services Commission (HHSC) had developed plans for a national community health scheme and women's and Aboriginal health centres fitted comfortably into the framework. Officers of the commission helped, as far as possible, to overcome the obstacles put in place by sub-national bureaucracies and by antagonistic vested interests. Dr Sidney Sax, Chairman of the HHSC, had a strong background in primary health care. Along with Dr Gwen Greenman, his wife, he had provided medical services for poor people in South Africa. The two had set up a large community health centre in Alexandra Township, a violent, overcrowded settlement on the edge of Johannesburg (Royal Australasian College of Physicians web site). After arriving in Australia, Dr Sax participated in work to develop community health services for New South Wales, and, in his senior health policy position for the Whitlam Government, he was well placed to support strong primary health care, including separate women's health centres. This policy direction was also championed by some members of the Labor Government. The reform ideas being articulated posed a major challenge to both health system structures and society's wider institutions.

When the Whitlam Government lost office, there were six funded women's health centres and 21 refuges approved for funding. The first national women's health conference had been held in Brisbane in 1975 and was opened by the Prime Minister. The first Commonwealth funding had been provided for Aboriginal-controlled health centres and a network of community health centres had been set up. The period of the Fraser Commonwealth Government (1975–83), however, brought severe cuts in community health program funding under which most women's health centres were supported. The centres were forced to turn to State governments for funding—a long process but one that eventually bore fruit.

Despite the unfavourable political climate at the Commonwealth level after 1975, the women's health movement continued to expand and to campaign for policy reform on a number of fronts. Several State and Territory governments took positive action in the 1980s, developing women's health policies and strategies. The movement staged a second national women's health conference in Adelaide in 1985. Work at the grassroots level slowly percolated upwards, creating another policy opportunity when a second Commonwealth government willing to support women's health came to power. The Hawke Labor Government, elected in 1983, found that women's health, including maternity-care reform and occupational health and safety (OHS), was a major concern when it held consultations for its National Agenda for Women. Policy action was announced, a consultation and policy development process was undertaken and, in 1989, Australia became the first and only country to implement a national policy on women's health.

Australia's First National Women's Health Policy

The 1989 National Women's Health Policy (NWHP) is the high point of policy achievement for the movement. Indeed, the 1980s can be seen as the golden years of policy achievement. The NWHP identified six underpinning principles: a social view of health; a lifespan approach without undue focus on the reproductive years; participation by women in decision making as consumers and providers; women's rights as healthcare consumers, including privacy, confidentiality, informed consent and the right to be treated with dignity; the right to accessible information in order to make informed decisions; and the need for accurate data and research, including women's views about health. The seven priority issues selected were reproductive health and sexuality, the health of ageing women, emotional and mental health, violence against women, occupational health and safety, the health needs of carers and the health effects of sex-role stereotyping. The five key actions developed to advance the priorities were improvements in health services for women, provision of health information, research and data collection on women's health, women's participation in health decision making and the training of healthcare providers (Commonwealth of Australia 1989:78–81).

The development of affordable, acceptable, accessible and appropriate health services was to take place through a 'dual strategy'. A separate women's health sector would examine new issues and develop new models of practice in participation with women on a day-to-day basis in a 'comprehensive and accessible' network of primary healthcare services. Practice in the separate sector would lead by example, influencing the way the mainstream operated (Commonwealth of Australia 1989:82). During the consultations, women expressed strong support for separate women's services that would be low cost, multidisciplinary, holistic, located in one place and would provide illness-prevention information and advice. Women said they wanted to participate in decisions about health and treatment and they looked forward to being able to choose services that had been tailored to meet their needs. A separate women's health sector was essential to the improvement of mainstream services (Commonwealth of Australia 1989:60–1; Dwyer 1992a:213).

By the early 1990s, experience showed that changes had already been wrought. Feminist criticisms of inappropriate minor tranquilliser use, for example, had become respectable and were acknowledged in the mainstream after a decade of lobbying. Another example was that the work done in rape crisis centres had become a model for more appropriate policies and practices in mainstream services. In two decades, the 'movement had extended the territory' of what could be discussed 'in mainstream debates about how to care for women' (Dwyer 1992b:26).

The National Women's Health Policy and Program continued to advance women's health for years after its launch. Having the ideas and concerns of Australian women written in black and white in a national policy document not only increased their currency but also bestowed legitimacy. Policymakers and activists alike could refer to the principles enunciated and the evidence presented. The separate women's health sector was enlarged and a wide assortment of projects and programs was supported, creating a strong basis for innovation and political action.

The election of the neo-liberal Howard Commonwealth Government in 1996, however, ushered in more than a decade of antipathy towards the women's movement. In 1997, responsibility for the provision of women's health services was handed over to the States and Territories, although the national share of funding was maintained. Shortly after the Howard Government was elected, a delegation from the Australian Women's Health Network (AWHN) arranged a meeting with the Minister Assisting the Prime Minister for the Status of Women. Members of the delegation were taken aback when the minister opened the conversation by asking, 'Well, girls, is there anything left to achieve in women's health?'

In 2004, the Commonwealth made an unsuccessful attempt to exclude women's health services from the funding flowing through public health financing channels. During this period, the States and Territories, for their part, all maintained existing services, although no conditions requiring them to do so were attached to Commonwealth funding. Although the Commonwealth policy environment was hostile, at the sub-national level, women in government and outside were able to use the policy to support their arguments and claims.

From 1995 onwards, the women's health movement consistently called for revision and updating of the NWHP and for a resumption of Commonwealth responsibility but there was no policy response. A change in direction took place in 2007, however, when the ALP heard the message and committed itself to a new NWHP should it win the next national election. This was the only women-specific policy that the major parties took to the election—an indication of changing attitudes to women's issues and the importance of women's vote since the 1970s.

The Relevance of the 1970s for Present-Day Health Reform

The structural proposals developed in the 1970s have lost none of their relevance. Indeed, they might be even more relevant in the twenty-first century as lifestyle factors such as obesity increasingly undermine health at the same time as increasing the cost of hospital and medical services. Without structural change, a destructive spiral is created: more people suffer from more serious and chronic illnesses, the costs of treatment continue to climb, rendering the prospect of significant investment in primary health care and prevention increasingly unlikely.

Nor have women's health priorities lost their relevance. Violence, sexual assault and sexual and reproductive health problems persist. Preventive health and support services are still in short supply. Mental health—long the Cinderella of health issues and a major concern for women, as the NWHP pointed out—is at last receiving more policy attention but huge shortcomings remain. The community-based primary healthcare sector is small and fragile, after many years of neglect. Financial barriers to hospital and medical services are not as high as they were in the pre-Medicare 1970s but steadily increasing user charges are preventing people, especially low-income earners, from using services. Geographical access remains a serious problem: all services are scarce outside the cities, while access to culturally appropriate care is still a priority for non-Anglo-Australian women.

All the while, the international health research community, including the WHO, continues to produce evidence endorsing a social health perspective. The WHO released an influential report in 2008 that argues that daily living conditions—including a healthy environment, the availability of fairly paid work, economic security, a fair distribution of resources and power and access to a comprehensive range of services—are essential for decent health. Recommendations include political empowerment for the marginalised, gender equity[6] and greater equity in all public policies, including taxation. The report points to serious, avoidable health inequalities, not only between countries but also between different groups within single countries. It presents the astonishing example of a 28-year discrepancy in life expectancy between men living in different suburbs of Glasgow (WHO 2008a:32).

In keeping with this evidence, the social determinants of health are now more widely acknowledged in Australian policymaking circles. All the major policy

---

6 Gender, in contrast with biological sex, has been described as 'the array of socially and culturally constructed roles, personality traits, attitudes, behaviours, values, relative power, and influence that society ascribes to the two sexes on a differential basis' (Canadian Institutes of Health Research 2000).

documents of recent years recognise the structural causes of ill health, including acknowledgment of gender as an important determinant. A gender perspective, like a diversity perspective, recognises that differently placed people—in this case, men and women—experience health and illness differently and that different expectations and norms influence experience and behaviour. Similarly, it is recognised that socially and culturally determined roles and expectations influence outcomes for people, including those with disabilities and those from different income and ethnic groups. Moreover, discussion documents argue that preventable health inequalities can—*and should*—be reduced.

So why is it, then, that although the need for structural reform through investment in preventive primary health care is recognised, so little action is taken? The answer lies chiefly in the immense political power of opposing interests. In the first place, there are the vested interests of providers, who benefit financially from the system as it stands. As the biggest single industry in OECD countries, the health sector provides high incomes and profits and prestigious positions for large numbers of service and technology producers. In Australia, system arrangements directly augment incomes and profits through hefty public subsidies. Change is vehemently resisted when it threatens to disturb existing distributions of income and status (see, for example, Alford 1975; Evans 1998; Sax 1984). Another barrier, as mentioned, is the increasing cost to the public purse of expensive hospital and medical services. A related factor is that business-sector interests are a less direct but nevertheless powerful set of opposing forces. By promoting the value of balanced budgets, low taxation and a market distribution of goods and services, they make it politically difficult for governments to find new money for investment in areas such as primary health care.

Under the Rudd and Gillard Commonwealth Governments, a small window of opportunity for reform was opened. The Commonwealth has claimed health reform as a priority since 2007 and incremental responses based on the recommendations of recent inquiries are beginning to be introduced. Action includes a commitment to 'closing the gap' between Aboriginal and non-Aboriginal health outcomes, for which some funding has been allocated. Ironically, it is under the top-down Northern Territory Emergency Response that Aboriginal-controlled health services are being expanded. While it is too early to assess the impact of the changes, the Rudd and Gillard health reforms are discussed further in the concluding chapter.

About this Volume

This account of the history and politics of the Australian women's health movement traces its presence as an integral part of the wider reform movements of the 1970s, particularly the health reform movements. It provides a record of some of the work women have done and locates actions and events in the context of general political and social forces, including the opposing forces that have impeded the path to reform. It looks also at the way windows of opportunity for policy advancement opened in different jurisdictions at certain times, and offers an explanation of the reasons for this, with particular attention to the impact of feminist activism. Those readers who are primarily interested in the movement and its activism might wish to focus on the first six chapters. Those more interested in public policy and the influences that shape it will find this discussion from Chapter 7 onwards.

The story told here is only one among many possible accounts of the Australian women's health movement and its impact on public policy. It draws upon a rich tapestry of experiences, which is open to interpretation from a variety of perspectives. I anticipate that some readers will disagree with some of my arguments and with the emphasis placed on some events and issues rather than others. This is unavoidable given that the movement encompassed diverse perspectives from the beginning. Some women might wish to focus on the uniqueness of the movement's ideas. I have chosen to draw attention to the strong concordance between the principles of women's health and other sets of reform ideas, including those that predated the movement, those that were at the cutting edge in the 1970s and those that are on international and Australian political agendas in 2011. In making these connections, the overlap between the principles of women's health and those of the community health/new public health movements and the Aboriginal health movement is clear. What all these approaches have in common is a structural view of the causes of health and illness. Hence, they focus on improving the health of whole populations, especially those groups most at risk, through investment in community-based, preventive approaches, which would complement the system for treating individual episodes of disease. Persuading policymakers to adopt this comprehensive approach to the health system has been one of the major objectives of the women's health movement.

The health centre movement, the movements against violence and sexual assault, the maternity-care reform movement and the movement for reproductive rights have been selected for discussion. Activism to achieve women's reproductive rights[7] has been part of the work of all feminist groups. Initially, the women who set up centres and services were all feminists. Indeed, the movement 'has its ideological base in feminism' (Shuttleworth 1992:17). But as time went on, women who do not necessarily so describe themselves have promoted women's health. Because of space constraints, however, discussion will focus mainly on feminist work and action—the driving forces of the movement, especially in terms of advocacy for structural change.

From the late 1970s onwards, there was a remarkable proliferation of women's health groups—an indication of the strength of the movement. To name just a few in no particular order, groups for women with eating disorders, postnatal depression, HIV/AIDS and mental health problems have been established, alongside others focusing on lesbian health, maternity care, cancer support and the wellbeing of older women carers. Some work within an overtly feminist framework; others do not. While all are part of the modern women's health movement, it is clearly beyond the scope of a single volume to examine them all.

One important grouping that I have left to one side is Australia's network of Family Planning Associations, which have made a strong contribution to women's health. Family Planning Associations have, however, never branded themselves as part of the women's movement and they predate the second-wave movement.[8] In 1960, the Racial Hygiene Association changed its name to the Family Planning Association of Australia and in 1961 it opened its first clinic in Melbourne. Men, as well as women, have always been part of the active membership (Siedlecky and Wyndham 1990). Space constraints prevent even a cursory glance at this movement's multifaceted activities. The YWCA is another group whose work is not covered, despite having made a significant contribution. It works to facilitate community development and to provide support for young women and young families. Indeed, its focus on the many aspects of life that impact on wellbeing is consistent with a social health perspective. Moreover, the 'Y' has frequently worked with sections of the women's health movement on specific projects. Other women's groups that have worked to advance women's health include the Country Women's Association (CWA), the Catholic Women's League and the National Council of Women of Australia. These organisations do not, however, always support feminist goals and are not primarily concerned with health.

A focus on 'feminist' women's health groups raises the question of what I mean by the term in this book. There has never been a single feminism in Australia, as examination of serious disagreements in the following pages will show. Moreover,

---

7   Many Aboriginal and Torres Strait Islander women see reproductive rights differently—discussed further below.
8   For the purposes of this account, the 'second-wave' women's movement is the surge of feminist activism that took place in most OECD countries from the late 1960s onwards.

from the 1980s onwards, the existence of many 'feminisms' was recognised. Some versions have lost support and new perspectives have emerged, so that any definition has to be flexible and inclusive. I favour the kind of portrayal developed by the editors of the *Oxford Companion to Australian Feminism*, because it seems able to account for multiple strands of thought. 'Feminism', the editors propose, 'involves a sense of and concern with women's oppression, an interest and engagement in addressing, altering, or reforming it and a concern about women's claims to full citizenship and to recognise their social economic, cultural and political participation' (Caine et al. 1998:x). A feminist approach in women's health has been described as one where there is an

> emphasis on 'empowering' women rather than 'helping' them, of 'engaging' women in their own health care management, rather than 'fixing' them, and providing information so that women make their own informed decisions...the feminist/women-centred health model provides an active and equitable exchange where the health professional is recognised for her skill and expertise but the woman is recognised to be the expert in her own life and circumstances. (Cameron and Velthuys 2005)

What follows is a policy study, set in historical perspective, which seeks to answer major questions. Why is Australia the only country to have enacted two national women's health policies? Why is it also the only country to have attempted to establish a national network of community health centres? Why is it a leader, internationally, in developing public responses to domestic violence? What are the conditions that have come together at different times to create windows of opportunity for structural health reform? And what are the major obstacles? Why, despite the evidence, the hard work of so many groups of citizens and acknowledgment by policymakers, do the structures of the health system in 2011 remain much as they were 40 years ago?

The organisation of the book is as follows. The first chapter examines the women's health movement, the ideas that influenced it and that it developed further. It reviews feminist critiques of the conditions of women's lives and of the conventional medical system. The unique Australian debate about whether or not to accept government funding to help run services is examined, along with criticisms that the Australian women's movement is Anglocentric. Chapter 2 provides a glimpse of pioneering women in action at the grassroots level, as they organised, set up separate services and attempted to put women's health on policy agendas. Chapter 3 examines the consolidation phase, when more health centres were established and women moved to work in funded services alongside their grassroots sisters. Chapter 4 looks at the growth and strength of the movement as groups within it proliferated and traces the networks, formal and informal, that women formed. The extensive collaborations between groups, including inter-organisational action to advance occupational health and safety, are examined in Chapter 5. The struggle for reproductive rights, including maternity rights, is discussed in Chapter 6. State and Territory government responses to women's advocacy are examined in Chapter 7, and Chapter 8 traces Commonwealth policy responses, including the development of the two national policies. The ninth chapter is an analysis of broad policy determinants that have shaped responses to the movement. An evaluation of the social change and policy reform achieved is presented in the concluding chapter.

1. Concepts, Concerns, Critiques

The driving ideas and principles underpinning the Australian women's health movement have remained remarkably stable over time, which is counterintuitive given that the movement has always included women with a range of perspectives. As Stevens (1995:26) has argued, the context of the early years was not 'quiet conformity to an overarching ideology' but rather a time of 'great turbulence in the development of new ideas, forms of organisation and in the ways in which women related to each other'. Ideas were developed, changed and reformulated in line with experience and changing circumstances. For example, among those setting up early centres and services the question of whether to accept government funding was contentious. While opinions were strong and feelings ran high, the issue was resolved relatively quickly because agencies could not survive without financial support. Similarly, aspects of the feminist critique of conventional medicine lost some of their relevance as appropriate responses were put in place. Other parts of the critique, such as questions of unnecessary medicalisation and criticising the inadequacy of pharmaceutical safety evaluation, are as relevant as they ever were.

Priorities sometimes differed even when agreement was strong. Among Anglo-Australian women, there was general agreement on a number of central issues, including the harmful effects of Western gender roles, the shortcomings of conventional hospital and medical services, the gaps in available services, the need for information to make informed decisions about health and treatment and women's reproductive-health rights. In setting out to achieve change where it was vital, movement members were initially unaware that their concerns were not shared by all Australian women and that for some, racism and cultural insensitivity were higher priorities. Differences between women from divergent backgrounds gave rise to animosities and tensions, some of which remain but in working to improve women's health through multiple avenues many groups have nevertheless developed successful collaborations.

The unifying set of ideas around which the movement revolves is that which underpins a social view of health. The social perspective developed early and took deep root, creating common ground between women from diverse backgrounds. There is wide agreement among feminists with its underlying principles, which include social justice, holism, respect, empowerment and participation. Immigrant women applied these principles in the services they established and Aboriginal women seem always to have known about the social determinants of health.

Women and Healthcare Provision through the Ages

> Legislators, priests, philosophers, writers, and scientists have striven to show that the subordinate position of women is willed in heaven and advantageous on earth. (de Beauvoir 1972:22)

Second-wave women's health activism, in Australia and elsewhere, was cast by many as radical in the early years. Throughout history, however, women have struggled to gain and retain a respected voice in healthcare decision making. Direct action in support of women's health rights is recorded as early as the third century BC when Agnodice was arrested and tried for practising gynaecology and obstetrics, allegedly without formal training—a forerunner to modern accusations that some women's health workers are not properly trained. The leading men of Athens found her guilty but her patients demonstrated in her support, forcing men to change the law and allow women to train and practice.[1] Since then, women have struggled against repeated attempts made on religious and other grounds by churches, governments and male members of medical professions to exclude them from medical education and to preclude independent midwifery practice.

Women have provided health care for their families and community members as nurses, unlicensed doctors, pharmacists, herbalists, abortionists, counsellors and midwives since ancient times (Ehrenreich and English 1973:3; Willis 1983:94). Records have it that a midwife was present at the birth of the prophet Mohammed in 570 (Giladi 2010:190). Khaldun, a Muslim historiographer who died in 1406, dedicated a chapter of a large history to midwifery, arguing that midwives were better acquainted with obstetrics than others and better able to treat children's ailments than male physicians (Giladi 2010:185). In Europe and the Middle East, women continued to practice both as midwives and as obstetricians, despite opposition and sometimes in contravention of the law. In England, the term 'man-midwife' first appeared in the seventeenth century but, until the twentieth century, childbirth was almost exclusively women's business (Willis 1983:94–6).

Aboriginal women played an important role in Australian history as midwives in their own communities and for non-Aboriginal women in country areas. They also played a role in caring for non-Aboriginal women when they were ill. Women from the Wiradjuri tribe, whose country is central New South Wales, are reported to have delivered as many white babies as black babies (Gaff-Smith

---

1 Whether Agnodice was a historical figure has been questioned; however, even if she were not, the recorded struggle was clearly part of ancient experience. The story is eerily similar to modern attempts to keep women out of medicine.

2003:20). A settler's wife has told an illuminating story of being called to assist at a premature birth. The distressed husband read from a medical book outside the room and shouted orders, while the Aboriginal midwife, Fanny, ignored him and the settler's wife and quietly did what needed to be done. A premature baby girl 'so tiny she would have fitted into a pint jug' was safely born (Holthouse 1973:85–6). Childbirth is still women's business for many Aboriginal women, with mothers passing knowledge from generation to generation and assisting daughters during birthing (Webb 1986:1–3). Similarly, a century ago in rural New South Wales, my own great-grandmother was midwife at my mother's birth and the births of my uncles and aunts. She was midwife also for extended family members and anyone in surrounding communities who chose to call for her. I am not aware that she had any formal training, nor are there written records of her work; Australian midwives left very few accounts of what they did (Willis 1983:94).

Women's Health Reform Movements

In the United States, Weisman (1998) has identified what she calls a women's health 'megamovement' over the past two centuries, comprising several 'episodes of intense public attention to women's health'. Women were prominent in the social health movement of the 1830s and 1840s, which advocated what is now called primary health care[2] and set up training and information sessions (Baldry 1992). Women physicians and social reformers took leading roles in a subsequent wave of women's health action in the concluding decades of the nineteenth century—a struggle partly about reproductive rights. This period coincided with the women's suffrage movement in North America and Europe, Australia and New Zealand. A later women's health activity phase, between 1900 and the 1920s, focused on maternal and child health, sex education and birth-control rights. Margaret Sanger, a public health nurse and reproductive-rights activist, founded the American Birth Control League in 1921, after witnessing shocking loss of young life for want of appropriate information and care. The organisation became the Planned Parenthood Federation of America in 1942. It played a major role in the struggle for medical abortion in the United States, which was legalised in September 2000. The fourth stage of the women's health 'megamovement' is the grassroots movement that began in the late 1960s (Weisman 1998:37–92).

---

2   There is a distinct difference between primary health care and primary medical care. Whereas primary health care focuses on the provision of a comprehensive range of community-based services, including prevention, primary medical care is mainly concerned with the delivery of conventional treatment services to individuals. The distinction is important because, as Keleher (2001:57) argues, primary health care can make a difference to health inequalities in the population as a whole whereas primary medical care treats individual episodes of disease.

Australia, too, has seen several waves of women's health activism. A women's movement, at least partly concerned with health, has been present since the nineteenth century. Marilyn Lake (1999) has shown that the women's movement did not disappear after that 'first wave' but that women remained active through the twentieth century, struggling for a range of rights and freedoms, including equal pay, reproductive rights and sex education. At the end of the nineteenth century, Australian women agitated for special women's health services. Women-only hospitals run by and for women were established in capital cities. Demand for these services was overwhelming. For example, women are reported to have come 'in droves from all over Victoria' to the Victoria Hospital for Women, which was opened in a small church hall in 1896 (Robertson n.d.). In an early example of Australian women taking a social health perspective, the Women's Progressive League, founded in 1900, initiated discussion groups and courses on matters that included health and diet, and they lobbied for reform of factory, health and prison legislation (Baldry 1992).

The contraception and abortion-rights movement developed late in Australia, however, hampered by elite concern about declining birth rates in an empty continent. Following a drop in the birth rate after 1890, a royal commission was established in New South Wales in 1903. Its report is said to have influenced Australian policy for half a century. It regarded the use of contraceptives as a national problem caused by the growing selfishness of women and a love of luxury and social pleasures. In the years that followed, all States extended their laws restricting the availability of contraceptives (Browne 1979:24–8). The birth rate fell again between 1928 and 1935, provoking another round of official concern and 'invocation of the twin spectres of physical decline and national powerlessness' (Hicks 1978:158). As Pringle (1973:19) has argued, the ideology that was imposed on everyone displayed 'total contempt for actual attitudes and behaviour or for the rights of women to seek fulfilment outside narrowly defined roles'. Under these circumstances, family planning organisations were not formed until the 1930s and abortion-rights groups became active only after World War II (Siedlecky and Wyndham 1990:9–31).

The most recent wave of women's health activism emerged at roughly the same time in the United States, Australia, Britain, Canada and New Zealand and a little later in Ireland and South Africa. These are, of course, the major English-speaking industrial countries. There were, however, no comparable mobilisations in non-English-speaking capitalist democracies. Feminists in Norway, for example, were intrigued when I inquired about a Norwegian women's health movement in the 1990s. They answered that they saw no need for a specific focus on women's health, as the mainstream system could be influenced to respond appropriately. The reasons women's health movements were formed in one set of countries and not in others are touched on in Chapter 7 but thorough analysis must wait for another study.

The Modern Women's Health Movement in Australia

The second-wave women's movement in Australia—at first called women's liberation (WL)—emerged as feminist groups formed in capital cities and quickly proliferated. Sydney WL began in January 1970 and within a year groups had formed in every major town. Melbourne alone had 34 different groups by 1971 (Kaplan 1996:32). Although originating in 'new left' politics, WL groups encompassed a range of perspectives. At first, there was reliance on material heavily imbued with socialist ideas, primarily from the United States and Britain. In some States, the movement was initially a people's liberation movement. In South Australia, for example, men participated in women's meetings for the first several years (Kinder 1980:30–54). In other States, however, the movement was partly 'a revolt against New Left men' who, while concerned about imperialism, oppression in the Third World and against minority groups, were nevertheless happy to dominate and exploit new left women (Curthoys 1984:162). Groups in different parts of the country quickly communicated with each other which brought a level of consensus. As time went on, theoretical analyses of women's oppression were developed. New left ties meant that socialist ideas were strong so that women's oppression was often explained as a product of capitalism and patriarchy (Curthoys 1984:162).

Health, especially reproductive health, was a major issue from the beginning. Sex-role stereotyping and media exploitation of women were other early concerns (Kinder 1980:30–54). The more centrist Women's Electoral Lobby (WEL) was formed in 1972. Initially, an uneasy tension characterised relations between the two: whereas WEL focused on working within state institutions (an approach called liberal or 'reformist' feminism), WL aimed to achieve a radically restructured society—a project some women thought would be scuttled by working through existing structures (Kinder 1980:104–8). Despite the differences, the two groups cooperated and marched together on International Women's Day (IWD). In some settings, including Western Australia and the Australian Capital Territory, collaboration appeared to come easily and some women participated in both groups.

Initially, WEL adopted the six demands that WL had formulated: equal pay, equal employment opportunity, equal access to education, free contraception, abortion on demand and free twenty-four-hour child care. This list expanded to include other policy areas and soon recommendations were being made about taxation, the structure of work, paid maternity and parental leave, access to justice and the public–private dichotomy. The notion that particular issues were women's issues was abandoned and most Australian feminists soon argued that all areas of public and private life were important to women.[3]

By 1973, groups whose primary interest was health began to form. In Melbourne, for example, the Women's Health Collective and Women against Rape were set up. In Adelaide, all segments of the women's movement were concerned with aspects of health. A group called The Body Politic, largely comprising nurses and trainee doctors, was formed in 1972, absorbing an existing abortion-rights group. It was concerned with a wide range of women's health issues and emphasised the need for sex education, producing an information sheet called 'How not to get pregnant, how to find out if you are and what to do about it', which was distributed widely and became the subject of vice-squad inquiries. A member of the group subsequently graduated in medicine and became one of the founders of Adelaide's first women's health centre. Even within feminist health reform groups, however, rape as a health issue was rarely mentioned (Kinder 1980:88–9), indicating the strong taboos around the subject. Sydney women celebrated IWD in 1973 by holding a commission over a weekend at which women shared their experiences. Health, especially the inadequacy of hospital and medical services, emerged as the main topic. At follow-up meetings, groups were formed to work on various issues and one was to focus on health services for women (Cooper 2003). Similar developments took place in Melbourne.

The Struggle for Health Information

Simone de Beauvoir helped to lay the philosophical foundations for modern women's health activism when she argued in *The Second Sex* (first published in 1949) that women had limited control over their bodies, their minds, their lives and their destinies. 'Woman is determined not by her hormones or by mysterious instincts', she argued, 'but by the manner in which her body and her relations to the world are modified through the action of others than herself' (de Beauvoir 1972:734). While professionals monopolised health information, women could not participate equally in treatment and care decisions or attempt to control their own bodies.

The quest for knowledge and information emerged as a key issue in the consciousness-raising (CR) groups of the 1960s in the United States. Members of the pioneering Boston Women's Health Collective, for example, realised in 1969 that they knew very little about how their bodies worked. They undertook to research topics, found they could understand medical and scientific writing and

---

3 Separatist feminists, whose ideas include the view that women need to live separately from men, do not necessarily share this opinion.

decided to put together an information course for women. These efforts resulted in the book *Our Bodies, Ourselves*, first published in 1971, later translated into a dozen languages, adapted to suit different countries and now in its sixth edition. From the late 1960s onwards, a feminist information-dissemination effort took place in the United States, particularly in the cities (Lipnack 1980; Ruzek 1978). At the same time, in Britain, a feminist health education movement emerged, in which women produced information materials and other resources, together with lists of speakers, to facilitate knowledge dissemination (Doyal 1983:22).

Information was a central issue at the first Australian national women's health conference, held in 1975. One major recommendation from the gathering was that 'a federal commission be set up to investigate all aspects of health education' (Commonwealth Department of Health 1978:3). Women reported finding it extremely difficult to get the information they needed from medical practitioners, particularly if there were additional obstacles, such as language barriers. For example, in the late 1970s, widespread misinformation was found among immigrant women in Melbourne by Women in Industry, Contraception and Health (WICH), a newly formed grassroots non-governmental organisation (NGO). WICH discovered women who were taking the contraceptive pill without knowing it was a contraceptive and others who had had intrauterine devices (IUDs) fitted that had not been changed for years (Caddick and Small 1982). Even where there were no language barriers, women often found it hard to find out what they wanted to know. A young woman, Susan Waide, told me about her unsuccessful efforts to extract information from her doctor during her first pregnancy in the 1970s. 'Y'know how it is', she told me, 'Pat you on the head and kick you out the door'.

The early women's health centres aimed to fill some of these gaps, both inside and outside their walls. Activities included discussion sessions, coffee gatherings and self-help meetings. As in the CR movement, group meetings were recognised as valuable mechanisms for exchanging information, ideas and experiences. Women aimed to 'get to know themselves, reinterpret their biological function, question their role in society' and 'regain control over their bodies. And their lives' (Sandall 1974:89). Feelings of frustration and powerlessness associated with inadequate information were closely related to dissatisfaction with conventional hospital and medical services.

The Feminist Critique of Conventional Medical Care

At one end of a spectrum were straightforward expressions of anger about the attitudes of medical practitioners and the inappropriateness of many treatments.

At the other end, sociological and political analyses of modern medical care drew on social theory and the 'limits to medicine' perspective discussed above. As Dorothy Broom (1991:43) explains, women were dissatisfied with medical services, critical of many of the professionals who delivered them and had a vision of a radically different society, in which women would be no longer subordinate, would be proud of their bodies and would enjoy life conditions that would enable them to be responsible for their own health and health care.

Social institutions are a product of their time and place and, in medicine in the 1960s and 1970s, women were seen primarily as wives and mothers, rather fragile creatures (nevertheless capable of long hours of unpaid work, without recreation, and sick or weekend leave), who spent most of their lives in the recesses of the private sector taking care of others. Founding members of the Boston Women's Health Collective identified four prevailing cultural notions of femininity that they found restrictive: woman as inferior, woman as passive, woman as beautiful object and woman as exclusively wife and mother (Boston Women's Health Book Collective 1976:18). Such ideas were conveyed to medical students in gynaecology texts, which adhered tenaciously to views of women as frigid and sexually unresponsive, long after contrary scientific evidence was available (Broom 1991:38–9; Scully and Bart 1973). An Australian bureaucrat's view of single, middle-aged women, as expressed in a Commonwealth Minute Paper in the 1960s, captures a perspective not uncommon at the time: 'A spinster lady can, and very often does, turn into something of a battle axe with the passing years. A man usually mellows' (Commonwealth of Australia 1963).

The Subordination of Women in Health Care

At a fundamental level, many women have a strong sense that health care really is women's business, given the long history of involvement, and many were dissatisfied with a system in which women constituted the bulk of health professionals but medical system decision making was heavily dominated by men. In Australia, organised medicine had long worked to marginalise women providers. It had campaigned against the introduction of any service, such as baby health centres and school health services staffed by nurses, which might be a threat to the size of private medical markets. By the middle of the twentieth century, these campaigns had successfully sidelined female professionals, leaving hospital and medical systems dominated by men, with doctors filling most key positions (Gray 1991:60–2; Willis 1983; Wyndham 1983:28–30). The division of labour resembled that in wider society: women did the low-status, low-paid caring and support work while men in high-status, well-paid positions made the all-important decisions. Pringle and Game (1983:94) argue that 'in no other workplace are power relations as highly sexualised as they are in hospitals.

Bureaucratic domination is directly reinforced by sexual power structures.' They also found that increases in the number of male nurses and female doctors had not changed basic power relations. A similar situation prevailed in Britain (Doyal 1983:27).

Women still make up a majority of the health workforce in Australia. More than 90 per cent of nurses were women in 2006 (AIHW 2009:31). Although women constitute an increasing proportion of doctors, at 33.7 per cent, only 21.6 per cent of specialists are women (AIHW 2006:8, 16). Male dominance in health system decision making has many untoward consequences. For example, unpaid care giving is rarely recognised as a women's health issue. Primarily a cost-cutting exercise, policies promoting shorter acute hospital stays and de-institutionalisation in the mental health, disability and aged-care sectors have transferred responsibility to predominantly female carers, significantly increasing the burden of unpaid work and undermining women's capacities to achieve economic and other forms of independence (Armstrong et al. 2002).

Medicine's Role in the Subordination of Women

The male-dominated medical system of the 1970s, it was argued, not only reflected the views about women held in wider society but also played 'a particularly strategic role in actively creating these stereotypes and in controlling women who may deviate from them' (Doyal 1983:26). The views about women presented in medical textbooks, for example, masqueraded as scientific fact when, in fact, they were (male) socio-cultural interpretations. Feminists claim that unscientific medical discourse of this kind is really social and political action that helps to sustain the status quo (Braun 2003:5–10). In this and other versions of the narrative, medical personnel operate as agents of the establishment (reviewed in Broom 1991:44–7), constructing 'deviance' through interpretation and labelling processes and controlling it through medicalisation and other avenues, such as population policies. Men become experts on women's bodies and medicine is involved in the construction of a particular view of the 'nature' of women, labelling and treating 'normal' and 'abnormal' femininities. Broom (1991:53–7) suggests that the word femininity itself conjures up notions of illness and disease because women and sick people share characteristics, such as weakness, passivity and dependency.[4]

---

4 Similarly, some semiologists argue that the word 'woman' is infused with inerasable meanings of weakness and subordination or even that it simply means reproductive capacity. Simone de Beauvoir (1972:35) wrote: 'Woman? Very simple say the fanciers of simple formulas: she is a womb, an ovary; she is female—this word is sufficient to define her.'

Feminists argue that these influences are particularly apparent in mental health systems, where therapeutic models perpetuate gender stereotypes, pathologise women's anger and maintain their lack of power (Ussher 1991:209). From the beginning, women's emotional health and wellbeing were major issues in women's health centres (Schofield 1998:1–9). The view that women suffer more mental ill health than men because they are subjugated, distressed and unhappy was put forward in the early years. On entering the psychiatric system, women are confronted with a view of mental health that is inherently sexist: women's distress is pathologised rather than validated. The impact of violence and trauma is not given full weight, the social conditions of women's lives are not examined and women's control is further undermined because information about treatment choices is not readily available. Research on women's mental health remains sparse and there is insufficient recognition that women and men might experience conditions, such as stress, differently. An interactionist model, it is argued, needs to be developed, which examines social conditions and psychical factors as they occur together. In this view, the traditional therapy model of dominant professional and submissive client must be replaced with an egalitarian approach (Hodges 1997:22–30).

Superior–Subordinate Relations

The Women's Commission was told in Sydney in 1973 that doctors' attitudes towards women were often experienced as patronising and judgmental and sometimes as degrading and humiliating. The commission was a two-day gathering of some 500 women organised by WL as part of the 1973 IWD activities. Patronising doctor–patient interactions could occur in any setting: in the 1980s, a newly retired State Minister for Health, needing minor surgery, asked a question about the procedure, to which her doctor replied, not with an answer, but with the admonition: 'Now you are going to be a good girl, aren't you?'

Women reported especially distressing experiences when seeking abortion services. Jean Taylor (2003) remembers the concerns expressed in the early 1970s during her volunteer work with a new Melbourne WL information service:

> Many women were looking for a sympathetic doctor so they could have an abortion and the Women's Abortion Action Campaign (WAAC) was set up in 1972 to campaign for the repeal of anti-abortion laws…We encouraged women to let us know what their experiences had been… so we could have a resource file of doctors who could do abortions or other medical procedures or consultations in a sympathetic way. In the same way we also had a file on doctors who were less than sympathetic

or downright incompetent and dangerous. We were challenging sexist attitudes and ways of looking at the world. Doctors and other professionals were often quite sexist and wouldn't give women information, so we were encouraging women to ask their doctor questions and find out what was happening about treatment. From this, women started to be involved in their own health care.

Women also identified a lack of sympathy for victims of violence and a lack of concern about what women themselves wanted and needed (Siedlecky 1977:30). Many felt unable to discuss problems with their doctors. The tragic consequences that can result from ineffective communication and inadequate training to deal with issues such as domestic violence are illustrated in the case of Heather Osland, who was convicted for her part in the murder of her violent husband. Osland had attended her doctor regularly for 10 years prior to the killing, with recurrent cystitis, and vaginal and pelvic infection and inflammation, resulting from marital vaginal and anal rape. She had taken her children, who displayed serious behavioural problems and sometimes physical injuries, to the same doctor. Her husband also attended the practice. Osland was treated with antidepressants, tranquillisers and antibiotics and although there were discussions with her doctor about marriage problems, these discussions were not included in her records nor were the problems connected with her medical conditions (Taft 1999:64). This might be an extreme case, in terms of both the oversight and its consequences, but it illustrates the way non-medical and even medical problems, major and minor, can slip through the net in the absence of information and training.

Another major issue for 1970s women was that their health problems were frequently trivialised, regarded as exaggerations, not believed and/or passed off as emotional reactions or overreactions. Endometriosis, for example—a painful condition—often went undiagnosed for years. Women felt that menstrual problems, pelvic infections and the like were not given appropriate attention and were meant to be 'suffered in silence' (Broom 1991:37). Indeed, as late as 1990, the menstrual cycle had not been studied in depth (Doyal 1995:17). Chest pain, long-term chronic pain, headache and dizziness were other conditions women felt were often not taken seriously. Moreover, research shows the same symptoms were taken more seriously in men, who received quite different treatments. For example, chronic pain might be treated with painkilling drugs in men but with tranquillisers or even shock treatment in women. Other studies showed female prisoners were far less likely to receive conventional medical treatment, and women with heart disease were treated differently from men with the same condition (Wyndham 1983:29).

Unnecessary Medicalisation

Women complained and continue to complain about the unnecessary medicalisation of life events, such as menstruation, pregnancy, childbirth, menopause and mental ill health. Social and emotional problems, in particular, are often treated medically. The women's health movement quickly identified the heavy prescribing of tranquillisers as highly inappropriate. In 1984–85, 70 per cent of the six million prescriptions written in Australia for benzodiazepines were for women. Estimates were that between 30 and 40 per cent of these women would become addicted both physically and psychologically. Women from non-English-speaking backgrounds were particularly likely to be prescribed tranquillisers (Crawford and Elliott 1994:143). The safety of many treatments was questioned. The untoward effects of drugs, such as Depo-Provera, and of devices such as the Dalkon Shield, were discovered and publicised. The use of the contraceptive pill came to be seen as a massive experiment on women: dosage levels were the subject of trial and error and use became widespread before longer-term effects could be known.

More recently, the use of hormones has become highly controversial (Boston Women's Health Collective 2006). After millions of women had been prescribed hormone replacement therapy (HRT), evidence appeared that implicated it in either causing or exacerbating a range of cancers, including lung cancer, leading one researcher to question its use in medicine in any form (Ganti 2009:1218). Researchers argue that the HRT experience reaffirms the importance of mandatory randomised trials. Recent work to develop a 'female Viagra' for women with supposedly low libidos is seen as an attempt to create a new disease, called 'female sexual dysfunction', and so establish a new and potentially lucrative market. The work has been strongly criticised by feminists and others (Moynahan 2003).

Gender Bias in Medical Research and Practice

The priorities and methods of medical research have attracted criticism since the early 1980s. Even within the biomedical model, research on women was the exception rather than the rule. Until the 1970s, 'women's health' was thought of as comprising reproductive issues and gynaecological diseases but even these were seriously under-researched (Doyal 1995:17–18). Women were heavily under-represented in clinical studies, which primarily studied men and then applied the findings to both sexes (Keville 1994). In Australia, funding for women's health research constituted a 'tiny fraction' of the total until 1990 (Broom 1991:38). Inquiries of the National Health and Medical Research Council

(NHMRC) and the Australian Institute of Health and Welfare (AIHW) in 2010 failed to establish what proportion of total health research was specifically devoted to women. The NHMRC collects data only on the research it funds itself, not on the total Australian research effort. In 2010, however, $82.3 million of a total of $730.1 million, or approximately 11 per cent, was identified as being for 'women's health' (NHMRC Research Funding Dataset 2000-2010). Inquiries of the AIHW were less satisfactory. In reply to my questions[5] and follow-up questions, I received the following reply by email: 'I passed your enquiry around to colleagues specialising in areas that your questions were around. The general consensus was that we are unable to answer the questions, this is due largely to [the fact] that we try not to differentiate between sexes in our reports.'

Given that the importance of collecting sex disaggregated data and the need for gender analysis has been acknowledged for many years, it is astonishing AIHW staff seem unaware of the arguments.

By the 1990s, it was acknowledged in overseas medical research circles that clinical trials on diseases that affect both men and women should include both men and women as subjects (Cohen and Sinding 1996; Keville 1994). US responses include the establishment by the Institutes of Medicine of a committee to consider ethical and legal issues surrounding the inclusion of women in clinical studies, which recommended that women be included 'wherever possible' (Mastroianni et al 1994). The US Congress passed legislation in 1993 stipulating that women must be included in clinical trials in sufficient numbers to obtain 'a valid analysis' of differences in the way women and men respond to drugs, therapies and treatments. Later research, however, suggested that companies were disregarding aspects of the legislation (Pear 2000).

Similarly, the Medical Research Council of Canada issued a paper in 1994 drawing attention to the need for gender balance in research. In Australia, the NHMRC's *National Statement on Ethical Conduct in Human Research* (2007) does not reflect these concerns, referring only to 'women who are pregnant'. Its recently revised *National Ethics Application Form*, however, which researchers must use to apply for ethics clearance, asks applicants about the ratio of males to females that will be recruited and whether the ratio accurately reflects the distribution of the disease, issue or condition within the general community. Research published in a high-profile international journal in 2010 showed continuing gender bias and prompted leading women's health NGO Women's Health Victoria (WHV)

---

5 The questions asked were: 1) What proportion of total Australian health research funding is devoted to studying women's health? 2) What proportion of women's health research is devoted to areas other than reproductive and sexual health? 3) What are the rules about the inclusion of women in clinical trials for diseases that affect both men and women, such as cardiac disease? 4) What proportion of research on cardiac disease is conducted specifically on women?

to issue a media release calling on the Australian Government to develop and enforce a set of national guidelines to ensure that medical research takes account of gender differences (WHV 2010).

Biased research results in biased approaches to care. Until recently at least, drug and alcohol rehabilitation policies and services in Australia centred on the needs of men with little recognition that these differed from the needs of women. Almost all the research that had been undertaken investigated men's experiences (Morgain 1994:175–6). There were few women-only alcohol and substance-abuse centres where women who, because of past experiences, were afraid to use mixed-sex services could go, and there was virtually no provision for women with children. Similarly, few professionals were trained to deal with the effects of abuse and violence on women and children. Moreover, awareness of the need for cultural sensitivity was low.

Gender Bias in Treatment

Biased medical research leads to biased treatment, with women less likely to receive 'accurate diagnosis and appropriate treatment' (Bönte et al. 2008; Keville 1994:129). We do not know whether inappropriate treatment is less common than it once was but we do know that serious problems remain. Rosenberg and Allard (2007) found 'a pattern of overestimation of benefit and underestimation of harm' for women being prescribed statin therapy. A large study in the United States found that women are 30 per cent less likely than men to receive the kind of stroke care that limits brain damage (RedOrbit News 2009). A number of studies show that women with cardiac disease are treated less appropriately than men, even after accurate diagnosis and hospitalisation. For example, research in Germany, the United Kingdom and the United States found that 'primary care doctors' behaviour differed by patients' gender in all three countries'. In Australia, recent research by the AIHW found that although cardiovascular diseases (CVDs) are a major health threat for Australian women, awareness of this threat is low. Both the severity and the number of episodes per woman can be reduced, the report argues. An 'enormous potential' exists, according to the AIHW 'to improve the risk profile of Australian women and therefore reduce the numbers of women and families affected by CVD' (AIHW 2010b).

To summarise the feminist critique, in the male-dominated medical system, men are not only experts on women's bodies, they are also experts on women's healthcare needs and make crucial decisions on services and treatments. Women have been subordinated as health professionals and, in many other respects, medical practice perpetuates the inferior status of women. Unnecessary medicalisation and gender bias in research and practice result in suboptimal health outcomes. From the social health perspective, a wide range of primary health and community services is seriously undersupplied. Like Aboriginal Medical Service (AMS) workers, women identify the need for more holistic, preventive, community-based services.

The Integrity of Medical Research

Concerns have emerged about the scientific integrity of medical research, following changes in the way it is funded. Whereas in the 1960s most research was publicly funded, by 2006 approximately three-quarters was funded privately. Moreover, until the 1990s, most drug company-funded research was undertaken in universities; however, research has moved to for-profit locations, where fewer checks and balances operate. Pharmaceutical companies can now select the research designs most likely to produce the results they want, they can terminate studies if the findings contravene their interests and they can fail to publish results altogether. The fear is that private research is 'far more likely to produce results that support the sponsor's interests' (Boston Women's Health Collective 2006). Three Australian oncologists caused something of a stir in 2010 when they pointed out that 27 of 32 authors of research published in *The Lancet* had declared financial links to the drug company that had funded the research. The authors, it was argued, had a potential conflict of interest (Medew 2011).

In recent years, the pharmaceutical company practice of employing ghost writers to write reports for medical journals has raised concerns about skewed findings. Experience validates such concerns. A study of court documents in the United States, for example, showed that 26 medical journal articles between 1998 and 2005 'emphasised the benefits and deemphasised the risks' of HRT. All had been drafted by a medical communications firm paid by a major pharmaceutical company (Singer 2009:A1). Allegations have also been made about biased reports on antidepressants and diet drugs and, more recently, about cancer and haematology drugs. A recent analysis of reviews of a new drug for type-two diabetes found that experts who were paid by the drug's manufacturer were more likely to report favourably on efficacy and safety. Investigation was prompted by sharply conflicting conclusions in published scientific work, some of which had warned about significant risks (Bakalar 2010). Medical journals have been forced to abandon the honour system of disclosure and introduce 'ghostbusting' measures in an effort to reduce industry-financed writing assistance (Singer and Wilson 2009:B1).

A Social View of Health

A person's physical health is like a frozen moment taken from the social and economic environment.

— Stephanie Bell, 2001, Director, Central Australian Aboriginal Congress

Australian women did not need epidemiologists to tell them that the conditions of their lives had important ramifications for their health. According to Laurie Gilbert, Director of the Women's Health Unit in the then Commonwealth Department of Health in the 1980s, Australian women understood and subscribed to a social view of health before they had heard the term. Laurie Gilbert was a member of the team, headed by Liza Newby, which consulted with women about their health needs for the 1989 NWHP. As the NWHP argues, a 'major reason for the acceptance by so many women of the social health perspective is their understanding, often from personal experience, of the links between poverty, type of employment, education, access to housing, and health' (Commonwealth of Australia 1989:10).

Another reason so many women take a social view, it has been suggested, is that they are more likely to use, or want to use, the health system for health reasons, whereas men use it mostly for illness. Aboriginal women have been keenly aware that life conditions affect health outcomes for a very long time. And although Aboriginal, immigrant and Anglo women often had different priorities, they were in agreement on most aspects of the social perspective. As Broom (2001:98) argues, 'women of all racial and ethnic backgrounds were united...in their call for a voice in personal health care decisions and in the formulation of health policy'.

A social health perspective is an extension of the feminist critique of conventional medicine in the sense that it argues that a treatment focus is narrow and misses a great deal that is crucial for human health. When women talk about gaps in services, some of the things they are noticing are the paucity of prevention advice, counselling and support.

In a social view of health, the focus is on population rather than individual health. It is concerned with 'the causes of the causes'. Outcomes emerge from complex interactions between social, economic, cultural, environmental and biomedical factors rather than arising from biological determinants alone. Furthermore, feminists argue that biology is not given and unchangeable, as it tends to be in the medical scientific view, but is influenced by multiple factors. Therefore, biomedical processes cannot be understood out of context. In this view, as Hammarstrom (1999:243) argues, 'there is a close interplay between social and biological factors, which means that biology must be problematised'.

There is no clearer association in the epidemiological evidence than that between poverty and inferior health outcomes; however, the poor are not the only ones who are affected. There is a definite social gradient in health, which shows that everyone's health is less robust than it might be, perhaps affecting even those at the top of the socioeconomic scale. Health outcomes consistently improve as socioeconomic status improves, with the biggest differences obviously found between those at the top and those at the bottom. It follows therefore that comfortable, middle-income people, for example, have poorer health outcomes than they might have (WHO 2003:10–11). Recent research suggests that levels of inequality, material and social, can explain the social gradient. Countries with the largest gaps between rich and poor experience more mental illness, more drug and alcohol-related problems, more obesity, higher rates of teenage pregnancy, poorer educational performance and literacy scores and higher rates of homicide (Wilkinson and Pickett 2009).

Inequality works to undermine health, it is suggested, by increasing stress right across society. Stress, medical research shows, produces a range of diseases and behavioural problems. In heavily unequal societies, the rich fear the poor and the poor suffer from status anxiety and shame, making everyone's health poorer than it might be. In more equal societies there are higher levels of trust and lower levels of stress. Low status, low levels of respect and feelings of low self-esteem, rather than material deprivation per se, contribute most to poor health and help explain the social gradient (Wilkinson and Pickett 2009). Such arguments fit with the findings of earlier studies. For example, Kawachi et al. (1999) studied men and women across the 50 American States and found that both smaller wage gaps between the sexes and higher levels of women's political participation were 'strikingly correlated' with lower female *and male* morbidity and mortality. Status, the authors conclude, reflects 'more general underlying structural processes associated with material deprivation and income inequality'. Such findings corroborate the arguments of Aboriginal people who point to the devastating health consequences of colonisation and racism.

Returning to the health of the most disadvantaged, the close association between poverty and very poor health outcomes holds both between countries—some rich, some poor—and within countries, whether they are OECD countries or those that are less well off (WHO 2008a). Women are everywhere over-represented amongst the poor.[6] Australia's gender pay gap, for example, contributes to economic insecurity, increasing the number of low-income families, especially female-headed families, with a negative impact on health, including that of

---

6 This is not generally the case for Aboriginal women, who point out that they often have better jobs and higher education levels than Aboriginal men.

children. It also contributes to financial vulnerability for women, especially women in retirement. The effects of the pay gap are exacerbated by socially prescribed caring responsibilities.

Violence is another major 'cause of the causes' of poor health. While the underpinnings of violence are complex, there is wide agreement that intimate partner violence, in particular, is firmly embedded in gender inequality. Violence is detrimental to women's health in many ways. A major WHO study found that violence had a negative impact on women's physical, sexual, reproductive, psychological and behavioural health, as well as having fatal consequences in cases of AIDS-related mortality, maternal mortality, homicide and suicide (Krug et al. 2002).

Post-traumatic stress disorder (PTSD) is more prevalent among women who have experienced violence, along with neurological disorders as a result of head injuries and attempted strangulation. Women who have experienced violence have more sexually transmitted and urinary tract infections, more migraine headaches, more chronic pain and poorer reproductive health outcomes (Coker 2005:1; Taft et al. 2003). Moreover, studies show that the health consequences of abuse can persist for years and that the more severe the abuse, the greater is the detrimental impact on health, with multiple episodes having a cumulative impact.

Workplace conditions can give rise, directly and indirectly, to poor health outcomes. Discrimination or harassment in the workplace, for example, might lead to anxiety, depression and other mental health problems and economic insecurity—all closely associated with reduced life chances and poorer health. The Canadian Women's Health Strategy (Health Canada 1999) identified 12 key social determinants of women's health: income and social status; employment status; education; social environment, including social support and social exclusion; physical environment, including access to food, housing, transport, clean air and the like; healthy child development; personal health practices and coping skills; access to health services; social support networks; biology and genetic endowment; gender; and culture. Indeed, each of these categories is an umbrella for more specific determinants.

A biomedical perspective of health, in contrast, is narrower. It focuses on the immediate or direct causes of ill health, which are seen as located in individual bodies in interaction with outside causal factors, such as germs, toxins and injuries. The human body is seen as a set of interdependent but contained systems, and ill health is treated as a failure of one of the parts. Disease unfolds within individuals. Day-to-day interactions with broader social and physical environments are outside the scope of inquiry (Doyal 1995:15–16).

Very different views of appropriate public policies flow from these distinct perspectives. If the causes of ill health are predominantly biomedical and largely outside human control, the role of public policy is limited. In an 'old' public health framework (as discussed in the Introduction), the range of responsibilities is relatively narrow but includes provision of clean water, sewage disposal and health regulations. Public authorities might also provide relevant health information and enact legislation to restrict the activities of commercial enterprises if health concerns are at stake. Importantly, people in wealthy countries now agree that good-quality hospital and medical services should be made accessible to citizens, and public policies are required to regulate access.

In contrast, where a social determinants view of health is taken, extensive public intervention is the rational response, both inside and outside health systems. If the 'causes of the causes' can be known and understood, it follows that health and public policy should focus on prevention as well as cure. A social determinants perspective requires substantial investment in primary, community-based health care to complement medical and hospital services, as well as investment in economic security, physical security, affordable housing, accessible education, food security and so on.

While the women's health movement has championed a social view of health and illness, this is equally relevant to men's health. Gender, which is one of the social determinants, helps shape the conditions of men's lives, just as it does those of women. Male gender roles might work to undermine health by encouraging physical risk taking and, perhaps, the denial of emotions, physical discomfort and pain. The expectations held about what is required of breadwinners might induce men to work in stressful, dangerous occupations or to work unhealthily long hours. Risk-taking behaviour can have untoward effects on the health of both men and women, particularly in relation to sexual activity. We might not be able to tell for sure whether women suffer more morbidity than men (Broom 1991:47–52), but a social health perspective tells us for certain that many men and women suffer high levels of avoidable ill health as a consequence of the constraints and requirements of masculine and feminine gender roles.

A Peculiarly Australian Debate: To accept or reject state funding?

The question of whether women should collaborate with 'the state' (or government) was a strongly contested issue in the early Australian women's health movement. The problem arose when the movement established its own services and public funding support was a real possibility. Conflict and bitter disagreements ensued and in some cases permanent ruptures followed.

Demand for the services women's health centres provided was strong and placed a heavy load on volunteer and low-paid service providers. Some workers felt frustrated, wishing to devote more of their time to broader, change-seeking action, but often found their energies consumed by day-to-day service provision (Broom 1991:120–2). Thus, some found the prospect of financial support attractive. Whereas social liberal (social democratic) feminists were generally comfortable working through government institutions, women oriented towards socialist, anarchist, radical, cultural and lesbian-separatist feminist perspectives generally held reservations. Divergent perspectives are nicely illustrated in a letter written by Beatrice Faust, the founder of Melbourne WEL, to Biff Ward, convenor of Canberra WL in 1972. 'Does Canberra Women's Lib plan to establish a second branch of WEL?' Beatrice asked. She went on to suggest: 'If you believe the democratic process is useless, perhaps you could pass this on to someone who still has hopes of it' (reproduced in McCarron Benson 1991).

In the 1960s and 1970s, many feminists were preoccupied with analysing the nature of 'the state', which was a reflection of the strength of socialist feminist thinking at that time. In the Marxist tradition, the institutional apparatus— which includes government, the economic system, the legal system, the education system, the military, the police and so on—is referred to as 'the state'. The state is regarded as an instrument of oppression, used by the ruling class to prevent a revolution from below that would benefit the more numerous working class. Socialist feminists, therefore, work within a tradition that is highly suspicious of the state. Distrust of public-sector institutions also emanated from women's lived experiences. Because there was relatively low female participation in the public sphere, the state could be seen as male in character, with institutional arrangements, practices and processes that were alien to women.

Another strand of thinking analysed the state as male dominated or patriarchal. In Kate Millett's view, for example, patriarchy is a universal phenomenon and patriarchal government is an institution under which 'half of the populace which is female is controlled by that half which is male' (Millett 1977:25). Patriarchy is deeply entrenched and runs through all the political, social and economic institutions of all societies. In this perspective, as Randall (1988:10–11) argues, 'the state has remained a bastion of male power', controlling women's freedom, restricting creativeness, denying autonomy and 'withholding from women large areas of society's knowledge, power, opportunity and resources'. Government, some feminists suggested, was conducted as if men's interests were the only ones that counted (Pringle and Watson 1992:57).

Theorists also developed critiques of government bureaucracy—an arm of the state—which went beyond conventional complaints about red tape, goal displacement and empire building. Whereas behaviour, attitudes, structures and processes are seen as gender neutral in conventional organisation theory, feminist theorists argue that masculine values and assumptions underpin and reinforce the systems of sex stratification typically found in organisations. According to Ferguson (1984:4), the bureaucratic organisation of public life directly controls the work of most women employed outside the home. Further, because of its hierarchical nature, bureaucracy affects the entire society in a way that is antithetical to the goals of feminist theory and practice and antithetical to democracy. Clearly, such structures are not appropriate channels through which to pursue the liberation of women.

With these ideas in mind, some women searched for new ways of working, inspired by visions of a society based on empowerment rather than domination. In alternative structures, it is argued, women can work towards their own emancipation through processes in which they support and value each other and where the conditions for empowerment and skill development are present. In Australia, as elsewhere, feminist collectives were set up and were the chosen management form for many health centres, rape crisis, domestic violence, sexual assault and abortion counselling services (Outhwaite 1989:203–5). Non-hierarchical power structures in women's health were felt to benefit both workers and clients. In keeping with a radical democratic focus, Jocelyn Auer (2003:7) argues that hierarchical decision making in women's health reduces the power and information that workers have and this deficit is felt by clients.

As it developed in Australia, feminist theorising about the state produced different positions, with some accounts suggesting the possibility of meaningful improvement in the status of women through collaboration (see, for example, Allen 1990; Yeatman 1994). One strand of the 'reformist' view was that while seeking equality through the state might offer only limited prospects, the alternative of purchasing equality in the marketplace offered even less cause for optimism (Dowse 1984:143). Women were aware that accepting government funding would involve, at the very least, keeping records, writing reports and possibly complying with unacceptable conditions, such as restrictions on modes of operation and/or on the selection of clients. In practice, such restrictions quickly became reality. Marian Sawer (1990:50) notes the tensions created when women's health-sector workers became 'caught up in bureaucratic procedures', requiring them to produce business plans, job descriptions, policies and procedures. Collective-management models had to be modified and sometimes abandoned.

Controversy over state funding appears to have been stronger in the women's health movement than in the mainstream women's movement. It has been argued that there was scarcely a debate in the wider women's movement (Dowse 1984:146). An alternative view is put by Dorothy Broom (1991), who documents vigorous and sometimes bitter debates and irreconcilable conflicts. For example, differences between radicals and reformists in Brisbane's Women's House

Health Centre 'broke out into open warfare' in the mid-1970s, resulting in the centre losing its funding (Broom 1991:16). According to Broom's central thesis, working with the state in women's health involves women in a fundamental contradiction—the contradiction of 'using the system to change the system'. In this view, very briefly, both medicine and the state are patriarchal institutions that prop up a social order that makes women sick. These institutions must be reformed if the underlying social conditions that give rise to avoidable illness amongst women are to be eliminated. The dilemma was expressed very clearly by the Women's Liberation Halfway House Collective just after accepting government funding in 1975:

> Whether we can threaten the relations of power and control that form the basis of this society while being financed by the system which maintains them, and how far we can use government funding to develop the potential of the Halfway House as a political weapon are the most important questions. (Quoted in Alley et al. 1980:10)

The movement has always been very clear that the relations of power and control need to be changed, both inside and outside the health system; disagreement centred upon the best way forward. Both Broom's work and my own research for this book suggest that opposition to cooperation with the state was much stronger among women's health advocates than in the mainstream women's movement. In interviewing activists from the 1970s and 1980s in the 1990s, I more than once heard the view that the kinds of policy changes that women were pursuing were insufficient to make even a dent in power relations.

Two points might help to explain the divergence between the women's health movement and the women's movement more broadly. First, it has been argued that radical feminists, rather than liberal or reformist feminists, have been a particularly important force in the women's health movement (Kenway 1992:111; Outhwaite 1989:202). Radical feminists are especially concerned about sexual subordination and violence against women and have been highly active in the refuge movement. A second point of explanation is that in keeping with the feminist critique of medicine, the state is heavily implicated in supporting the mainstream medical system. Therefore many activists thought that collaboration would ineluctably lead to being asked to work within the conventional medical framework, with the accompanying displacement of goals. At Hindmarsh, in Adelaide, for example, the area providing medical services was organisationally cordoned off from the rest of the centre because feminists feared contagion from a medical hierarchy in their midst.

Whatever the reasons, diametrically opposed attitudes to cooperation with the state were a reality and a destructive force in several women's health centres. In a number of settings, the issue was not resolved, even if compromises were found. Joyce Stevens (1995:17) describes differing perspectives at the Leichhardt Women's Community Health Centre (LWCHC), Australia's first women's health centre:

> [S]ome thought that they should take advantage of the more favourable situation to try to build some permanent outposts for women, such as women's services controlled by women. Others thought that the movement needed to maintain its radical and oppositional stance without the support of government funding or interference. The tensions between these positions were not resolved and they often coexisted in a type of unhappy marriage within projects, including LWCHC, where defiance and acquiescence were twin progeny.

In South Australia, tensions over how far to go in engaging with the state continued into the 1980s, along with concerns about losing touch with the grassroots feminist movement (Auer 2003:8). Most groups providing services, however, wherever they were located, accepted government funding from necessity, which created very real difficulties for many movement members interviewed for this book. Women reported that relationships with the state were 'always fraught'. Many thought that a level of separation was necessary to retain critical independence and pursue feminist goals; securing survival through the state risked submerging the reform agenda.

With the passage of time, the 'revolution–reform dilemma' that Broom (1991:128) noted became less apparent. Today, women's health workers are far more likely to be concerned about the sufficiency, indexation and security of public funding. Awareness of threats to independence is still keen, however, and radical health reform is still a major objective. In the early days, the decision to accept government funding undoubtedly weakened the movement by costing it members. Sarah Maddison has argued that an 'unintended consequence of state engagement' was the exclusion of many radical, socialist and anarchist feminists from the women's movement, with a subsequent decline in energy and activity (Maddison 2001). State engagement certainly alienated many radical feminists who distanced themselves from reformist activity. Moreover, antagonisms were such that continued cooperation would have been very nearly impossible. The decision of some to accept public funding, however, did not prevent radical, socialist and anarchist feminists from continuing their own preferred forms of activism and there is no clear causal link between engagement with the state and the decline of the women's movement as a whole.

An Anglocentric Women's Movement

The Australian women's movement, like sister movements elsewhere, has been described as centred upon the dominant group, or, in the Australian case, centred upon Anglo-Australian women. It has also been criticised consistently by women with disabilities for neglecting their issues. Early second-wave feminism is said to have taken a 'coherent, fixed, singular and unitary' view of the position of women. In this reading, women are everywhere subjugated to patriarchy—a condition that gives rise to similar experiences for all women everywhere. An all-inclusive feminism of this kind, as postmodern analyses point out, ignores differences between and within groups of women and ignores differences in preferences and priorities. By ignoring differences, positions outside the mainstream are marginalised: a unitary, single-perspective feminism cannot take into account the experiences of black women, immigrant women, refugee women, women with disabilities or lesbian women, to name just a few. Second-wave feminism, critics argue, is dominated by white, middle-class women, whose focus on their own issues marginalises the concerns of 'others' (Larbalestier 1998:150).

This is not the place to discuss Australian feminist discourses (see, for example, Bulbeck 1997; Larbalestier 1998), but portrayal as fixed and singular overstates the case. A diversity of views was always present, acknowledging a variety of 'feminisms' and cultural differences. Mary Kalantzis (1990:40–1), for example, has described Sydney meetings of an ethnic women's network, which included women as different from each other as Muslim women in *purdah* who wished to reform working conditions to allow traditional prayer sessions, and women from South American backgrounds who saw Australian women's organisations as politically backward.

While single-perspective feminism never existed, the theoretical position that dominated in the early years did not take account of the perspectives of all women, including Aboriginal, Torres Strait Islander, immigrant and refugee women. Goodall and Huggins (1992), for example, identify key differences between Aboriginal and non-Aboriginal women. They point out that, in many ways, Aboriginal women are in a better position than Aboriginal men, holding positions of power within their own communities—the reverse of the general situation for Anglo-Australian women. Moreover, Aboriginal women are generally better educated than Aboriginal men and often have higher-status jobs. Whereas Anglo-Australian women were demanding rights to abortion and contraception, Aboriginal women were fighting against unwanted sterilisation and the loss of children to various agencies. Thus, many of the demands of non-Aboriginal women were irrelevant to Aboriginal women and some were contrary to their wishes (Burgmann 1984:37). The major issue for Aboriginal women has been the white feminist movement's refusal to acknowledge the extent and depth of racism and the priority many Aboriginal women give to supporting Aboriginal men and to building healthy families and communities. Without recognising 'the full horror of racism in Australia', 'white women simply invited Aboriginal women to join the movement' (Goodall and Huggins 1992:401–2).

Feminists have also been guilty of attempting to speak 'for' Aboriginal women, rather than inviting Aboriginal women to speak for themselves. Perera (1985) recounts the story of a women's housing conference where Anglo women told Aboriginal women about their housing needs. The Aboriginal women present walked out in protest, giving rise to consternation and feelings of guilt. In the process of 'reconciliation' that followed, Anglo women learned something about the requirements of effective consultation and inclusion. Bronwyn Fredericks (2010) discusses the many barriers that still preclude effective cooperation between Aboriginal and non-Aboriginal Australian women.

Immigrant women, too, have charged the movement with racism and with relegating immigrant women's activism to the sidelines (Larbalestier 1998:148–58; Murdolo 1996). As with Aboriginal women, here, the main issues are often different and include problems of racism, poverty, language barriers, isolation, discrimination by supervisors at work, unfamiliarity with workplace rights and cultural disadvantage. Also, even though refugee women often find themselves with 'the dirtiest and most dangerous jobs on the factory floor' (Fraser 2008), unions have been slow to recognise their problems. As Kaplan (1996:125) argues, 'the right of participation was questioned even in the workplace'. Access to services was also fraught with problems. For example, immigrant women returned to violent relationships more frequently than Anglo women, leading refuge workers to believe this pattern constituted a safety risk for workers and other residents. According to Fraser (2008), the predominantly Anglo-Australian workers lacked 'the knowledge—or sometimes the desire—to help women from other cultures'. Another obstacle to identifying with the Anglo-Australian feminist movement was 'a pervasive stereotype' of immigrant women as 'uneducated, unskilled, under the thumb of a dominating father or husband, and uncomplaining' (Fraser 2008).

Immigrant and Aboriginal women have pointed out that they were politically aware, active in campaigns and active in setting up organisations and services to meet the problems they experienced. As Burgmann argued in 1982, 'there *is* a black women's movement—it is just that white women know virtually nothing about it' (1982:37, original emphasis). There is also an Aboriginal women's health movement, as the activism described in the following chapters demonstrates.

Consequently, the work of Aboriginal and immigrant and refugee women has often been left out of 'mainstream' accounts of what is erroneously labelled 'the' Australian women's movement (Murdolo 1996). Despite limited opportunities and heavy oppression, Aboriginal, Torres Strait Islander, refugee and immigrant women have certainly been part of an Australian movement to improve the conditions of women's lives. Immigrant women set up a number of their own associations and services from the 1970s onwards.[7] For example, the Migrant Women's Association was set up in 1973 in Sydney and the Migrant Women's Refuge was established in Melbourne in 1978. The new centre could not meet demand so a way around the problem was found by setting up the Refuge Ethnic Workers Program (REWP) in 1981. This service provided language and advocacy services for immigrant and refugee women in Anglo-Australian refuges and became a model for service provision. In its current form as the Immigrant Women's Domestic Violence Service (IWDVS), it is funded by the Victorian Government. It offers services in many languages and engages in prevention work, training and community education (Fraser 2008; IWDVS web site).

At the same time, Aboriginal women were establishing their own separate services. Aboriginal women's work in the founding of community-based health services has been mentioned and, in the early 1980s in Perth, a woman headed the AMS. The Council for Aboriginal Women of South Australia was set up in 1966 and, while not focusing specifically on health issues, it was concerned with women's and children's services, welfare and race issues (Grahame and Prichard 1996:37). The National Council of Aboriginal and Island Women was founded in 1970, concerned with health, race, welfare, children's issues and legal rights. The Victorian Council of Aboriginal and Island Women was active in the 1970s and the 1980s (Grahame and Prichard 1996:122). Among the council's activities was supporting the establishment of the Aboriginal Health Service, Fitzroy, in 1973 and an Aboriginal girl's hostel in Melbourne. Murawina Aboriginal Preschool and Women's Hostel was established in Chippendale, Sydney, in 1972. Mimbingal Violet (Vai) McGinness Stanton, of Kungarakany and Gurindji descent, was one of the founders and later coordinator of the Foundation of Rehabilitation with Aboriginal Alcohol Related Difficulties (FORWAARD) in 1976 (Grahame and Prichard 1996:42).

The Aboriginal Women's Centre was set up in Darwin in the second half of the 1970s and refuges were established in many places, including Melbourne and Moree, New South Wales. The last provided services for non-Aboriginal women as well. The founders of Cawarra Aboriginal Refuge, established in

---

7 According to Kaplan (1996:124–5), as well as experiencing racism, immigrant women were not helped by ethnic organisations. She points out that the first national conference held by the Federation of Ethnic Communities Councils of Australia in 1979 had one female delegate and no women on the executive. 'Neither ethnic community organisations nor the government gave enough weight to migrant women's concerns', she argues. See also Sawer (1990:107–39).

Sydney in 1979, had originally tried to locate it in the suburb of Penshurst but lost council approval due to racist reaction. (Grahame and Prichard 1996:28). The Western Women's Council was formed in Wilcannia, New South Wales, in 1984, concerned with caring for the land 'in the broadest sense' and opposing the establishment of an army base on 'fragile desert land east of Wilcannia'. Health was a concern, along with racism, imprisonment, police harassment and violence. The Federation for Aboriginal Women was formed in Victoria in 1982, with a number of aims including 'consolidating and strengthening of Aboriginal women' and promoting 'universal cooperation and friendship with all women's organisations' (Grahame and Prichard 1996:45).

Early Cooperative Ventures

For all the understandable distrust that many Aboriginal, Torres Strait Islander, refugee and immigrant women felt and still feel towards Anglo-Australian women, there are examples of collaboration and evidence of a slow coming together. A group called Joint Women's Action began in Canberra in 1972. It focused on 'justice for blacks and whites' and put together a leaflet dealing with the interracial rape of Aboriginal women and girls, which was co-authored by black and white women (Grahame and Prichard 1996:63). In Alice Springs, WL helped to campaign to protect a women's sacred site from being flooded to create a recreational lake (Grahame and Prichard 1996:9). The Alice Springs Women's Centre—part refuge, part health centre—provided services for both Aboriginal and non-Aboriginal women, and women from different backgrounds participated in management.

Living in small communities seems to be conducive to breaking down barriers between women of difference. Women in Broken Hill, New South Wales, founded the Multicultural Women's Resource Centre in 1986. Originally an initiative of the Filipino Women's Association, it received early funding from the Commonwealth Department of Immigration and Ethnic Affairs. The centre is managed by a committee of women from several ethnic groups, including Aboriginal and Anglo-Australian women, and it provides services, including health information and outreach, for all women in the area.

The cooperative effort that went into founding a women's refuge at Bourke, New South Wales, demonstrates that cultural differences do not necessarily prevent women from different backgrounds working together. Over more than a decade, work by Aboriginal, Anglo and Indian women, with the help of some men, enabled a centre to become established without government funding. This story of cooperation and perseverance has been summarised as follows: 'In an otherwise racially divided community, we have managed to have Aboriginal and non-Aboriginal women work together for the common good. Many women who would have never met have come together and made friends' (Alvares 1992:183).

A number of writers acknowledge the 'well-meaning concern' of many Anglo-Australian feminists towards non-Anglo groups (Fraser 2008; Goodall and Huggins 1992; Kalantzis 1990). Goodall and Huggins (1992:402) argue that the Australian women's movement learned about difference 'slowly and somewhat painfully' over the first two decades. Tensions continued, however, because both the way that 'racism shapes sexism' and the needs of Aboriginal women to strengthen their communities were not sufficiently understood. Goodall and Huggins note, however, that supportive and productive relationships did sometimes develop.

In summary, Anglo-Australian concerns dominated the early women's movement but, gradually, feminists established links with women from different cultural backgrounds and learned more about their issues. For their part, some immigrant and refugee women, as well as some Aboriginal women, began to find value in working with some Anglo-Australian women. The collaboration that became possible is illustrated by the work of two immigrant women living in Queensland in the 1980s. Raquel Aldunate and Gladys Revelo both worked at the Brisbane Migrant Resource Centre but, as well, they belonged to the Women's Health Centre, the Community Health Association of Queensland, the Migrant Women's Network, the Australian Social Welfare Union, the Women in Trade Unions Network, Radio 4EB, the Chile Solidarity Committee, the Latin American Centre and others (Aldunate and Revelo 1987:40).

Women's Health Services and the Needs of Non-Anglo Women

This discussion of difference and exclusion would be incomplete without taking into consideration the efforts made by women's health centres, refuges and sexual assault centres to meet the needs of the non-Anglo women who live in surrounding communities. From the beginning, despite ignorance and racism, many workers in women's health centres sought to discover what local women needed and wanted. They attempted to provide culturally appropriate services and, where possible, assisted groups to set up their own services. Most women's health centres were deliberately established in areas of high need, where low-income, immigrant, refugee and sometimes Aboriginal women lived (Auer et al. 1987:77; Broom 1991:3). They aimed to be accessible to disadvantaged women and some focused specifically on the needs of migrant and/or Aboriginal women (Broom 2001:101). The work of LWCHC serves as an example.

LWCHC, like most sister centres, was located in the midst of a large working-class and immigrant population. From the beginning, 'before the concept of multiculturalism had been invented' (Stevens 1995:48),[8] almost one-third of the women using the centre were immigrants. Ways of delivering appropriate services were explored and, within a year, information and services were being provided in three languages. In the second year, bilingual and multilingual workers were employed. Visits were arranged to factories and hostels and a publicity campaign on immigrant radio and in the press elicited an 'overwhelming response'. Italian women became members of the collective.[9]

Throughout its 38 years, LWCHC has continued to provide services for immigrant women, altering direction and focus in response to demographic changes. The factory-visits program was expanded towards the end of the 1970s and became an established Factory Project in the 1980s. Information brochures were translated. In 1983, LWCHC and the similarly located Liverpool Women's Health Centre, which had been doing its own research into women's industrial health problems, set up the Health in the Workforce Factory Project, which operated for more than a decade. The project employed women from Yugoslav, Chilean, Greek, Turkish and Vietnamese backgrounds. Between them, members of the group spoke 16 languages.

Outreach work uncovered the stressful lives of women working at home. In addition, immigrant women, it was found, often had little information about their health. Many had never had a pap smear and, as a group, they were frequently prescribed tranquillisers. Outreach work in factories and shopping precincts became a standard part of LWCHC's work. By the mid-1980s, the managing collective included South American, Italian, Thai, Turkish and Polish women. Information brochures in Italian, Spanish, Polish, Turkish, Greek, Arabic and Vietnamese were produced. In the early 1990s, Vietnamese and Chinese women joined the staff, and services were developed for newly arriving Pacific Island women. LWCHC continues to provide a range of services for the immigrant women who live nearby.

Mary Dimech, writing in 1982, recognised the efforts that many Anglo feminists had made to address the problems of immigrant women, pointing to the activities of workers' health centres, women's health centres and some refuges. She argued that women's movement campaigns for equal pay, the right to work,

---

8　Stevens might be right about the timing of the introduction of the concept of multiculturalism. Certainly, the term was not widely known or well understood in 1974. About this time, however, the Minister for Immigration, Al Grassby, worked to win support for multiculturalism from the Australian community.
9　It soon emerged that there were significant cultural differences between women from different parts of Italy.

child care and abortion were all of benefit to immigrant women as were the efforts of teachers' unions to promote appropriate language-teaching services for migrants, particularly women (Dimech 1982:16).

Working with and for women from different cultural backgrounds was not, however, achieved without tensions and difficulties. LWCHC programs did not (and probably could not) provide for the needs of all clients, leading some immigrant women to feel 'that they were outside the real experience and discussions of the collective' (Stevens 1995:53). Anglo women struggled to understand the problems immigrant women faced and many wrestled with the fact that some immigrant workers had little knowledge of feminism and were not committed to its principles. For example, one worker is reported to have had problems with the collective mode of organisation and with the propagation of the 'Women's Libbers' creed'. As Stevens (1995:53) has recorded, 'it was often difficult to decide how and if it was possible for feminism to incorporate an understanding of all these experiences'. Most members of the collective, however, were strongly committed to providing services for all women who lived locally.

Many other women's health centres made similar efforts. Loddon Campaspe Women's Health Service and North-East Women's Health Service in Victoria developed factory projects soon after opening in the 1980s. Although the board was Anglo-Australian, women from non-English-speaking backgrounds were employed at the Hindmarsh Women's Health Centre, Adelaide, from the early days. The staff of Liverpool Women's Health Centre came from diverse cultural backgrounds, including three Aboriginal staff members employed in 1984. Funding limitations, however, prevented Liverpool from reaching all the groups that were known to have needs (Edwards 1984:22). In 2008, staff members of Women's Health Care House, Perth, spoke 14 different languages and arrangements were in place for interpreters in other languages to be present at appointments or to speak with clients on the phone. In some centres, lesbian-focused programs have been developed (Cameron and Velthuys 2005). This list is far from exhaustive.

In summary, racism, ignorance and lack of understanding, along with a heavy focus on the priorities of Anglo-Australian women, were, and possibly still are, part of the women's health movement experience. Some successful joint ventures have, however, been developed and women's health movement workers, within the resources available to them, have made efforts to respond to diverse health needs. The value of collaboration, where it proved possible, was recognised by Raquel Aldunate and Gladys Revelo, when, at a community and environmental health conference in 1986, they acknowledged 'the support of our friends, companeras, mainly Anglos, who cared enough to get beyond their guilt, and or ignorance, and therefore beyond their own racism' (Aldunate and Revelo 1987:41).

Conclusion

Women with divergent views and from many cultural backgrounds have been part of the Australian women's health movement and while there have been disagreements and differing priorities, a core set of ideas, around which there is considerable agreement, serves as a guide for action. The question of whether community-based service-providing groups should accept public funding has long been settled, not to everyone's satisfaction, and for many years the task has been to acquire sufficient resources to be able to respond to women's expressed needs and pay workers decent wages. A great deal of learning has taken place as Anglo-Australian movement members realised that not all women shared their concerns, priorities and ways of doing things. While it is as misleading to talk about the Anglo-Australian women's health movement as one homogenous whole as it is to talk about 'all Aboriginal women' or 'all immigrant women', understanding has been developed between these different groupings and collaborative and fulfilling working partnerships have been formed.

The critique of curative medicine, developed in Australia and other English-speaking countries, was a crystallising force in the early years and continues to be relevant. Unsatisfactory encounters with the medical system were common enough for large numbers of women to identify with the critique. Some modification of medical practice has taken place, particularly in relation to the provision of information as a basis for effective informed consent. Serious concerns remain, however, including continuing medicalisation, gender bias in medical research and treatment, questions about the safety and appropriateness of pharmaceuticals and the paucity of prevention advice and support services.

The social view of health, which is an elaboration of feminist criticism of the undue focus on treatment in conventional medical care, takes into account the impact of life circumstances on health outcomes. Developed from everyday experience in a context of support for structural health reform, it forms the centrepiece of the movement's ideas. Outside the movement, the concept has gained legitimacy, as supporting evidence of its validity accrues. Within the movement and in the public health and Aboriginal health movements, it is strongly endorsed. Achieving structural change in the health system and in the unequal conditions of people's lives is the task that the Australian women's health movement set for itself.

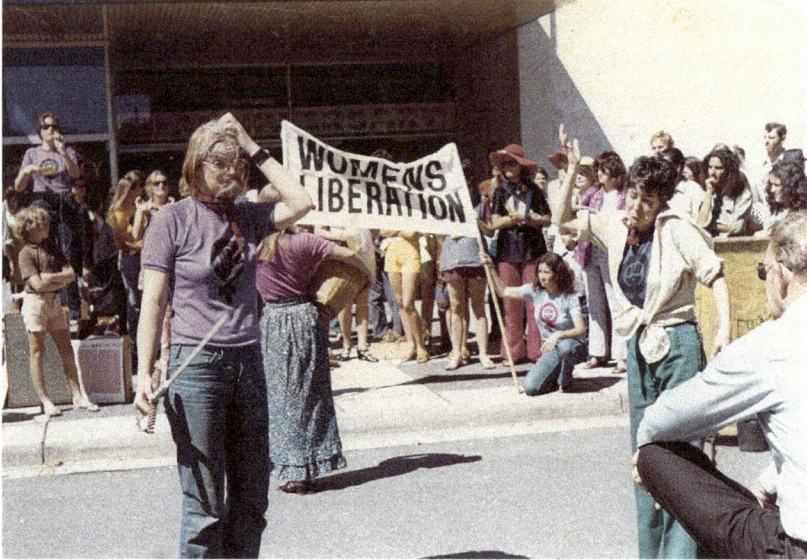

Canberra Women's Liberation presenting street theatre, International Women's Day, 1972.

Photo: Property of WEL History Project

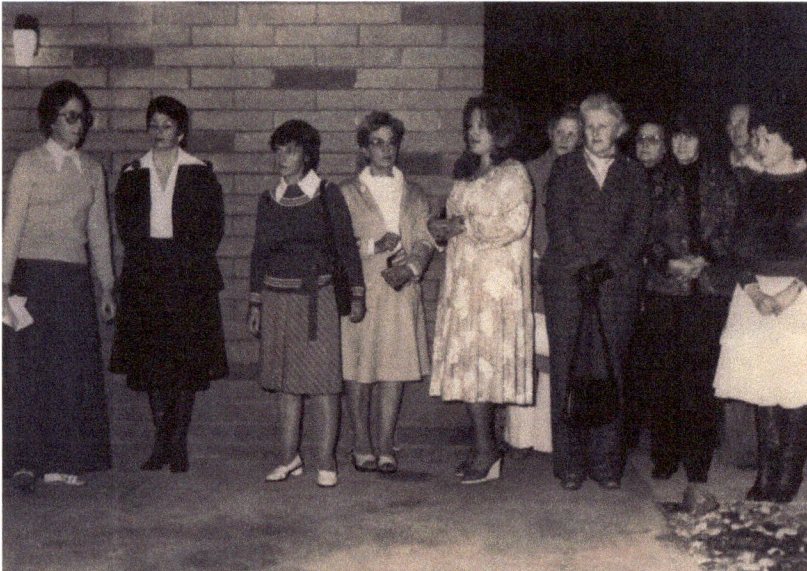

Opening Warrina Women's Refuge, Coffs Harbour, New South Wales, July 1978. From left: Salvation Army Capt. Gail Rogers, Betty Craft, Director, Jan Ireland, Mary Curran, Joan Dunkley, Bel Weise, Patricia Degens, Shirley Jones, Valerie Furniss.

Photo: Pat Degens

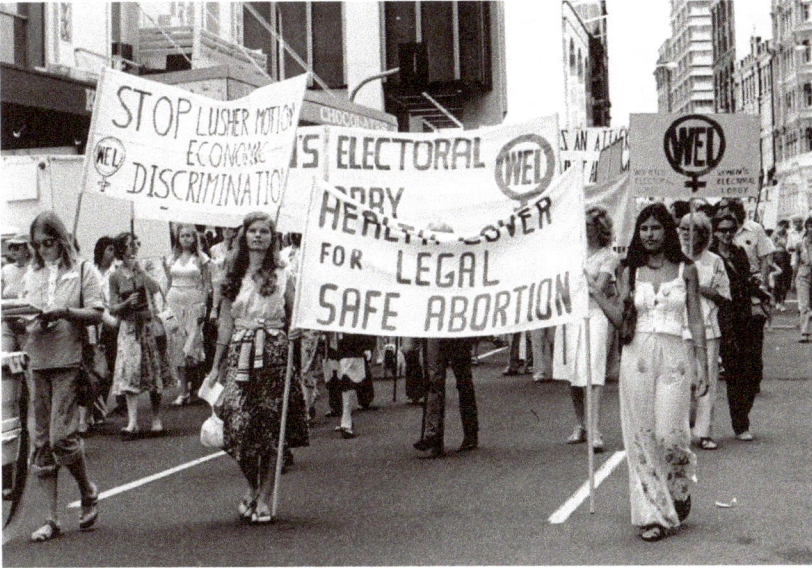

WEL-NSW members marching against the 'Lusher Motion', a Bill moved by MP Stephen Lusher in the House of Representatives to restrict the payment of medical benefits for termination of pregnancy, International Women's Day, 1979.

Photo: The Search Foundation, Mitchell Library of New South Wales

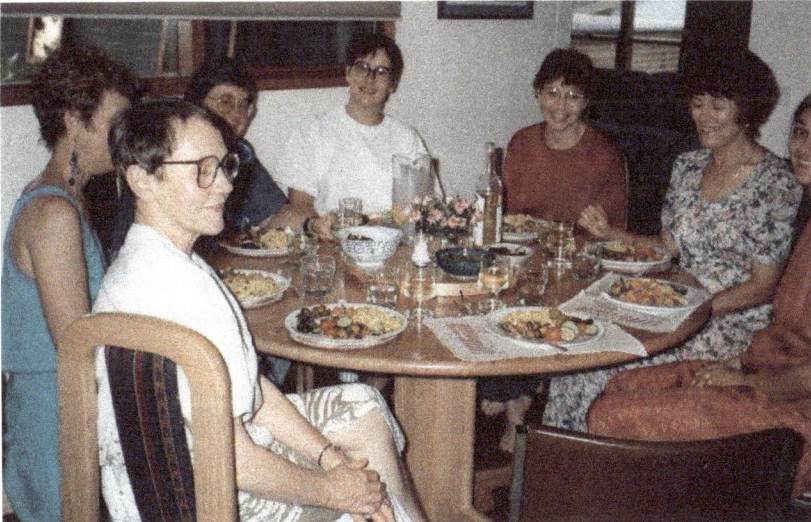

ACT Women's Health Network members enjoy lunch at Romaine Rutnam's home, 1995. From left: Dorothy Broom (obscured), Mary Sexton, Ann Smith, Karen Nienaber, Charlotte Palmer, Gwen Gray, Romaine Rutnam (obscured).

Photo: Manoa Renwick

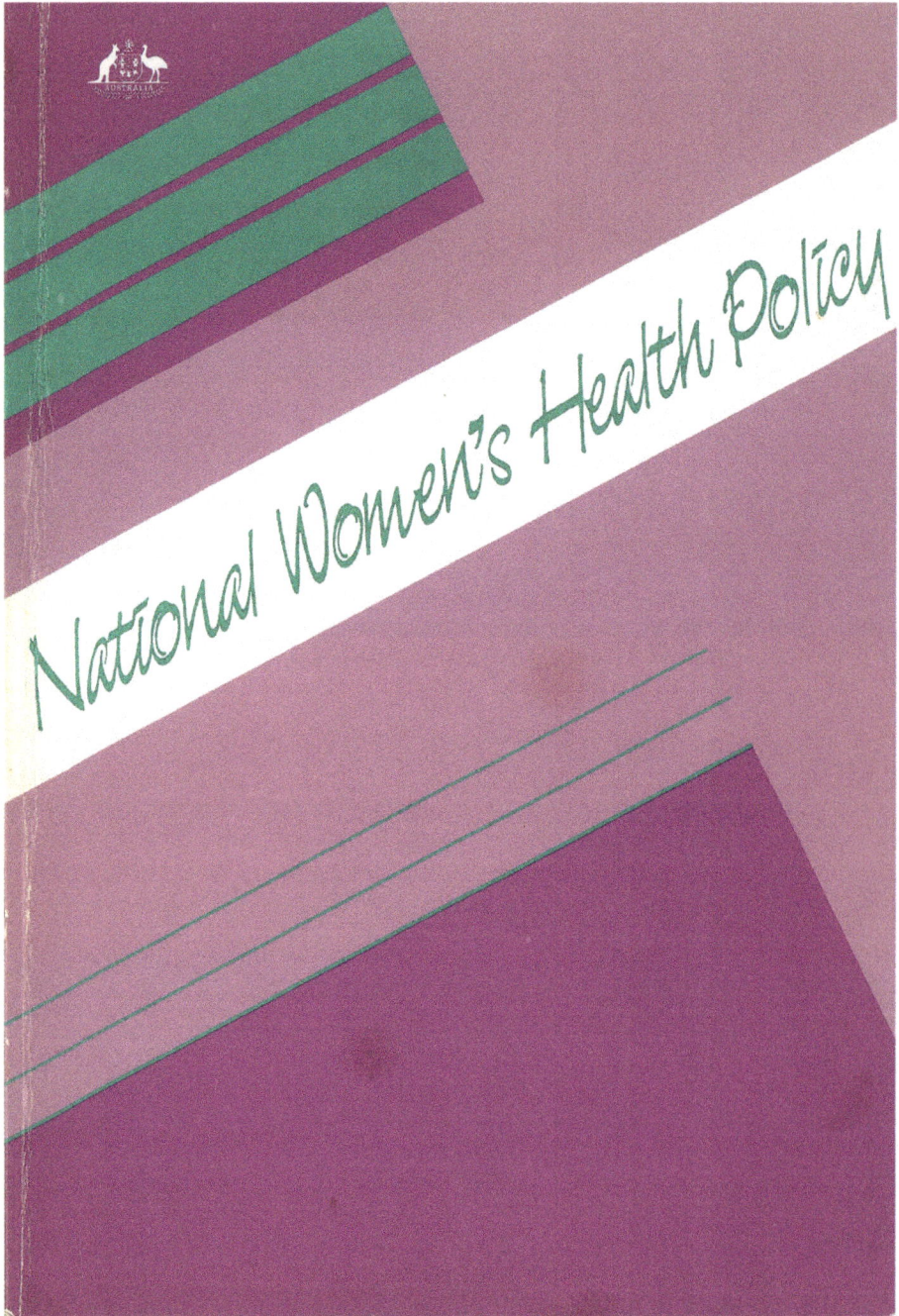

The National Women's Health Policy, 1989.

2. With Only Their Bare Hands

We had no one on our side, no political parties, no governments, no armies, no police, no trade unions and no religions. All we had were ourselves—women.

— Zelda D'Aprano (in Robertson n.d.:Ch. 16)

The Australian women's health movement embarked on a journey of discovery in the early 1970s, knowing little more than that the existing system was causing deep pain and was not meeting women's needs. Members had scarcely any money and often knew little about health, the health system or how government worked. However, as they listened to each other's experiences and formulated their critiques, they developed two aims: first, they wanted to change the power relations of society that placed women in a vulnerable, subordinate position, and second, they wanted to support the women they were hearing from, many of whom were desperate to find compassionate medical services. In order to politicise the problems they saw, they needed to articulate a set of concerns. This task was not an easy one, not only because it was virgin territory but also because criticism of science, medical science and the medical profession was uncommon at the time and practically unheard of from women! Moreover, they had to speak out in public about unmentionable topics that opened them to portrayal as extremists—easy targets for ridicule. Rape and incest were completely taboo subjects and even domestic violence was hardly mentioned at the time, even within the counselling community.

Initially, women's attention focused on reproductive health issues where the gaps were glaring; however, a broader approach, a social view of health, soon developed from the stories and experiences that were shared. In the process of working for the structural reforms that follow from a social perspective, women faced formidable opposition: from the medical profession, from the religious right and its institutions, from bureaucracies bent on doing things the way they had always been done, and from governments that had no feeling for holistic health perspectives and often lacked the political will to confront powerful opposition.

This chapter presents a sketch of the political and service-providing activities of the early years. Because Broom (1991) has provided a detailed account of the establishment of Australia's first dozen 'founder' women's health centres, only a summary is presented here. The second part of the chapter examines the establishment of the first refuges and services for women who had experienced sexual assault. Setting up separate services was radical action, especially for women without resources, and is a distinctive feature of Australian activism.

In other countries with strong women's health movements, relatively few such services were established and even fewer have endured. The separate women's health sector is testimony to the strength of the Australian movement and to the dedication of its members.

Women's Health Centres and Services

The 1970s was a 'period of ferment and hope that the world could be a better place' (Auer 2003:3). As in the United States, women in Australia met in consciousness-raising (CR) groups in the late 1960s where one of the aims was to unlock the silence about women's personal experiences and to draw out the political implications. Women also found these processes therapeutic (Orr 1994:209). Issues were discussed and evaluated in small groups, with a particular focus on the effects of traditional female roles, such as responsibility for caring. Women acted as each other's sounding boards; 'old inhibitions and superstitions about women's physiology and psychological natural impediments were realised for the crap it was' (Melbourne University Consciousness-Raising Group 1974:46). The disruption of conventional views about the female role and the development of new norms about what constitutes femininity emerged from these processes. Many groups attempted to work systematically and to devise new practices to replace the old, especially in relation to households, sexual relationships, raising children and participation in public life (Connell 1987:30–1).

Jean Taylor (2003) describes her CR/WL experience in Melbourne as follows:

> From the moment I joined the Brunswick CR group, I was completely involved. The Women's Liberation Centre was set up, with a telephone for information and support and also as a meeting place for unfunded activist groups. I started doing roster there. The centre was basically a large meeting space at 16 Little Latrobe Street. So women could either drop in, if they were in the city, and pick up the latest position paper… or subscribe to the *Women's Liberation Newsletter*…so much was being published and written about and women were ringing in about all sorts of things. Domestic violence was rife and by the mid-1970s referrals to refuges became crucially important.

CR and WL groups were being established at the same time. Mass gatherings were held in an atmosphere that was peaceful but often radically confrontational. For example, thousands of women, with their children and dogs, attended the 1972 International Women's Day (IWD) march in Sydney, playing havoc with traffic. They carried flags and banners, sang and chanted. There were Hyde Park picnics, concerts and street theatre depicting the stages of women's lives. A few women removed their T-shirts in protest against double standards and were protected by others when police tried to move in. A man from the New Theatre, wearing a bearskin, was arrested for wheeling a model of a giant penis through the streets in a barrow—a send-up of prevailing masculinist views. IWD Sydney made a profit from the day, which was used to rent the first WL House in the city (Stevens 1985).

In CR and WL groups, health emerged as an urgent issue but activists initially had no idea how to respond. As Zelda D'Aprano (in Robertson n.d.) describes the situation:

> Answers had to be found and found fast, for many of these women were desperate. Quickly we had to gather information and pass it on. Off we went to find sympathetic doctors; to talk to nurses we knew; and to read everything we could find. Off to seminars, conferences, into courses to find out how the healthcare system worked; into jobs within the system; calling public meetings to see if what seemed wrong, really was. We found it was much worse.

The wish to support women who needed services that were unavailable is easy to account for but the determination with which women set about establishing their own health centres and crisis-support services with so few resources is not so easily explained. Not only were women short of money, they were also inexperienced politically. They knew little about lobbying, conducting advocacy or dealing with bureaucracy. As Lyn McKenzie (1979), a founding member of the Melbourne Women's Health Collective, recounts, few members of the collective had any experience in writing submissions or seeking funding and few had 'access to the manner in which the bureaucratic maze could be successfully tackled' (McKenzie 1979:40).

Reproductive health and, to a lesser extent, mental health issues were early priorities. Adelaide WL recognised the need for easily understood information about contraception and in 1970 planned a pamphlet called *What Every Girl Should Know about Contraception*. Run off in early 1971 and reprinted several times, it was distributed widely to schoolgirls, working women and university students, among others (Kinder 1980:49–51).[1] In its 1971 manifesto, Adelaide WL declared that women had the right to control their own bodies and called for publicly funded birth-control education, the abolition of the 27.5 per cent sales tax on contraceptives and the establishment of community-based birth-control centres.[2] It argued that local health centres should provide services for

---

1   The pamphlet inspired the highly controversial Sydney publication *What Every Woman Should Know*, first printed in July 1971 (Stevens 1995:15).
2   While WL took action on reproductive health issues, including contraception, from 1970 onwards, the newly formed WEL was directly responsible for having the luxury tax removed. WEL made a submission in the middle of 1972 to the tariff review being undertaken by the Tariff Board. As a result, the ALP promised

psychological disorders and that free abortion on demand should be available. Mental health issues and 'dealing with doctors and psychiatrists' were priorities when the Adelaide Women's Health Group formed in 1973. By the time planning for the Hindmarsh Women's Health Centre was under way in 1975, a social view of health was being articulated. The new centre was to 'provide a coordinated community-based service which would cover the physical, psychological and social aspects of women's health care'. Preventive primary health care and health education would be made available and women's health research and community action would be promoted (Radoslovich 1994:14–17). Such a broad agenda was at the cutting edge of ideas at the time. The following list provides a summary of the main services established in the 1970s.

Selected Women's Health Centres and Services Established in the 1970s

1972

- Children by Choice, Brisbane, family planning and abortion information service.

1974

- Adelaide Women's Shelter, also known as Naomi Women's Shelter.
- Bonnie Women's Shelter, Sydney.
- Collingwood Women's Health Centre, Melbourne.
- Elsie Women's Refuge, Sydney.
- Hobart Women's Shelter.
- Leichhardt Women's Community Health Centre, Sydney.
- Nardine Women's Shelter, Perth.
- Rape Crisis Centre, Melbourne.
- Sydney Rape Crisis Centre.
- Women's Health and Community Centre, Perth.
- Women's Liberation Halfway House, Melbourne.

1975

- Alice Springs Women's Centre, primarily a refuge, Northern Territory.
- Blacktown Community Cottage, Sydney.

---

to remove the luxury tax on contraceptives, make the contraceptive pill free through the Pharmaceutical Benefits Scheme and support the development of family planning networks. Action on all areas was taken as soon as the Whitlam Government gained office (Sawer 2008b:37–8).

- Bringa Women's Refuge, Dee Why, Sydney.
- Brisbane Rape Crisis Centre.
- Canberra Women's Refuge.
- Darwin Women's Health Centre.
- Hindmarsh Women's Health Centre, Adelaide.
- Hunter Region Working Women's Centre, now Hunter Women's Centre, New South Wales.
- Launceston Women's Shelter, Tasmania.
- Liverpool Women's Health Centre (which later participated in establishing Sunshine Cottage, a local childcare service, Amberley Single Women's Refuge, Rosebank Sexual Assault Service, Dympna House, an incest counselling service, Campbelltown Women's Health Centre and Jilimi Aboriginal Women's Health Centre, now Waminda), Sydney.
- Women's House Health Centre, Brisbane.
- Women's Health and Community Centre Rape Crisis Centre, Perth.

1976

- Adelaide Rape Crisis Centre.
- Central Coast Women's Health Centre, Gosford, New South Wales.
- Christies Beach Women's Shelter, South Australia.
- Marrickville Women's Refuge, Sydney.
- Marty House, Woolloomooloo, Sydney, for women with substance-abuse issues.
- Sexual Assault Resource Centre, Perth.

1977

- Bankstown Women's Health Centre, Sydney.
- Bessie Smyth Feminist Abortion Clinic, Sydney.
- Cawarra Women's Refuge Aboriginal Corporation.
- Women's Health Care House, Perth.
- Women in Industry, Contraception and Health (now Multicultural Centre for Women's Health), Melbourne.

1978

- Anne Women's Shelter, South Australia.
- Geelong Rape Crisis Centre, Victoria.
- Warrina Women's Refuge, Coffs Harbour, New South Wales.

1979

- Elizabeth Hoffman House, emergency accommodation and support for Aboriginal women and their children, Melbourne.
- Sexual Assault Service, Queen Victoria Medical Centre, Melbourne.
- Wagga Wagga Women's Health and Support Centre, New South Wales.
- Working Women's Centre, Adelaide.

New South Wales

Australia's first women's health centre was established in Leichhardt, Sydney, in January 1974. The preparatory work was done by members of Control, a grassroots abortion referral service. The need for the centre was amply demonstrated when the first client arrived before the furniture and, within six months, a 10-day wait for an appointment developed (Broom 1991:4). Women came from all over Sydney—17 per cent travelling from the outer western suburbs—which alerted staff to serious unmet need. It was decided to apply for funding to establish another centre in Parramatta. In the meantime, a group of women had begun to meet in Green Valley. They wanted a multipurpose women's centre and a refuge. They learned that Leichhardt had plans for a western Sydney centre and successfully petitioned to have it located in Liverpool (Liverpool Women's Health Centre web site).

Liverpool Community Women's Health Centre was opened in April 1975, the premises having been painted and prepared by the women themselves. Leichhardt Women's Community Health Centre (LWCHC) also established the Bessie Smyth feminist information, counselling and abortion facility (Broom 1991:1–14). Following a community-development approach, these centres helped to establish more agencies, including Sunshine Cottage, a local childcare service; Amberley Single Women's Refuge; WILMA, a women's health centre in Campbelltown; Rosebank Sexual Assault Service; Jilimi, now Waminda, Aboriginal Women's Health Centre on the South Coast of New South Wales; and Dympna House, an incest counselling service. The Leichhardt centre was also involved in the establishment of the Workers' Health Centre in Lidcombe, by way of its interest in occupational health and safety (OHS) issues. Both Liverpool and Leichhardt were inundated with inquiries from groups wishing to set up their own centres, demonstrating the urgency of the need being expressed. Staff supported initiatives in Bathurst, Wagga Wagga, Bowral and Nowra.

The Bessie Smyth Foundation provided supportive, holistic, non-judgmental services, delivered in a setting intended to be homely rather than clinical. Clients were able to bring their children if they had no-one else to care for them. A charge was necessary to make operations viable but it was recognised that even a small charge was beyond the capacity of some women. Bessie Smyth staff therefore set up the Powell Street Clinic in Homebush in 1977 to provide information and counselling support on the basis that no woman should be turned away because of inability to pay a user fee.[3] Information was provided in 13 languages plus English, both over the phone and face-to-face.

After 25 years, Powell Street became financially unviable and was sold to Marie Stopes International in 2002.[4] As well as providing 42 000 safe, affordable abortions and countless counselling and support services, Bessie Smyth provided training for health professionals and student placements. Clients came from all walks of life and included marginalised and disadvantaged women, 'illegal' migrants, sex workers, women in prison, women leaving prison and women with drug and alcohol-related problems. With the funds from the sale of the Powell Street Clinic, the foundation continued to provide counselling, referral, information and support services for destitute women. Repeated efforts were made to secure funding for the establishment of a State-wide information service, similar to Queensland's Children by Choice (of which more below). In 2008, operations ceased, although the foundation was retained, in case a 'window of opportunity' should emerge for the establishment of a new women's reproductive health service.

Another early New South Wales centre is the Working Women's Centre, near Newcastle, set up in 1975, as a multipurpose centre, providing health, legal aid, counselling, information, employment and childcare services. An enormous amount of work was involved in setting up and maintenance because funding had to be secured from a variety of separate sources (Broom 1991:15–16)—a situation that continues in 2010! The centre, now the Hunter Women's Centre, has been unable to obtain the services of a doctor since 2003. It provides short, medium and long-term counselling, undertakes casework and outreach where resources allow and runs support groups and health-related activities, including dancing, Tai Chi, massage and meditation.

---

3   A user fee, charge, co-payment or out-of-pocket expense—terms used interchangeably in Australia— comes about when there is a gap between the Medicare rebate and the fee charged by the provider. User charges constitute a serious financial barrier to the use of medical services.
4   For the same reason, Sexual Health and Family Planning ACT transferred its abortion service, Reproductive Health Services, to Marie Stopes in 2004.

Victoria

> The concept of worker control and the principle of collectivity was alien to the members of the HCC [Hospitals and Charities Commission]. (McKenzie 1979:41)

Two issues dominated the overflowing speak-out organised by WL, the Union of Australian Women and the YWCA in Melbourne in 1973: poor health care and lack of information. Women gave testimonies about poor-quality services and about services they could not find or could not afford. The Melbourne Women's Health Collective was formed after the meeting, supported by a donation of $490 from an abortion trust fund that had recently closed. Premises were rented for the Collingwood Women's Health Centre and furnished from donations and small grants. Within a few months, the centre had five doctors, several nursing sisters, a naturopath and a dietician. Service provision was voluntary, although after Medibank, the Commonwealth's new national health insurance scheme, came into operation, medical services could be bulk billed. Demand was heavy, as in New South Wales, and evening sessions often lasted until midnight (Hull 1986). Dorothy Broom (1991:12–14) has described the funding difficulties experienced as a result of federal processes and State-level political intransigence but, briefly, Commonwealth funding was to have been channelled through the Victorian Hospitals and Charities Commission (HCC) in 1975. The commission, however, imposed conditions that were unacceptable to the collective, including that services be provided for both men and women, that men be allowed to join the collective and that doctors be paid by fee-for-service rather than salary or other means. Compliance was unthinkable. The Melbourne Women's Health Collective closed its doors for clinical services at the end of 1975 and requested that the grant money be returned to the Commonwealth (Hull 1986; McKenzie 1979).

South Australia

> The health bureaucracy appears to have had an unfavourable view of the women's health centre from the start. (Quoted in Auer 2003:5)

As in Victoria, in South Australia, the health bureaucracy strongly opposed separate women's health centres. Opened in 1976 after operating from the house of one of its doctors, the Hindmarsh Women's Health Centre was the first in South Australia. The founding collective hired an old building and renovated it, assisted by volunteers, male and female. Expectations were high: a comprehensive, women-centred, child-friendly service would provide comprehensive services including relationship support and would help women to reach their potential

(Radoslovich 1994:15–16). Commonwealth funding was temporarily blocked in the Health Department but Hindmarsh became established and operated successfully for four years. In 1980, however, disagreement broke out between women who thought the centre had lost its independence and vision through its close alignment with government and those of a more moderate persuasion. An unsympathetic government lost no time in withdrawing funding and appointing an administrator. The Women's Adviser to the Department of Premier and Cabinet was a key player in trying to salvage something from the ashes, and the Health Minister, Jennifer Adamson, was supportive. In response to vigorous grassroots lobbying, the minister was able to preserve the funding for another centre. Shortly afterwards, Adelaide Women's Community Health Centre was established in North Adelaide and most of the Hindmarsh staff moved to work there. The original collective, however, decided to continue operations, providing some medical services, workshops, herbal treatments and massages (Broom 1991:19–21, 93–101; Radoslovich 1994:19–21).

Western Australia

In Perth, women formed the Women's Centre Action Group, which met weekly at the WEL premises from October 1972 onwards. Establishing a refuge was chosen as the top priority. Preparatory work proceeded through 1973 and the Nardine women's refuge was opened in July 1974. Shortly afterwards, the Women's Health and Community Centre at Glendower Street began operating on a voluntary basis and was officially opened in 1975 after it received Commonwealth funding. The focus was on providing services for all women on the grounds that women from all income groups suffered discrimination and stereotyping in the medical mainstream. A split between radicals and moderates—described to me as 'an implosion'—led to the withdrawal of funding in 1976. Again, the money was preserved for another centre, and Women's Health Care House opened in 1977 (Broom 1991:14–15). The small premises led workers to feel they were operating from 'a resurrected sardine tin' but the centre was able to move to its present location at 100 Aberdeen Street in 1989 (Stroud 1989:3). Medical, counselling, information and postnatal depression services are provided along with support and advocacy for women suffering mental health problems and women experiencing domestic violence. Community-development projects and workshops are held, child care is available for clients and development and training are provided for health and social welfare professionals.

Queensland

At a time when State politicians were telling women that everything they could possibly need was being provided in hospitals, grassroots women set up Women's House Health Centre in Brisbane in 1975, as part of a multipurpose centre. Participants remember it as 'a hotbed of dispute' between women with different feminist orientations. Differences were not just between radicals and reformists but also between women of different sexual persuasions. Early management committees did not keep accurate records so the auditor was unable to produce an audited set of accounts and the centre lost its funding after less than two years. A variety of fundraising activities was used to survive. Some services, mainly refuge services, continued on a voluntary basis but the centre had to move to save money. The second set of premises was in poor repair but was nevertheless full to overflowing with women needing shelter. At this time, Premier, Joh Bjelke-Petersen, said there were no homeless young people in Queensland and returned $14 million to the Commonwealth Department of Housing.

The centre was eventually funded under the National Women's Health Policy (NWHP) in 1990 (Broom 1991:16–17). Among the 'memorable moments' of the early years was the arrest of Women's House workers for singing *Lest We Forget* for women raped in war.

Northern Territory

In Darwin, local WEL women, supported by general practitioner Lyn Reid, wrote a health centre funding proposal to the Health and Hospitals Services Commission (HHSC) in 1974. Darwin Women's Health Centre, a combined health centre and refuge, was opened in 1975, having been delayed for six months, this time not by the local bureaucracy but by Cyclone Tracy. Divisions among members and identification with radical elements gave the NT Government an opportunity to withdraw funding in 1980. In Alice Springs, too, WEL women were behind the establishment of a women's centre, which was primarily a refuge and was opened on a volunteer basis in an old house in 1975. It provided crisis counselling, referrals and emergency accommodation, but it too lost funding in 1980, and although volunteer workers tried to continue, the service was closed and the house bulldozed (Broom 1991:21–2). Local women, however, worked to re-establish a centre and 14 months later Women's Community House was opened as a refuge in an old building which was intended to be temporary. It took a further nine years to arrange for specific-purpose accommodation and a renamed Alice Springs Women's Shelter opened in 1991. The service has expanded, gaining a children's support worker, an outreach worker, a domestic violence counsellor and a community-development and training worker. An outreach service for women and children who do not want to stay at the shelter and transitional housing arrangements operate at other locations. The service, which is jointly funded by the NT and Commonwealth governments through the Supported Accommodation Assistance Program (SAAP), is open to women from all cultural backgrounds.

Refuges, Shelters and Houses[5]

> The needs of women and children escaping domestic violence are as complex and varied as the many kinds of violence that are being escaped from. (Pateras 1997:4)

The Australian refuge movement has been a major force in having violence recognised and accepted as a serious women's health issue. The political pressure generated at the local level slowly percolated upwards, in due course finding expression in national policies. Violence against women has deep historical roots. In eighteenth-century Britain, the law still allowed men to beat their wives, and nineteenth-century English and Australian laws regulated violence rather than outlawing it. It was a major issue for first-wave feminists: Louisa Lawson wrote with outrage about it in *The Dawn* in 1891 (Spinney n.d.:1; Weeks and Gilmore 1996:141). Despite more than a century of activism, however, the National Council to Reduce Violence against Women and their Children (hereinafter referred to as the National Council) (Commonwealth of Australia 2009a:20) found that one in three Australian women still experience violence at some time in their lives. The majority of perpetrators are men, and women are mostly assaulted in their own homes, often repeatedly, by men they know. Violence is a major cause of homelessness for women and children. In 2003–04, the Australian Institute of Health and Welfare (AIHW 2005a) found that 33 per cent of women in SAAP-funded services were escaping violence, along with 66 per cent of accompanying children.

Violence is a major cause of ill health: intimate partner violence was the leading contributor to death, disability and illness for Victorian women aged between fifteen and forty-four years in 2004, ahead of well-recognised risk factors such as high blood pressure, smoking and obesity. Intimate partner violence contributed 8 per cent of the total disease burden for Victorian women aged between fifteen and forty-four years and 3 per cent of the burden for all Victorian women in

---

5 'Refuge' is the term generally used in Victoria, New South Wales and Western Australia, while 'house' or 'shelter' is more common in Tasmania, South Australia, Queensland and the Northern Territory (Weeks 1994:44).

that year (VicHealth 2004). Violent relationship experiences are associated with allergies and breathing problems, pain and fatigue, bowel problems, vaginal discharges, eyesight and hearing problems, asthma, bronchitis, emphysema and cervical cancer (Loxton et al. 2006). This major health risk factor is not easily or effectively addressed in the conventional medical system.

The magnitude of the problem emerged early in CR groups and phone-ins (Smith 1985:26; Weeks and Gilmore 1996:143). Women sought refuge from violence and sometimes because their children were being sexually abused (Geddes 2007:2). With almost nowhere for women to go, collective members often provided accommodation in their own homes; however, the problem was too big to be solved in this way and feminists knew that prevention required that the issue be taken out of the private sector where it was invisible and debated publicly (Orr 1994:9–10). Elimination would require fundamental changes in societal values, in public policy, in the conduct of relationships and in the status and economic independence of women. Sustained political action would be necessary.

Feminist refuges were established to provide immediate support and to lobby on key issues, such as public housing, income support, employment, education and child care. Refuges also supported women after they moved on, where necessary (Orr 1994:210). One of the first attempts to establish a refuge 'by women for women' was in 1971 when Joyce Johnson and Elizabeth Hoffman set up a facility for Aboriginal women and their accompanying children in Melbourne. Both women worked at the Aborigines Advancement League, where women who needed crisis accommodation often presented. 'Aunty Joyce' and 'Aunty Liz' also took women into their own homes. The original attempt failed and the facility was taken over by a hostel (Smith 1979) but the two women continued to work towards a refuge. In 1979, under the auspices of the Aborigines Advancement League, they established a service that later became Elizabeth Hoffman House. A community-controlled organisation, with a management committee and elected office bearers, the house was incorporated in 1984, when it secured independence from the League. The underpinning philosophy is that Aboriginal people have a right to self-determination and self-management and that each community is best able to identify its own needs and develop and monitor its own programs. It provides emergency accommodation for Aboriginal women and children, counselling and support services (Elizabeth Hoffman House web site).

In 1974, non-Aboriginal women established refuges in Sydney, Melbourne, Adelaide, Perth and Hobart. The story of the way Elsie, the first permanent 1970s refuge, was set up and maintained in Sydney has been told in detail by one of the founders, Anne Summers (1999:315–26). Briefly, a refuge working group of the Sydney Women's Commission, looking around for appropriate premises, noticed that the Church of England held unused buildings in Glebe.

The group wrote to the church, hoping to negotiate to rent a house for a modest sum but the church refused to meet with them. Outraged, the group decided to squat in one of the houses. Having let themselves in by forcing a window, they found that the house next door was also vacant and shared the large backyard. They then contacted television networks and announced that Australia's first feminist refuge had opened.

Premises are one thing. Operational money is another. The rundown houses were soon crowded, women and children often had only the clothes they stood in and there was no money for food and electricity. Summers relates the struggle to obtain government funding, the compassion of women who came to help, the generosity of local Glebe merchants, who often gave what was needed, and the lengths that were taken to survive. She recounts the determination to continue political action as well as provide a service for women. Elsie survives today, one of 83 refuges for women and children in New South Wales.

In Melbourne, more than 100 WL members became part of the Halfway House Collective formed in April 1974. The group met for months, writing letters, funding submissions and a manifesto and attempting to gain media coverage. Following Elsie, they considered squatting, since public authorities, churches and private developers all owned empty houses. The idea was rejected, however, on grounds that stability was needed for women and children already in precarious circumstances. Instead, efforts were made to persuade owners to allow empty houses to be used (Women's Liberation Halfway House Collective 1977:13).

Eventually, a community woman offered the use of a house for a year and WL Halfway House opened in September. The collective had a flat decision-making structure, with both service users and workers involved in planning strategies and running of the house. A roster was organised in four-hour shifts, with one woman remaining overnight, along with transport and babysitting rosters. Jean Taylor (2003) describes her experience:

> I became involved in roster work...That was amazing...I had no idea, really, what I was doing. I went along because some of the Brunswick CR group volunteered at a public meeting to become members of the committee...it was very difficult to get funding because the government wasn't funding refuges...We just kept putting in submissions.

Within two months, the centre was running out of space and money. It survived on donations and proceeds from fundraising events, such as jumble sales. WEL assisted by setting up a trust fund to pay for electricity, rates and phone. Besides running costs, residents needed money to set up new accommodation in order to move on. In early 1975, modest Commonwealth funding was obtained and the collective was able to pay its workers. The first employees were a diverse group, including 'a mother of six, a counter-culture freak, a Toorak lady, a heavily feminist dyke, a dedicated resident intent on bringing fun to the Women's Movement, a trained statistician that never was and one that defies all attempt at description' (Women's Liberation Halfway House Collective 1977:113).

Working conditions were onerous and a division threatened to open up between paid workers and the rest of the collective. One ex-worker has left a record of her feelings: it helped in the job to have 'no heart' to avoid emotional involvement, to enjoy being a hermit because there was no time for social life, to be able to function well on minimal sleep and to own a truck to carry around 'all the necessary papers, speeches, cards, articles and files' (Women's Liberation Halfway House Collective 1977:115).

When the original house was sold, another round of letter writing, lobbying, speaking to the media and searching for premises began. The HHSC grant included only $50 a week for rent. A former private hospital was located on the outskirts of the city. After the move in April 1975, however, it transpired that the lease was not renewable because the building was earmarked for demolition. Another frustrating search began; no-one was prepared to consider letting to a feminist women's refuge. Suitable premises were eventually found and the house moved for the third time in 20 months.

Another problem was conflict with the Victorian Government about confidentiality of location. Collective members insisted on secrecy in order to protect women from angry partners. After a protracted struggle involving media debate and direct action, a compromise was reached: selected government women, who visited at least once a year and reported on operations, became address holders (Orr 1994:217; Women's Liberation Halfway House Collective 1977:32–3, 69).

Political action focused on housing shortages, income-support requirements and police handling of domestic violence. Direct action included a demonstration outside the Victorian office of the Commonwealth Department of Social Security in May 1975, which drew attention to the inadequacy and uncertainty of the pensions available to women who had no other means of support. Later that year, a campaign to increase the availability of low-cost housing included squatting in unoccupied Housing Commission flats. In the same year, the collective wrote a submission to a police inquiry on behalf of women who had used the house. It argued that women experiencing domestic violence found the police unsympathetic and unreliable and that distrust was common. A number of recommendations were made, including suggestions for police training, but the collective was told that the submission did not fall within the terms of reference of the inquiry.

In the 15 months until the end of 1975, Halfway House received accommodation requests from 907 women and 1949 children but only 202 women and 304 children could be accommodated. Places were found for 38 women and 52 children in private homes, leaving 667 women and 1593 children who had to be turned away. The collective estimated that the voluntary time devoted to Halfway House during the period was equivalent to that of 25 full-time workers (Women's Liberation Halfway House Collective 1977:5, 85).

The first Adelaide women's shelter was set up in June 1974 in response to phone calls from women who had nowhere to go. A small group squatted in a vacant house belonging to the Highways Department, then informed welfare agencies of their existence and called for donations of furniture and volunteer support. The group had already established contact with the local Bowden/Brompton Community Development Group and was hoping for ongoing support. The condition of the house, however, was poor: 'there was no laundry, the roof leaked, a wall was falling down, there was only an outside toilet and the yard was not closed off' (Otto and Haley 1975:11). Feminist activist Sylvia Kinder (1980:150) has described the project as a 'desperate attempt to alleviate a pressing need'.

Unforeseen problems quickly emerged. First, establishing trusting relationships with women staying temporarily was sometimes difficult. Second, housing-market obstacles often prevented residents from moving on so conditions became overcrowded, dirty and fraught with disagreement, instability and lack of privacy. Third, some clients were simply homeless rather than escaping violence and some had drug, alcohol and mental health problems. Providing support required skills and resources beyond the means of the group, members of which were on a steep learning curve trying to obtain information about welfare benefits, legal rights, hospital services, housing availability and the like. Fourth, residents had varying attitudes and needs, creating friction and difficulties. Some wanted their partners to be able to attend the shelter to facilitate negotiations; others felt the need for sanctuary from men. Since the address was not secret, men sometimes turned up looking for women to date!

As in other feminist establishments, at the Adelaide Women's Shelter, the founders did not have a uniform view on principles. Most favoured cooperative, non-hierarchical management structures but one, it appears, did not, and saw herself as matron/landlady. Within the first month, heated arguments broke out and after less than six months a serious rift developed (Otto and Haley 1975:12–16). Members of the Highways Department were drawn into the dispute but the compromises put forward were unacceptable to collective members, who eventually withdrew (Smith 1985:28).

Another Adelaide shelter, Christies Beach Women's Shelter, was established in 1976 by a group of women who had met in the women's studies department at Flinders University. Initially, one of the women opened a drop-in centre at her shop, to which a steady stream of women trying to escape violence presented themselves. Soon the chairs were replaced with mattresses. Clearly a shelter was needed and lobbying began. The Housing Trust was eventually persuaded to provide a house but women had to raise money to pay the rent. The St Vincent de Paul Society helped with furniture and provided food vouchers in emergencies. In 1977, ongoing funding was obtained from the State Government.

As mentioned, the Perth Women's Centre Action Group (WCAG), comprising WL, WEL and others, decided to give priority to a refuge because the three existing centres for homeless women in the city were overflowing. In July 1974, Nardine Women's Refuge was opened in a three-bedroom house, without public funding. A mixed group of more than 40 WCAG-trained community women provided a 24-hour service. Operations were financed from donations. The principles were feminist and included the provision of respectful support and empowerment through self-help and collectivity. As in other pioneering refuges, at Nardine, the floors were soon covered with extra mattresses and overflow families were accommodated in private homes. Even then, in the first year up to four families each day were turned away (Murray 2002:21–31).

In 1975, the refuge moved to much larger premises, by which time it had secured State Health Department funding; however, the new house soon overflowed as well. The adjoining property was taken over and in the late 1970s a third house was acquired nearby. Collective members lobbied ministers and bureaucrats, staged rallies, attended forums, presented papers and wrote submissions. Direct action included accompanying a group of women and children to a departmental office and refusing to leave until something was done. The political climate in the second half of the 1970s was unsympathetic and feminist refuges were seen as politically embarrassing. The Premier, Charles Court, said on radio that the recipe for a successful marriage was a tolerant and patient wife. The police responded to a call for help from Nardine in the case of a violent incident by raiding the place instead, in the belief that the women were drug-taking hippies (Murray 2002:31–45).

Initially, Nardine workers were largely from Anglo-Australian backgrounds, with little understanding of the lives of Aboriginal and immigrant women. As experience grew, however, the refuge began to facilitate cultural sensitivity training and it gradually gained a reputation among Aboriginal women as a safe and accepting establishment. Nardine also implemented a policy of affirmative action in the employment of Aboriginal workers. Over the years, half or more of Nardine's residents have been Aboriginal women and their children who, because of the difficulties of securing appropriate, affordable housing, sometimes remained at the refuge for long periods. The refuge worked politically to raise awareness of housing shortages (Murray 2002:46).

Nardine continues to operate as a feminist refuge, funded by State and Commonwealth grants and short-term project money. As well as operating a residential service, it provides outreach, counselling and advocacy services. It is managed by a small committee, supported by a broader collective. Political activism to achieve social change is still central to its work, along with education projects that promote zero tolerance of violence against women and children.

In Hobart, the Women's Action Group, which had a sister group in Launceston, was formed in 1972. In 1974, the Hobart Women's Shelter was opened, followed by the Launceston Women's Shelter in November 1975 (Magnolia Place Team 2007; Murphy 2006). Both centres were overcrowded, under-funded and subject to opposition and criticism from the beginning. As in other places, in Launceston, committee members disagreed about management principles. Stress was further increased because fundraising was a constant necessity. For example, in 1977, when the Launceston shelter needed larger premises, the Tasmanian Government agreed to provide 50 per cent of the money, leaving the committee to somehow raise the other 50 per cent. It succeeded.

The Canberra Women's Refuge Committee was formed in 1974 and the Canberra Women's Refuge was opened in a suburban house on IWD, 1975. Committee members visited both Elsie and the Adelaide shelter and talked with Melbourne feminists, seeking advice and information. As in other places, in Canberra, the guiding principles were feminist. The house, owned by the Department of the Capital Territory (the Australian Capital Territory had not yet gained independence from the Commonwealth), had sleeping accommodation for 16 women plus three cots—and one wardrobe! The lounge room was used as an office, relaxation room, play room and bedroom (Canberra Women's Refuge Collective 1976).

The Canberra committee undertook groundbreaking political work. In 1976, two major discussion papers were written, the first on women, violence and the law and the second, on women, violence and housing. These documents were distributed widely to local and national politicians and relevant others. The law paper argued that women and children had a right to live in the marital home and that consideration should be given to evicting violent partners. Police should inform women of their rights and refer them to legal aid, it was suggested, and interpreters should be employed, as necessary. The group met with the Registrar and other officers of the Family Law Court, talked with police and met with the Assistant Police Commissioner. Public attention was drawn to the fact that non-molestation orders were often flouted and the police were asked to provide better protection for women.

The discussion paper on urgent housing needs argued that if refuges were to be able to take new clients, there must be a reasonable turnover of women and accompanying children. Because interim housing was so scarce, bottlenecks were forming. It pointed to the absurdity that women who were joint owners of a marital home were ineligible for emergency public housing. Interim housing was necessary to cover the period between separation and the settlement of financial and custody matters. Nor were woman eligible for alternative accommodation if the home they had lived in was publicly provided. The paper also pointed out that two women, who might meet at a refuge and might want to split costs and help protect each other, were not eligible to share a government house. Moreover, single women with children were considered high-risk tenants in the private sector and rental bonds were out of reach of those surviving on public benefits. This paper was circulated to politicians, housing officials, the Real Estate Agent's Institute and other key groups. The committee met with the Commonwealth minister responsible for housing and gained certain concessions.

The Canberra group also undertook direct action. For example, members 'sat in' a government house with a woman and her children who were threatened with eviction, after a bungle between departments in relation to rent. The eviction was averted. The group also formed a coordination team for ACT and New South Wales refuges in 1977, as part of a campaign to secure stable refuge funding from the Commonwealth (Canberra Women's Refuge Collective 1977).

In New South Wales, Bonnie Women's Shelter was opened in 1974 and the Blacktown Community Cottage was opened in 1975, along with Bringa Women's Refuge, Dee Why, which was set up by a feminist collective with help from unions, the Salvation Army and community groups. It works according to the principle of 'women helping women' and still operates. Marrickville Women's Refuge was established in 1976 after a funding struggle and a battle with the local council over premises. Marty House, Woolloomooloo, was founded in 1976 for women trying to recover from substance abuse in a house supplied free by the Sydney City Council.

The quest for Commonwealth funding for refuges is a complicated and protracted story, involving disagreement and confusion about which bureaucratic portfolio should be responsible. There were debates about whether funding should come from homelessness agencies or whether it should be provided by the social security or health departments. After interaction between feminists inside and outside government, the Women's Affairs Section of the Department of Prime Minister and Cabinet put a proposal to the Prime Minister that refuges be funded under the Community Health Program, which was accepted in June 1975. At that time, 11 refuges were ready to be funded (Dowse 1984:139–49; Sawer 1990:12–13). As discussed, however, the Fraser Government slashed Commonwealth funding, resulting in protracted funding insecurity. The next phase of refuge development is discussed in Chapter 3.

Sexual Assault Services

Feminists in the 1970s were intent on extricating sexual assault from the recesses of the private domain and placing it on public agendas—an unenviable task. They politicised the varieties of sexual violence prevalent in Western countries and argued that it was a systemic problem rather than a problem arising from the behaviour of aberrant individuals. For centuries, the attitudes and practices of the dominant culture had kept it 'marginalised, secretive, pervasive and ignored' (Doyle 1996:44). Whereas the anti-violence movement gained political support and early policy prominence, the same level of attention was not paid to sexual assault (Carmody 1990:303). In contrast, rape had become a major issue in the United States by the early 1970s.[6]

One of the reasons that feminist analyses of rape were slow to gain acceptance appears to be the strength of longstanding myths and stereotypes. Rationalisations that condone or trivialise rape and place blame on women and sometimes children have been identified in most countries and can be traced back to ancient times (Yarrow Place web site). In Australia, justifications are said to be deeply embedded as a result of the country's 'strange beginning', when women were imported to provide sexual and other services. There is also a strand of thinking that sees Aboriginal women as 'sexually available' (Broom 2001:96). Sexual assault has been 'woven through our landscape' from the time of white settlement (Simmons 2009). As Shoebridge and Shoebridge (2002:1) argue:

> Australia, perhaps more than most, is a masculine country…whose European settlement was by British and Irish, mainly male, convicts whose presence was supplemented later by boatloads of women, brought to civilise disruptive unruliness and begin building families… The masculine norm continued, through the mythology built up by participation in several wars, dominant industries such as mining and stock farming, and cultural obeisance to the romance of 'the bush'—non-metropolitan Australia where men are men and women are incidental.

---

6   Despite early attention, however, the fictions around rape remain. 'Few crimes in the United States today elicit as much scepticism and victim blaming as do allegations of rape and sexual assault' (Weiss 2009:810).

That Australia is the country with 'the highest incidence of recorded gang rape in the world' (McFerran 1990:193) lends support to such analysis. In 2005, more than 950 000 Australian women reported being sexually abused before the age of fifteen—a horrifying statistic (Commonwealth of Australia 2009a:19). The 2005 Australian Bureau of Statistics Personal Safety Survey showed that 19 per cent of women over the age of fifteen had experienced sexual violence and that about one in three who were physically assaulted by partners were also raped (Commonwealth of Australia 2009a:19). A 17-country study in 2000 found that Australia was one of four countries with the highest risk of sexual assault (van Kesteren et al. 2000:4, 35–6).

Historically, women have been held responsible for preventing rape. Apart from not talking to strangers, they have been told not to dress 'provocatively', to travel in groups, to always carry money for a taxi and to stay home after dark. Elder (2007:133) records a recent case where a girl raped on a school trip was questioned in court about the length of the skirts she wore. The idea that rape is a woman's fault is so deeply ingrained in Australian culture that women's services have had to stress, regularly and repeatedly, that this is not so.

The National Council to Prevent Violence against Women and Their Children argues that 'sexual violence by male intimate partners remains one of the least recognised, underreported and consequently, least prosecuted crimes' (Commonwealth of Australia 2009a:19). The feminist argument that there is more danger from family members, friends, work colleagues and other known persons than from strangers is borne out by evidence: less than 10 per cent of attacks on young women are made by strangers. Sexual assault is more prevalent in rural and remote areas and among younger women, Aboriginal women and women with disabilities. Estimates are that less than 20 per cent of sexual assault crimes are ever reported. Of the small number that come to trial, less than 20 per cent result in the accused pleading or being found guilty (Commonwealth of Australia 2009a:17–20).

Feminists argue that sexual violence is a structural problem: men who commit sexual assault are tacitly supported by an unequal, male-dominated society in which women have inferior status. As in the case of domestic violence, feminists challenge power structures and argue that attitudes must change. The myths to be subverted include that women 'ask for' and enjoy rape, that children can be 'seductive', that only 'loose' women are raped, that women and children often lie about rape, that only bad, deranged or stressed men commit sexual assault and that men have uncontrollable sexual urges (Cook et al. 2001:1).

As in the health centre and anti-violence movements, the movement against sexual assault set about the twin tasks of providing support services and developing strategies to promote social change. The Sydney Rape Crisis Centre formally opened in 1974. A group of volunteer women had been travelling 'all over Sydney' picking up women who had been assaulted and bringing them to the centre for counselling and medical services. The centre was funded by the Commonwealth in 1974, allowing workers to be paid. Currently known as the NSW Rape Crisis Centre, it is funded by the NSW Department of Health and adheres to feminist goals. It is not-for-profit and community controlled and its overarching purpose is 'upholding the rights of women to live in a socially just and equitable society and the rights of all people to live free of violence' (NSW Rape Crisis Centre web site). It provides 24-hour, seven-day-a-week telephone counselling and support, regardless of when the assault occurred. Support and information are provided about safety, emotional impact, possible actions and the availability of long-term services.

In Brisbane, Women's House established the Brisbane Rape Crisis Centre in April 1975, followed by a refuge the following month. As discussed, Women's House lost its funding after operating for less than two years but women continued to provide services on a voluntary basis. On condition that it raise $2500 of its own, the management group received $10 000 from the Commonwealth for a refuge in 1978. Not until 1983 did it receive funding for the Rape Crisis Centre.

Adelaide feminists established a rape crisis centre in an old house in 1976. As well as services, the centre established a forum for discussing the multiple issues surrounding rape, including legal issues. The centre also operated as a safe drop-in place, where women could share their experiences, chat and read. Self-defence classes were offered and training modules for nurses, teachers and other professionals were developed.

A rape-crisis group was formed within Melbourne WL in 1973. It set about gaining information on key medical, legal and statistical issues. Some members found the issues too confronting, however, and the size of the group shrank. The following August, another group was called together by WEL, which included women from the original group. A 24-hour rape-crisis service was established and the name Women against Rape was chosen. Prevention was a priority. After meetings with police, and medical and legal professionals to disseminate information and suggest referral, the Rape Crisis Centre was opened in November 1974, operating from the premises of the Melbourne Women's Health Collective in Collingwood and funded by donations. Its establishment drew considerable media attention and women who had been raped were soon seeking services.

There followed a long and unsuccessful struggle to gain public funding. Because the centre was a long-term project, it was ineligible for International Women's Year funds. The Commonwealth Department of Health authorised funding in 1975 but in another instance of bureaucratic obstruction, the money was blocked by the Victorian HCC on grounds that the organisation's aims were unacceptable: it was a women-only collective that did not depend entirely on professionals. It was decided to give up the quest for funding in 1976 because it sapped too much time and energy, and to operate independently. Collective members turned their hands to fundraising and pledged their own money on a weekly basis (Hewitt and Worth n.d.; Women against Rape Collective n.d.). Political action was continued until the late 1970s from WL Centre in Little Lonsdale Street, including campaigns for legislative reform and reform of court, police and hospital practices.

The Women against Rape Collective established the Geelong Rape Centre in 1978, following the poor treatment of a woman who had been raped. It ran on voluntarism and donations from workers, but, in 1984, it succeeded in gaining funding from the Victorian Health Department. In 1995–96, it was offering therapy groups for children, young women who were incest survivors, mothers of sexually abused children and adult women who had experienced incest. It also ran a men's group. A community-development worker coordinated community education in schools and for professionals. Campaigns included a week of action against domestic and sexual violence and a child-protection week (Geelong Rape Crisis Centre 1995–96). In 1999, it was one of seven organisations funded under the national Partnerships against Domestic Violence (PADV) to develop a model of best practice for working with children affected by family violence (Hunder 1999:iii).

In its early days, WEL formed the Rape Study Group in Melbourne to work for law reform and better services. Its advocacy resulted in the Victorian Rape Study Committee being established in the Department of Premier in 1977, which recommended the establishment of a government-funded 24-hour counselling service. The Queen Victoria Medical Centre set up a sexual assault service in 1979—the first public sexual assault service in the State. Another Melbourne group, the Campaign against Causes of Rape, was formed in response to a double rape-murder.

In Western Australia, the Women's Health and Community Centre had set up a rape-crisis service at Glendower Street in 1975 but it did not survive. A new centre was opened at Sir Charles Gairdner Hospital in 1976 in response to feminist concern about the treatment of women who wished to report a crime (Deller et al. 1979:771). The women who set up the second service prepared for it by holding consultations with the police, the Office of the Under Secretary for Law, the Women's Health and Community Centre, a panel of women doctors, officials from the Sir Charles Gairdner Hospital and forensic experts. The main aims were to provide comprehensive support services for victims of sexual violence, to promote greater community understanding and awareness, to establish appropriate education for medical, legal, police and health personnel and to support and encourage research (Deller et al. 1979). When the original women's health centre reopened in 1977, it housed the local branch of the Australian Women against Rape group until 1985.

The operation of the Sexual Assault Resource Centre (SARC) became controversial in the early days as women's health activists expressed concern that a hospital setting might not be conducive to women-centred care. A compromise position was reached whereby the service remained part of the public hospital but was managed by an independent board. During its first 2 years, the centre saw more than 200 clients. SARC is now located at the King Edward Memorial Hospital.

Nationally, Australian Women against Rape, which had State-based branches, was established at the National Conference of Rape Crisis Centres in Sydney in 1976. The main objectives were raising public awareness of misogynist ideas, and law reform. The organisation argued for legal recognition of rape within marriage, for corroboration requirements to be dropped in rape cases, for the previous sexual history of victims to be inadmissible and for the legal definition of rape to be extended to cover oral and anal penetration and attempted penetration. In 1976, it organised a national demonstration in support of a Brisbane woman accused of making a false rape complaint and drafted model rape legislation (Grahame and Prichard 1996:16).

Other Early Women's Health Agencies

Women in Industry Contraception and Health (WICH), as it was known for many years, is a Melbourne service with a long and successful history, set up by a grassroots group of women. In response to a dire lack of information about contraception and related matters among immigrant women working in factories, a well-attended public forum was held, which resolved that family planning education should be taken out of the medical context and located within the workplace and the community. Two doctoral students, with a small group of immigrant workers and advocates, established Action for Family Planning in 1977. The founders developed a multilingual factory-visiting program, which took reproductive health education to women where they worked. Financial support came from the technical and further education (TAFE) sector and the Commonwealth, allowing multilingual workers to be trained. Another round of advocacy and lobbying in 1980, when funding was running out, brought support from the Victorian Health Department and the Department of Immigration. In 1982, the name was changed to WICH, reflecting decisions to move beyond reproductive issues towards women's health in its social context. Information dissemination and advocacy continued and regular newsletters were produced. The Factory Visits Program was expanded to include OHS, mental health and, in the recession of the early 1990s, work, retrenchment and stress issues. At that time, a funding boost was received from the NWH Program and work was able to expand again, targeting a wider range of cultural and language groups.

In the second half of the 1990s, however, State funding was reduced, requiring the organisation to contract but it continued to respond to the needs of newly arriving groups. In 2000, the name was changed again, to Working Women's Health—again reflecting changing priorities. Bilingual health educators were trained in increasing numbers of languages, as resources permitted, and health education was extended to community settings, some of them rural, and to prisons. A library and resource collection was put together, including 10 000 health information items in 96 languages.

In 2006, the name was changed yet again, to the Multicultural Centre for Women's Health (MCWH), its present name, which reflects the 'organisation's multifaceted and comprehensive approach to immigrant women's health'. Currently, health information is provided in 19 languages in diverse locations (MCWH web site).

Another major 1970s initiative with a long and successful history is the Children by Choice Association (C by C), formed in Brisbane in 1972 from what had been the Queensland Abortion Law Reform Association. C by C was established as a family planning and abortion information service. Like so many women's services, it was set up in an old house, sparking a blaze of publicity, during which bricks were thrown through the windows. In Queensland at the time, termination was deemed illegal, even in a case where a woman had contracted rubella. Vasectomy was also illegal.

In this context, C by C made arrangements for women wanting an abortion to be referred to Sydney hospitals and organised help with travel costs. It lobbied, made submissions to public inquiries, picketed parliament, wrote letters and presented petitions, calling for the repeal of the relevant sections of the Criminal Code. The voluntary workers were trained and saw more than 300 clients per month, referred to them by doctors. So controversial was the work in 1977–78 that more than 120 media news items were generated. C by C staff persisted through a succession of crises in the 1970s and 1980s, which included attacks on clinics. Partly as a result, Queensland legislation was modified in 1986 but abortion was not removed from the Criminal Code.

Unable to gain government funding, the association nearly had to close because of serious financial problems in 1987; however, a request for support to the Planned Parenthood Federation of America, which normally funds only agencies in Third-World countries, was successful. The association was then able to expand its services, move into rural provision and offer some paid employment.

After three years, the US donor had its own funding reduced and was forced to discontinue support. Fortuitously, about the same time, the ALP was elected to government in Queensland after more than 30 years in opposition. Public funding was obtained in 1991, after which outreach, counselling, information, education and library services were expanded.

These activities brought renewed opposition from anti-choice forces, in the face of which the Goss Government shelved its election promise to remove abortion from the Criminal Code. Indeed, when a 'comprehensive' review of the Criminal Code was instigated in 1990, abortion laws were specifically excluded, even though one of the aims of the exercise was to ensure that the criminal law reflected contemporary attitudes. In response to a letter of objection from a women's group, the then Attorney-General replied that he would be acting improperly if he were to allow abortion laws to be reviewed because the Parliamentary Labor Party had unanimously decided that the subject 'was not on the agenda' (McCormack 1992:40). On Labor's defeat in 1996, the association lost its funding. Services were continued by volunteers but the hours of opening had to be reduced. Fundraising campaigns enabled the State-wide telephone counselling line to stay open. Labor's return to power in 1998, however, resulted in funding from Queensland Health, which continues.

C by C has been built on untold hours of unpaid and low-paid women's work and has provided extensive support services. It has worked steadily to raise public awareness about reproductive health issues and has lobbied and campaigned in support of legislative change. After almost 40 years, however, abortion remains in Queensland's Criminal Code, so powerful are the forces of the religious right and so reluctant are politicians to confront them.

Although it was not until the 1980s that women's health groups proliferated, a sprinkling of new groups formed in the 1970s to draw attention to needs in particular areas. The Women Behind Bars group was set up in Sydney in 1975, concerned with legal rights and women's health inside prisons. In Brisbane, the Women's Community Aid Association was established, taking up health and sexual violence issues and providing women with practical support. The Women's Health and Education Group was formed in Sydney in 1975 with the aim of contacting women outside the movement, especially rural women, young women and immigrant women (Grahame and Prichard 1996:154, 167). The Women's Information Centre Collective was formed in Townsville, which focused on rape crisis, abortion and women's services. Meanwhile, in far north Queensland, an Aboriginal welfare officer at the Cairns hospital, Rose Richards, became concerned that there was no halfway house for Aboriginal children brought to Cairns for treatment or for pregnant women awaiting the births of their babies. In 1976, she began to care for people in her own home, assisted by two other Aboriginal women, using their own money when necessary. This grassroots initiative became a successful halfway house in the 1980s.

Another 1970s grassroots undertaking about which little seems to be known was a second national women's health conference, held in Newcastle in 1977, organised by the Hunter Region Working Women's Centre (HRWWC). More than 100 women attended, along with half a dozen men. The main session streams reflected a social view of health: 'Becoming Healthy', 'Women at Work', 'Fertility and Sexuality' and 'Especially Disadvantaged Women'. A workshop considered the possibility of an Australian version of *Our Bodies, Ourselves*. Bridget Gilling, well-known feminist and campaigner, put forward a critique of the overemphasis on curative medicine. Alice Day, a sociologist, presented the now familiar argument that the nature of women's work makes them sick, particularly their inferior position in occupational hierarchies (Day 1977). Recent epidemiological evidence supports Day's analysis (Wilkinson and Pickett 2009).

Conclusion

It is evidence of both profound need and passionate commitment that women set up so many separate services in the 1970s. Looking back, their achievements are remarkable, given the minimal resources at their command and the strength of the forces ranged against them. Working often in the face of criticism and sometimes ridicule, women's health problems were identified and articulated. With little more than their bare hands, Anglo, Aboriginal and immigrant women set up health centres, reproductive health agencies, factory visitation programs, refuges and sexual assault centres to provide urgently needed services that were scarcely available elsewhere. Many episodes of extraordinary effort and personal generosity have undoubtedly been lost to history because women were too busy campaigning and providing services to produce written records.

Women of the early years succeeded in their twin aims of working at both the service provision and the political levels, supporting women and promoting women's health as a major political issue. A social health perspective, which has provided the movement with a solid set of foundational principles for 40 years, was worked out and voiced.

The new centres and services created an institutional foundation from which political action could more easily be orchestrated, although, as Broom has documented, the high demand for services always threatens to divert women from advocacy and social change work (Broom 1991:120–2). Despite the disagreements and implosions in Anglo-Australian women's health centres, activists were able to influence public policy when political circumstances were right. The campaigns around domestic violence and sexual assault brought hidden crimes onto the public agenda and paved the way for the extensive efforts of the 1980s and beyond. As Lynne Hunt (1994:390) has argued, the women's health movement worked outside the conventional health system, 'moved around' the medical profession and set up alternative services, creating a space from which to lobby for health system and societal change.

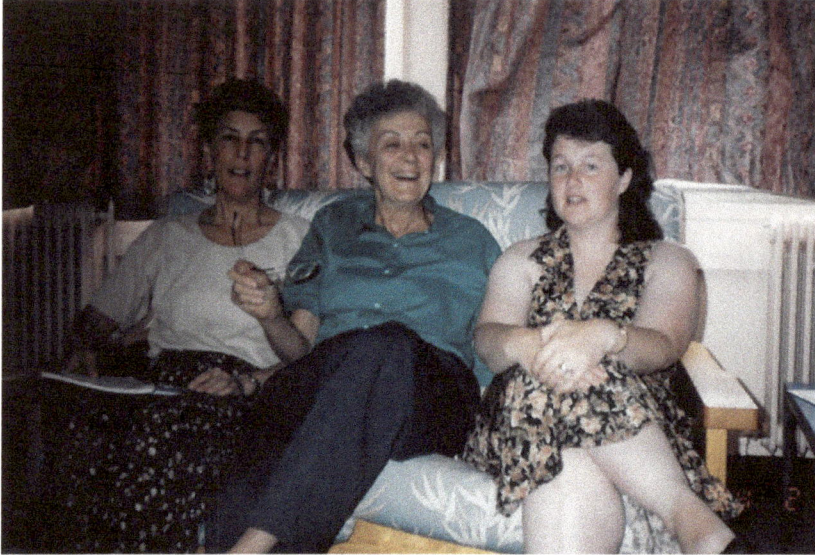

Movement members from all States and Territories gathered in Canberra in February 1994 to develop and write the AWHN Constitution. From left: Dorothy Broom (ACT), Manoa Renwick (ACT) and Sheryl Rainbird (Tas).

Photo: Julie McCarron Benson

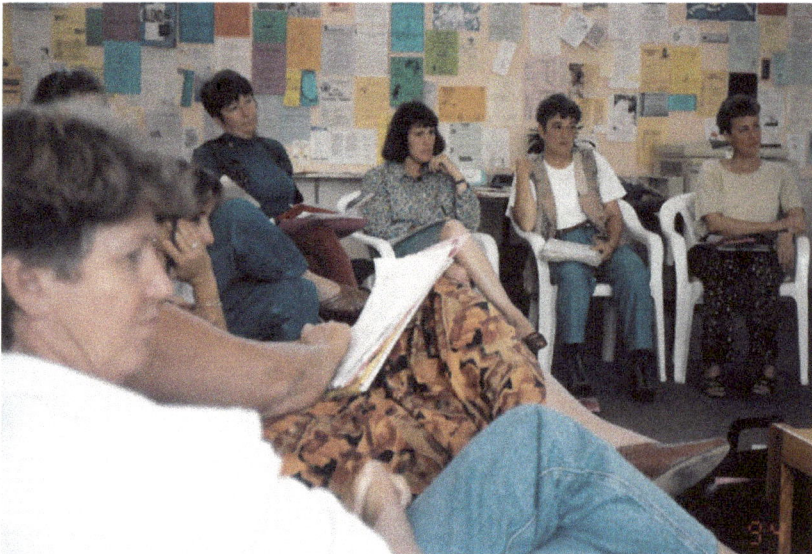

Carol Low (Qld), Annette Burke, partly obscured, (NSW), Keren Howe (Vic), Cate Mettam (SA), Nancy Peck (Vic) and Dorothy Broom listen to constitutional deliberations, Canberra, February 1984.

Photo: Julie McCarron Benson

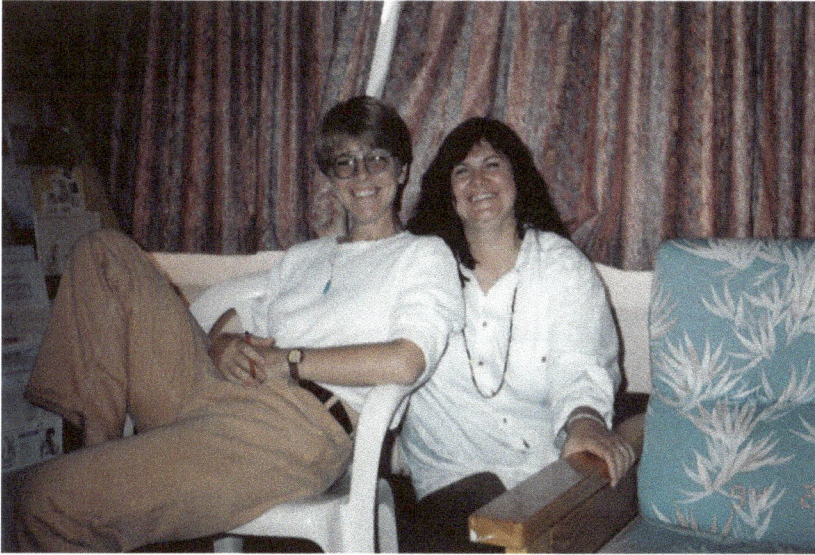

Annette Coppaola and Deborah Gough from the Northern Territory put on their best smiles at the AWHN Constitution meeting, February 1994.

Photo: Julie McCarron Benson

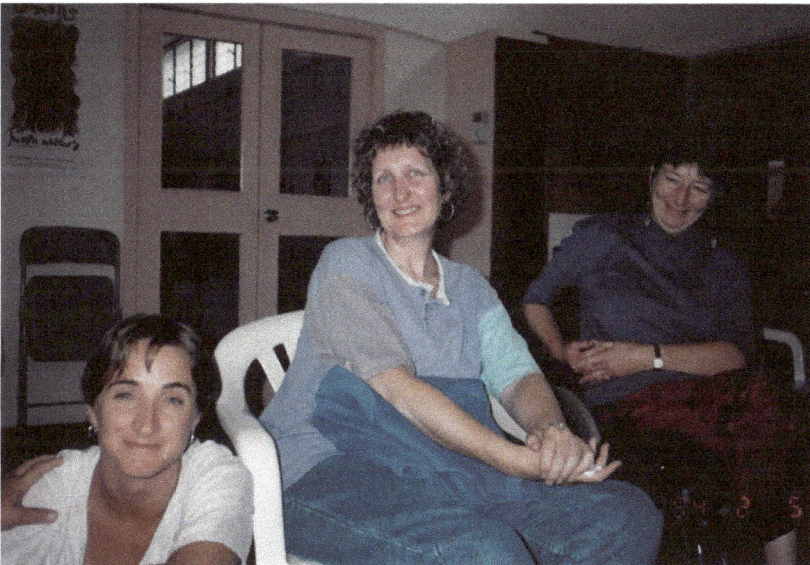

Annette Burke, Andrea Shoebridge (WA) and Keren Howe at the AWHN constitution development meeting, February 1994. Jan Darlington (Qld), Gwen Gray (ACT), Fiona Hillary (SA) and Marian Palandri from Port Headland, WA (whose fare was paid by BHP) were also present.

Photo: Julie McCarron Benson

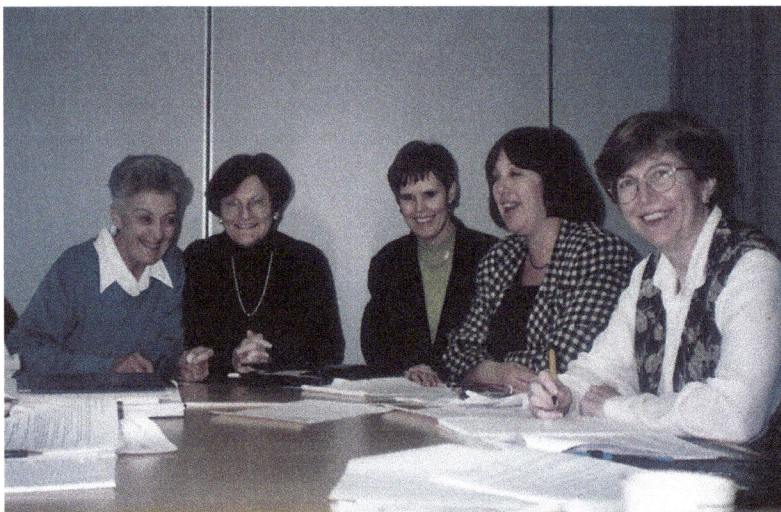

Meeting to discuss the evaluation of the National Women's Health Program, Juliana House, Canberra, 1996. From left: Manoa Renwick, Christine Purdon, Janette Gay, Barbara Gatler, Barbara Podger.

Photo: Manoa Renwick

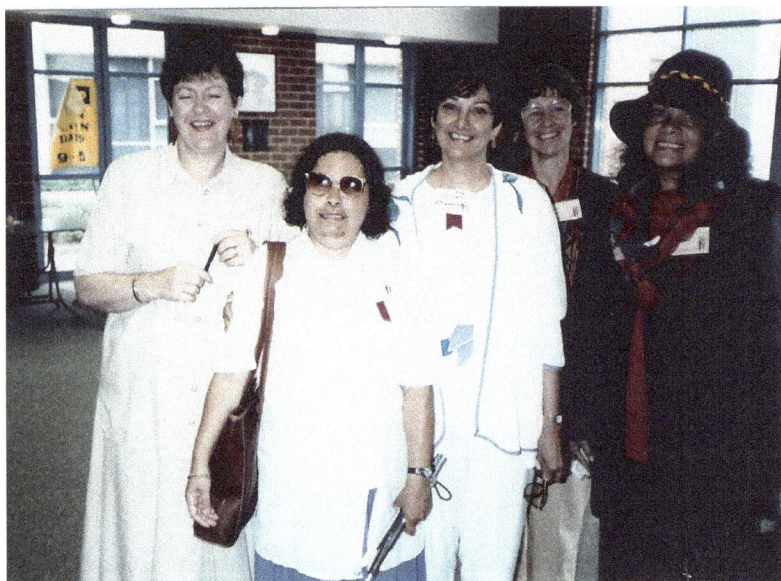

Some of the members of the organising committee for the Third AWHN National Women's Health Conference, Canberra, 1995. From left: Pam Neame, Roslyn Sackley, Romaine Rutnam, Debbi Cameron and Jilpia Nappaljari Jones (then Marjorie Baldwin-Jones).

Photo: Tony Adams

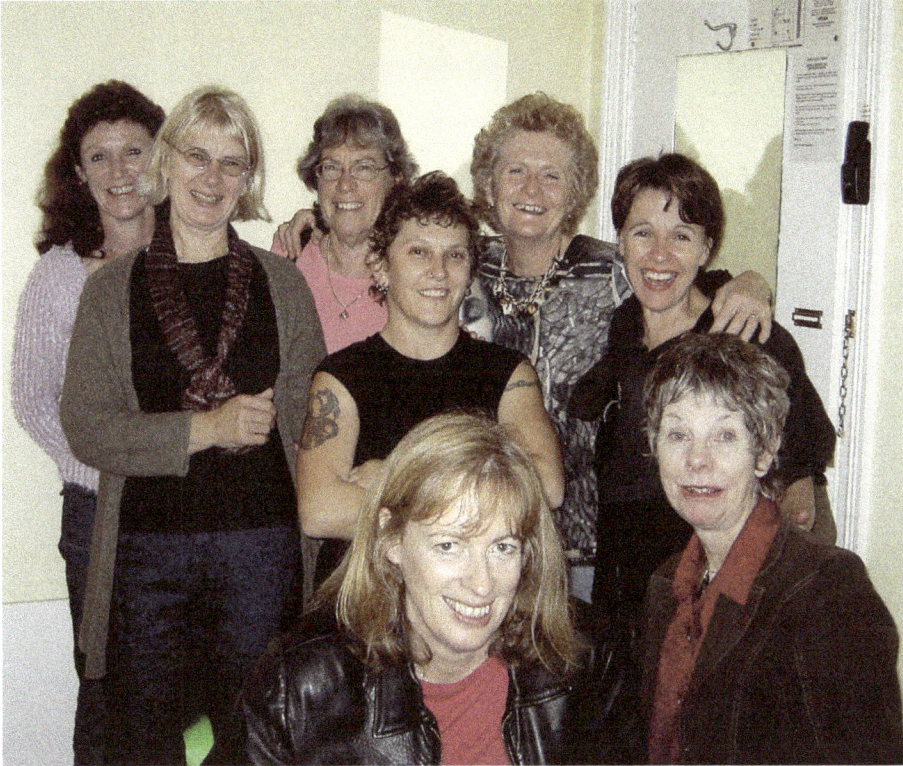

Tasmanian delegates at the Fifth AWHN National Women's Health Conference, Melbourne, 2005. Middle and back row from left to right: Karen Price, Yvonne Hardefeldt, Sally Riley, Tracey Wing, Joan Barry, Wendy Hartshorn. Front row: Morvan Andrews, Sue Moss.

Photo: Tracey Wing

3. Infrastructure Expansion: 1980s onwards

We bring women together to support each other and strengthen their sense of connection. Using a community development approach we involve women in a range of short or long-term health promotion activities within their own communities, including health festivals, support groups, resource production and more. (Women's Health West web site)

The two decades after the fall of the Whitlam Government can be seen as the high point of the women's health movement. A momentum had been generated that even unenthusiastic governments could not afford to ignore. The 1980s in particular was a period of intense policy development as the political advocacy of the previous decade began to bear fruit. Inquiries into women's health were held in most States and Territories and all produced women's health policies, plans or strategies. Similarly, in several jurisdictions, the first policies in relation to domestic violence and sexual assault were formulated. All governments set up women's health policy machinery in their bureaucracies during this time, in the form of either a women's health unit or a special women's health adviser. As a result, channels of influence became more diverse. Grassroots activists were able to interact more readily with women in the bureaucracy and opportunities were created to serve on government advisory committees and inquiries. At the Commonwealth level, the development and launch of the groundbreaking National Women's Health Policy (NWHP) was definitely the pinnacle of policy achievement.

Yet the movement faced a mixed policy environment, or series of environments, during the period. While no government after Whitlam's would be as strongly committed to structural reform of the health system, especially at the level of community-based health care, policy opportunities did emerge. These were all the more visible because they were interspersed with periods of resistance, sometimes bordering on overt hostility. During these years, members of the movement carried on their work in both the political and the service-provision arenas. Women from diverse backgrounds continued to establish new services to meet needs, sometimes in collaboration with each other, and although some centres waited years, in almost all cases funding was eventually allocated by one level of government or the other and sometimes by both. Staff in women-led services received training, often for the first time, and training packages were developed for relevant professionals, such as the police and lawyers. For mobilised groups in some States and the Australian Capital Territory, the NWH Program provided the funds with which to establish the health centres and services they had been planning for years.

By the end of the period, the Australian women's health infrastructure was largely in place; very few new centres or services have been established since the mid-1990s. Given the lack of Commonwealth policy interest since that time (notwithstanding the introduction of a second national women's health policy in 2010), the locus of action has largely moved to the sub-national level and sometimes involves local government as well. This chapter presents an overview of the movement's advocacy and infrastructure-building activities over the two decades, which are summarised in the list below. The policy responses of the period are examined in Chapters 7 and 8.

Selected Women's Health Centres and Services Established from 1980 Onwards

1980

- Adelaide Women's Community Health Centre.
- Dawn House, providing accommodation and support services, Darwin.
- Ngaanyatjarra Pitjantjatjara Yankunytjatjara Women's Council, provider of health and human services, South Australia.

1981

- Blue Mountains Women's Health Centre, New South Wales.
- Wirraway Women's Housing Co-operative, Moree, New South Wales.
- Women's Community House, Alice Springs, Northern Territory.
- Women's Place, for homeless or intoxicated women, Sydney.

1982

- Brisbane Women's Community Health Centre.
- Coffs Harbour Women's Health Centre, New South Wales.
- Dympna House, Sydney.
- Louisa Lawson House, Sydney.
- Women's Health Resource Collective, later Women's Health Information Resource Collective, Melbourne.
- Yinganeh Aboriginal Women's Refuge, Lismore, New South Wales.

1983

- Elizabeth Women's Community Health Centre, South Australia.
- Esther Refuge Collective, Sydney.
- Mookai Rosie Bi-Bayan, Aunty Rosie's Place, services for rural and remote Aboriginal women and children, Cairns, Queensland.
- The Women's Cottage, Hawkesbury District, Sydney.
- Toora Single Women's Shelter, now Toora Women, Australian Capital Territory.

1984

- Dale Street Women's Community Health Centre, South Australia.
- Illawarra Women's Health Centre, New South Wales.
- Immigrant Women's Support Service, Brisbane.
- Jilimi, now Waminda Aboriginal Women's Health Centre, Nowra, New South Wales.
- Migrant Women's Lobby Group, Adelaide.
- Refuge Ethnic Workers Program, Victoria.
- Southern Women's Health and Community Centre, South Australia.

1985

- Darwin Counselling Group, providing sexual assault services.
- Immigrant Women's Resource Centre, Sydney.
- Immigrant Women's Speakout Association, Sydney.
- Migrant Women's Support and Accommodation Service, Adelaide.
- Shoalhaven Women's Health Centre, New South Wales.
- Southwest Women's Child Sexual Assault Resource Centre, later Rosebank, Sydney.

1986

- Albury–Wodonga Women's Health Centre, Albury, New South Wales.
- Central West Women's Health Centre, Bathurst, New South Wales.
- Dympna Accommodation Program, Sydney.
- Goldfields Women's Health Centre, Western Australia.
- Migrant Women against Incest Network, New South Wales.
- New South Wales Women's Refuge Resource Centre.
- Sexual Assault Support Service, Hobart.
- Sexual Assault Referral Centre, Darwin.
- Women's Centre, providing sexual assault crisis services, Cairns, Queensland.

1987

- Blacktown Women's and Girls' Health Centre, Sydney.
- Campbelltown Women's Health Centre, also known as WILMA, Sydney.
- CASA House, Centre against Sexual Assault, Royal Women's Hospital, Melbourne.
- Congress Alukura, women's health, maternal and child health centre, Alice Springs, Northern Territory.
- Healthsharing Women, Victoria.
- Hobart Women's Health Centre.
- Immigrant Women's Health Service, Fairfield and Cabramatta, Sydney.
- Lismore and District Women's Health Centre, New South Wales.
- Penrith Women's Health Centre, Western Sydney.
- Ruby Gaea, providing sexual assault services, Darwin.

1988

- Domestic Violence Resource Centre, Queensland.
- Geraldton Sexual Assault Referral Centre, Western Australia.
- Gloria Brennan ATSI Women's Centre, East Perth.
- Sexual Assault Counselling Service, Alice Springs, Northern Territory.
- Waratah Support Centre, sexual assault and domestic violence services, Bunbury, Western Australia.
- Women's Health Service for the West, Victoria.

1989

- Laurel House, Launceston, Tasmania.
- Patricia Giles Centre, offering services for gay, lesbian, bisexual, transgender, intersex and queer (GLBTIQ) people.
- Whitfords Women's Health Centre, now Women's Healthworks, Western Australia.

1990

- Canberra Women's Health Centre, now Women's Centre for Health Matters.
- Cumberland Women's Health Centre, Sydney.
- Perth Women's Centre.
- Townsville Women's Community Health Centre, Queensland.

1991

- Geraldton Women's Health Centre, Western Australia.

- Rockhampton Women's Health Centre, Queensland.
- Wide Bay Women's Health Centre, Queensland.

1992

- Edith Edwards Women's Centre, accommodation and support services, Bourke, New South Wales.
- Ipswich Women's Health Service, Queensland.
- Logan Women's Health Centre, Queensland.
- Mirrabooka Multicultural Women's Health Centre, Western Australia.
- North-East Women's Health Service, Victoria.

1993

- Eastern Goldfields Sexual Assault Resource Centre, Western Australia.
- Goulburn North-Eastern Victoria Women's Health Service.
- Hedland Women's Health Service, Western Australia.
- Rockingham Women's Health Service, Western Australia.
- Women's Health Victoria, formed from amalgamation of Healthsharing Women and the Women's Health Information Resource Collective.
- Yarrow Place, incorporating the Adelaide Rape Crisis Centre.
- Yorgam Aboriginal Corporation, providing support services for people who have experienced violence, East Perth.

1994

- Gladstone Women's Health Centre, Queensland.
- Gosnells Women's Health Service, Western Australia.
- Gympie and District Women's Health Centre, Queensland.

1997

- Immigrant and Refugee Women's Coalition Victoria.

2002

- Aboriginal Family Violence Prevention and Legal Service, Victoria.

2005

- Women's Health Services, formed from amalgamation of Women's Health Care House and Women's Health Services.

The Context: Mixed political opportunity structures

The 1980s and 1990s saw both high and low points for the women's health movement, fluctuations that can be explained largely by the advent of favourable or unfavourable political opportunity structures. The defeat of the Whitlam Government ushered in a period of 'depleted political opportunity' for women's health at the national level, which was the first of two inauspicious periods in the life of the movement so far. Political opportunity structure is a term used to denote the political context in which social movements try to influence governments, and is held to be a key element in determining whether advocacy succeeds or fails. Opportunity structures can help to explain the rise, fall and transformation of social movements and can go some way to explaining different outcomes at different times within one country or in different countries (Meyer 2004:125-131; Tarrow 1996:81–99). Political opportunity structure interacts with other factors that influence policy, among which institutional arrangements are considered important (Gray 2008:55).

During the years of the Fraser Commonwealth Government, from the end of 1975 until 1983, opportunities for policy expansion, which had been wide open, all but closed. Moreover, most of Labor's health system reforms, which were of so much benefit to women and low-income earners, were steadily dismantled. The Fraser Government came to power promising to retain both the national health insurance scheme, Medibank, and the Community Health Program. Within months, it set up an informal interdepartmental committee to review the operation of national health insurance. No public consultation was ever undertaken nor was any report published, but over the next five years Medibank was steadily abolished.

In addition, Commonwealth funding for the Community Health Program, through which women's health centres and refuges were funded, was progressively slashed each year. In 1981, community health centre funding was completely absorbed into the general federal tax-sharing grants, absolving the Commonwealth of all policy responsibility. The previous grant conditions requiring that the remaining funds be used for the Community Health Program were lifted and Commonwealth monitoring ceased. Funding for the Aboriginal housing program was also drastically cut back (Dowse 1984:151). The one area where funding was not reduced in total was refuges, of which more below.

On the other side of the coin, as often happens in federations, political opportunities were relatively open in several sub-national jurisdictions. While there was sporadic support for women's health within the Liberal Party, particularly among women members, it was almost entirely under

Labor governments, national and sub-national, that significant reforms were implemented. Under National-Liberal Coalition or National Party governments, as in Queensland up to 1989, support for women's health was entirely absent. In jurisdictions where Labor had a significant share of office, reforms were introduced earlier. The South Australian Dunstan Labor Government, for example, passed Australia's first legislation making rape within marriage a crime, in 1976.[1] In New South Wales, the Wran Labor Government, which supported women's health, came to power in 1976 and was not defeated until 1989. Labor was elected in Victoria in 1982, re-elected in South Australia in the same year and elected in Western Australia in 1983, after being out of office for 11 years. In Tasmania, Labor lost power in 1982 and was not returned again until 1989, after which policy development moved ahead.

Opposition—and some support

All governments operated in a context where opposition emanated from the key player in health politics: the organised medical profession. The main doctor's union, the Australian Medical Association (AMA) has steadfastly opposed separate women's health services. Historically, it has taken a stand against all publicly funded services, such as baby health centres and venereal disease clinics in public hospitals because it feared such services might attract clients away from the private medical market. The President of one State branch of the AMA put the general case that separate women's health services are 'illogical'. Women are a majority of the population and consume a majority of the services. If they are not happy with the services, the services should be modified rather than supplied separately. The solution, the President suggested—missing the point that women would like more comprehensive services supplied by teams of providers—is to increase remuneration for general practitioners so they can afford longer consultations. Under the Medicare payment schedule, the 19-minute consultation is an economic disaster for doctors, the President told me. Publicly funded services are always unfair competition for the private sector,[2] he argued, especially in the face of what was seen as an oversupply of general practitioners in the 1980s and 1990s. In some States, AMA members actively campaigned against the establishment of separate women's health services. In Western Australia, where medical unions appear to be especially powerful, obstetricians from the King Edward Memorial Hospital for Women threatened to go on strike if the Government funded salaried midwives. For similar reasons, country general

---

1   Reform-minded governments are sometimes constrained by reform-resisting bureaucracies, as in South Australia in the 1970s and 1980s. This is discussed further in Chapter 9.

2   The claim to be part of 'the private sector' ignores the fact that approximately 80 per cent of 'private' medical incomes is drawn directly from the Commonwealth Treasury. It also ignores the reality that without a conduit to the public purse, the medical profession would be much smaller and its remuneration much lower.

practitioners and radiologists resented the introduction of mobile screening services. Indeed, Stefania Siedlecky, general practitioner, founding member of family planning, adviser to the Leichhardt Women's Community Health Centre (LWCHC) Collective and later Commonwealth women's health bureaucrat, remembers that some of the bitterest opposition to women's health centres came from female doctors, who asked that funding be withdrawn.

At the level of practice, however, general practitioners, even those who were initially suspicious, often found that there was little or no encroachment upon their markets. Indeed, many found that the work of the centres complemented their own. From the early days, LWCHC saw many women whose doctors had been unable to help them. At the Liverpool centre, acceptance was such that one gynaecologist developed the practice of having his female medical students spend time at the centre (Edwards 1984:22).

Although organised medicine was strongly opposed, many individual women doctors worked hard[3] over long periods as part of the general women's health movement, providing services in many of the early centres, usually on a voluntary basis. The contribution of Dr Janet Irwin from Brisbane is an example of dedication and hard work. Irwin, a long-time human rights advocate, campaigned strenuously on abortion issues, supporting C by C and early family planning initiatives in Queensland. She was director of student health services at the University of Queensland from 1974 to 1988, where she promoted student health and identified sexual harassment as a women's health issue. In 1982, the university was one of the first in Australia to establish procedures to deal with sexual harassment complaints. In 1996, Janet Irwin was appointed the university's first Sexual Harassment Committee conciliator. Among many other health-related activities, she served on the university's Status of Women Committee, where she fought for the rights of general staff members, almost all of whom were women, especially on OHS issues. She was also active in medical women's groups and is co-author of two books on raising female daughters, *Mom, I Got a Tattoo* and *Parenting Girls*. For her work in human rights and women's health, she was made a Member of the Order of Australia and awarded a Centenary Medal. Many other women were similarly dedicated.

Opposition sometimes came from unexpected quarters: in Sydney, it was suggested that a sexual assault counselling service should be set up at Rachel Forster Hospital for Women but the board decided that such a service was unnecessary. Another possibly unlikely opponent was the Parramatta Council, which objected to the establishment of a local women's health centre. In South Australia, the hospitals, as well as organised medicine and the bureaucracy, opposed both women's health and community health centres. Across the country,

---

3   Perhaps some men did also, although I have not uncovered written records.

general practitioner organisations opposed the appointment of women's health nurses. Finally, in some places, women opposed each other. In Tasmania, for example, some women consider that opposing positions within the movement in the 1980s and into the 1990s were at least as much of a problem as external opposition.

Women's Health Centres: Continuing expansion

Despite the forces standing against them and the scarcity of resources, community women continued to set up their own services. Aboriginal women worked together and through Aboriginal community health centres and Aboriginal resource centres, making their voices heard in a range of ways. Similarly, immigrant and refugee women continued to respond to expressed need.

Aboriginal Women's Initiatives

> To us, health is about so much more than simply not being sick. It's about getting a balance between physical, mental, emotional, cultural and spiritual health. Health and healing are interwoven.
>
> — Dr Tamara Mackean, Australian Indigenous Doctors' Association

A few examples of the various centres and services set up in different parts of the country by Aboriginal women are presented here by way of illustration. An impressive centre was established in Alice Springs under the auspices of the Central Australian Aboriginal Congress (CAAC). The major focus of the congress was health service provision from the beginning and the model adopted was comprehensive and community controlled, in keeping with the social health perspective. At the time, the NT Government was unsympathetic so Commonwealth support was sought, which enabled a general health service to be opened in 1974 (Rosewarne et al. 2007).

In the early 1980s, Central Australian Aboriginal women approached the congress about the need to respect traditional birthing practices and other concerns. As a result, the Birthright Research project was established in 1984 with financial support from the Commonwealth. The research team visited 60 communities and met with women from 11 language groups who were spread over 78 000 sq km. The research was followed up with the Women's Birthrights Conference, where the aims and objectives of a proposed new centre were worked out. A primary healthcare model was selected, to be based on traditional grandmothers' law, under which 'law, languages and culture' were to be incorporated into 'a women's health and birthing service' (Carter et al. 1987; Stuart 1995). The conference established the Congress Alukura Women's Council, which set up the Alukura Women's Health Program in 1985. Alukura means 'a woman's camp' in Arrernte, the language of the traditional owners of the Alice Springs area. The women's council is a subcommittee of the CAAC and has representative, advisory and decision-making roles in relation to women's law and practices. It set about the task of obtaining funding and was eventually successful. Congress Alukura opened as a pilot project with a midwife, a health worker and a liaison worker in June 1987 (Carter et al. 1987).

Alukura provides a range of health services for the city and surrounding regions, including comprehensive antenatal and postnatal care, shared maternity care, gynaecological services, a well women's clinic, sexual assault and domestic violence counselling and examinations, health education, transportation, health worker training and a bush mobile clinic. In 1994, Alukura was awarded a UN Human Rights Award for the development of its community health and birthing service. After 10 years of operation, the Acting Director was able to claim that 'we are one of the most experienced organisations in the country in Aboriginal women's health, a national leader in primary health care and a strong political voice for the health of our people' (Stuart 1995:179).

In the 1990s, some women were able to give birth at Alukura. In 2002, however, an agreement was signed under which Alukura midwives had visiting rights at the Alice Springs Hospital. For three years, babies were delivered at the hospital by Alukura midwives but in November 2005, due to staffing shortages and other issues, birthing services were suspended. Some of the special projects carried out by Alukura include a three-day Women's Health Conference in 1997, attended by more than 700 women, the production of a grandmothers' law video, which preserves cultural information, a cooperative research project on antenatal health, the development of the *Women's Business Manual* and the Young Women's Community Health Education Project (CAAC 2004–05, 2006– 07; Carter et al. 2004).

Concern about the lack of appropriate health services for Aboriginal women and their families emerged on the South Coast of New South Wales in the early 1980s. There were financial barriers to accessing mainstream services, which, in any case, could be insensitive to cultural needs. In 1984, the Aboriginal Women's Health Centre was set up under the auspices of Jilimi, the Shoalhaven Women's Health and Resource Corporation. A change of incorporation brought into being the South Coast Women's Health and Welfare Aboriginal Corporation and a change of centre name to Waminda in 1990. Understanding and valuing Aboriginal culture are fundamental at Waminda. Other principles are a holistic, family and community-as-a-whole approach to health and respect for women's agency and participation in decision making. Primary healthcare programs include the Women's Health Program, providing a health and sexual health clinic, screening services, support groups for grief and loss, physical activity groups, health promotion and information. A domestic violence support program is responsible for education, awareness and community-development projects, healing camps and court support. There is a drug and alcohol support program and a Koori Girls School Program, which aims to empower girls and young women and help them make informed, healthy lifestyle choices. A Koori Women's Playgroup supports mothers in relation to health, welfare, housing, finances and social and emotional wellbeing. An early childhood nurse and a dietician are employed, along with other children's service providers. The Family Support Program operates workshops for women and their children in skill development and strength building and identifies family needs in relation to housing, finances, social and emotional wellbeing and health. A parenting program aims to build stronger families and the Aboriginal Women Artist Cooperative promotes personal growth and empowerment through art and craft, as well as the development of business and information technology (IT) skills.

Aboriginal women in Cairns set up a women's and children's health centre in the early 1980s. An Aboriginal welfare worker from the Cairns Hospital, Rose Richards, aware that Aboriginal children from rural and remote areas were returned home before they had fully recovered because there was no appropriate Cairns accommodation, began to take children to her own home. With help from other women, including registered nurse and midwife Jilpia Nappaljari Jones, she eventually obtained funding to set up a halfway house. Later relocated, it became known as 'Rosie's Farm'. It was also apparent that transitional accommodation was needed for women who came from remote locations before the births of their babies. Secure funding was obtained and Rosie's Farm moved to its present location, where it is known as Mookai Rosie Bi-Bayan, or Aunty Rosie's Place. It provides services for women and children, including accommodation, transport, recreational activities, health support and advocacy, access to counselling, cultural and emotional support, reproductive health care, pre and postnatal care, nutrition and environmental health education, a playgroup and other educational activities. Anecdotal evidence from Mookai Rosie health workers suggests a reduction in the number of children who fail to thrive, an increase in breastfeeding, a drop in premature births and an improvement in infant health (Mookai Rosie Bi-Bayan web site).

Another Aboriginal women's centre, the Gloria Brennan Aboriginal and Torres Strait Islander Women's Centre, was established in 1988 by the Aboriginal and Torres Strait Islander Women's Congress of Western Australia to provide health and childcare information. Located in eastern Perth, it is a multipurpose centre. As well as health information, it provides assertiveness training and conducts courses in problem solving, conflict resolution, letter writing, management and communication skills and meeting procedures. It runs cultural education programs and provides support, counselling and referral services. Among its political projects has been the 'Stop the Abuse' campaign against sexual assault (Weeks 1994:86, 99).

The Ngaanyatjarra Pitjantjatjara Yankunytjatjara (NPY) Women's Council, which covers parts of Western Australia, South Australia and the Northern Territory, was formed in 1980 when women felt that their needs were not being addressed in relation to land rights. The council, incorporated in 1994, soon became a major provider of human services, juggling advocacy work with casework. It takes a holistic approach to issues such as domestic violence, aged care, emotional and social wellbeing, nutrition and disability needs. The Cross Borders Domestic Violence Service covers 350 000 sq km across the three jurisdictions (NPY Women's Council web site).

In other places, Aboriginal women work for health through local Aboriginal Controlled Community Health Services (ACCHS), or in cooperation with government-employed health workers. The *Aboriginal and Islander Health Worker Journal* provides a record of multiple health-improvement projects undertaken by Aboriginal women over three decades. For example, Lajamanu women, who live in an outback area of the Northern Territory, participated in a project designed to address alcohol and violence issues in their community in the late 1990s. The women painted their stories on calico, which was made into wall hangings and displayed in various public places, conveying their messages to their community. A banner, in English on one side and Warlpiri on the other, and a video were also made. The Lajamanu women insisted on involving men in discussions. Evaluation showed that alcohol and violence issues and strategies to overcome problems were more openly discussed in both family and women's groups. The principles on which the project was based demonstrate traditional views about the importance of community:

> Mobilising communities or even groups within communities has long been acknowledged as the most successful method of empowering people to take responsibility for their own health and well-being. Ensuring that the client group has ownership and direction of the program, in cooperation with an outside agency to support and help resource the activities is a virtual guarantee of a positive outcome for the community. (Clarence and McDonald 1998:2)

Storytelling has also been used by Aboriginal women as a method of health promotion. Drawing on the tradition of oral narratives and on aunty/niece and grandmother/granddaughter relationships, information about female sexual and reproductive roles and practices has been disseminated in several Sydney communities. In 1993, a group of Koori women elders, in cooperation with

Aboriginal academics and other women, made video recordings, in which the need for healthy lifestyles was stressed and information was provided about cervical cancer and coronary heart disease—two of the big illness issues for Aboriginal women. The Aboriginal women involved were empowered and affirmed in their roles as carers and health-promotion information was made available to be passed on to others (Newman et al. 1999:18). Other projects have used art to help women dealing with social and emotional issues and mental illness to feel safer and to bring women together for mutual support (Aboriginal and Islander Health Worker Journal 2002:12). These examples serve to illustrate the keen interest Aboriginal women take in improving the health of their communities.

Immigrant and Refugee Women's Initiatives

Similarly, immigrant and refugee women continued to set up their own centres and services, within the limits of the resources available to them. Gradually, collaboration with the Anglo-Australian women's movement grew. In most places, immigrant and refugee women sought to work with government departments and to gain representation on relevant boards and committees. Like the rest of the women's movement, the immigrant women's community lost human resources to bureaucracies, as women moved into newly created positions.

In most jurisdictions, from the early 1980s onwards, immigrant and refugee women were active around issues of health, culturally appropriate services, language barriers, isolation, the scarcity of interpreters and issues concerning overseas qualifications. Activism was easier in some States than in others. In Queensland, women had to work extremely hard to gain support for health issues. They tried to get appointments with relevant ministers, attempted to get representatives onto relevant advisory committees and tried to persuade the government to take responsibility for interpreting services. Progress was slow, however, under the National and National-Liberal governments that held power through the 1980s.

Brisbane women established the Immigrant Women's Support Service in 1984 with Commonwealth SAAP funding. The centre is multipurpose and community based and adheres to feminist principles. In 2004, it was providing services for women from 72 different countries through its two main programs, which focus on domestic violence and sexual assault. The service is now funded jointly by the Commonwealth and Queensland governments.

The Multicultural Women's Health Centre was established in Fremantle, Western Australia, by a group of women in 1985, spearheaded by the extraordinary efforts of one woman, Ronelle Brossard (Broom 1991). As well as providing for

101

the needs of immigrant women, the centre was soon also providing services for local Aboriginal women. Also in Perth, the community-based Ishar Multicultural Centre for Women's Health, formerly the Mirrabooka Multicultural Women's Health Centre, began operation in 1992. Its philosophy is grounded in a social model of health and, as well as core staff, it is supported by a band of volunteers. In 2009, Ishar collaborated with a neighbouring women's health centre, Women's Healthworks, supported by the Western Australia Department for Communities, to consult with more than 100 women on their views about issues of concern for the new national women's health policy. The centres wrote a combined submission to the Commonwealth.

In 1987, the Immigrant Women's Health Service was established in western Sydney, with centres in Fairfield and Cabramatta. It provides a comprehensive range of preventive and clinical services and information and referral services for women from diverse backgrounds and it adjusts its programs to changes in cultural demography. Special events are staged regularly, including cooking demonstrations, food sharing and well-known feast days.

Multipurpose immigrant women's centres and associations generally feature health as one of their priorities. The Immigrant Women's Speakout Association, community based and managed, was formed in New South Wales in 1985, following a successful speak-out gathering in 1982. The NSW Immigrant Women's Resource Centre was established at the same time. The association's priorities include health, domestic violence, child care, education, and workplace, legal and equity issues. It undertakes community-development projects and is particularly concerned about the needs of disadvantaged women. Speak-out gatherings were also organised in Brisbane and Adelaide in 1983.

The Migrant Women's Lobby Group, established in Adelaide in 1984, is a peak body for immigrant women's groups. Health issues are a major focus. Another such group is the Australian Vietnamese Women's Association, formed in Victoria in 1983. More recent groups include the Filipino Women's Support Group, New South Wales, formed in 1998, and the Victorian Immigrant and Refugee Women's Coalition, set up in 1997. The Migrant Women's Support & Accommodation Service (MWSAS) is a not-for-profit, community-based organisation, established in 1985 in Adelaide. It is a specialist provider of emergency and short-term accommodation and crisis and support services for women and children escaping violence. It operates an outreach service and conducts community education workshops. The organisation aims to promote the basic human rights of women and children from non-English-speaking backgrounds 'so they may live free of domestic violence' (MWSAS web site).

Anglo-Australian Initiatives

The second half of the 1970s was a period of serious funding insecurity for established women's health centres, while there were few financial opportunities for those that were trying to set themselves up. State and Territory governments were being asked to shoulder the costs of the Community Health Program and other programs as the Commonwealth withdrew its funding. Thus, even where sub-national governments actively supported women's health, money became scarce as the Whitlam Government's largesse came to an end. At the best of times, Australian federalism is characterised by severe financial imbalance, as discussed. This general situation was exacerbated by the balance-of-payments problems of the late 1980s and the recession of the early 1990s. At that time, the Commonwealth Labor Government drastically and unilaterally cut its grants to the States and Territories in order to curtail public spending, resulting in straitened financial circumstances at the sub-national level (Summers 2006:142–3).

In the late 1970s in New South Wales, where most of the women's health centres were located, women waged a time-consuming and discouraging battle for several years to maintain funding. They were assisted by femocrats and women in the ALP. Under the new arrangements, funding levels were reduced so that, for example, the workers at LWCHC received no pay increases during the first eight years.

Survival on minimal funding was one thing but the new centres that were trying to establish themselves from the mid-1970s onwards had an even more difficult time. Most opened and survived on a mix of volunteer labour, donations, the proceeds of fundraising and small, short-term grants. The Central Coast Women's Health Centre in Gosford began in 1976, staffed by volunteers. After two years, it succeeded in obtaining minimal funding but, until the mid-1980s, it relied heavily on donations and volunteers (Broom 1991:18–19). In 2011 it has satellite services in Woy Woy and Wyong. The establishment committee for the Bankstown centre in south-western Sydney was involved in four years of intense work before it received a small grant in 1978. The Wran State Government 'firmly refused' to fund it fully, in what was believed to be a strategy to discourage the formation of new centres (Smith 1984:5). Eventually, it received enough funding to allow it to expand in the mid-1980s (Broom 1991:23).

The Wagga Women's Health and Support Centre (New South Wales) was opened in 1979 after a long period of activism. The centre enjoyed relatively high levels of material support from the local community, despite the founders having to endure a deal of disparagement (Roberts and Stewart 1999). The feminist, community-based Women's Community Health Centre in the Blue Mountains was set up in 1982. In the Coffs Harbour area of New South Wales, the local branch of WEL researched women's health needs in 1973. Priorities were a refuge, opened in 1978, and family planning services. The Women's Resources Centre was opened in 1982, providing information and support and, later, family planning services. When funded in 1986, it became the Coffs Harbour Women's Health Centre. At that time there were health fears about the use of agricultural chemicals. Within hours of opening, appointments were booked out for three months.

The Illawarra Women's Health Centre (New South Wales), a feminist, community-based organisation, was opened in 1984. It houses a lesbian safe place, the Illawarra Lesbian Health Project, which provides health information and services for lesbians. Shoalhaven Women's Health Centre was opened in 1985. Another organisation, The Women's Cottage—not strictly a women's health centre—opened in the Hawkesbury district in 1983, funded by the Department of Community Services to be a resource centre. The cottage now functions primarily as a feminist women's health centre, helping to address considerable unmet need in its local area.

In 1985–86, women's health centres in Wollongong, Wagga Wagga, Campbelltown, Penrith and Blacktown received funding for the first time, as a result of the recommendations of the NSW Women's Health Policy Review Committee. In Bathurst, the Central West Women's Health Centre was opened in 1986. A feminist, community-based organisation, funded by the NSW Department of Health and the Department of Community Services, it aims to make its community safer, fairer and more supportive for women and children. Blacktown Women's and Girls' Health Centre was opened in 1987, after years of lobbying by a group of feminists. Initially funded by the Commonwealth, it works from a social determinants framework and is cognisant that many of its clients have low incomes. In the same year, Penrith Women's Health Centre and Lismore and District Women's Health Centre were opened. In 1990, the feminist Cumberland Women's Health Centre began to operate, with a particular focus on combating violence against women. It employs complementary health practitioners and an Aboriginal women's health worker. The Women's Health Centre in Albury–Wodonga is very unusual in that, instead of having to work long and hard for funding, it happened that money became available before women had fully mobilised (Broom 1991:143–4).

Other States have fewer women's health centres than New South Wales. Between the closure of the Brisbane Women's House Health Centre in 1977 and when the next centre was funded in 1990, a group of volunteers struggled to provide a rudimentary service. Over the years, hundreds of women belonged to the group and many came, left and joined again. By the early 1980s, the volunteers were despondent and their energies depleted. They had been unable to secure meetings with Health Minister, Brian Austin, and, indeed, he is said to have ridiculed and trivialised women's issues in public statements. Only three of the original group remained committed and such funding as they had derived mainly from a pledge system and from performing street theatre! A women's health centre group in Hervey Bay was mobilised and, in Rockhampton, a women's information centre was run by volunteers from donated premises in a shopping centre. Despite efforts across the State, there were limits to the community effort and interest that could be maintained in the face of a staunchly conservative government.

In 1982, however, a new collective formed in Brisbane, which opened Brisbane Women's Community Health Centre in Woolloongabba in early 1983. The centre was supported by project funding from the Commonwealth Community Employment Program (CEP). At the end of 1983, enough money was raised to employ Carol Low as a fundraiser and submission writer. Workgroups and subcommittees were formed and fundraising included staging a women's health day. A submission to CEP in 1984 produced funds to employ seven full-time and two part-time workers but when the funding finished, staff were reduced to three and survival again became dependent on a pledge system and small amounts of temporary funding. About this time, another group of women, sensitive to trade union issues without being trade unionists, began to meet in the Union of Australian Women offices. A Queensland branch of the Australian Community Health Association was formed and energy for a women's health centre was mobilised again, supported by the newly established Workers Health Centre and the Migrant Women's Speakout. A way was found to have Commonwealth money channelled through the Australian Community Health Association to the Queensland branch and then to the Brisbane Women's Health Centre, which received Commonwealth funding in this way for three and a half years. Hard work and strong commitment brought a modicum of success: Helen Abrahams, then a participant, now a Brisbane City Councillor, is of the view that anything that survived in Queensland during the years of government hostility is strong, like a desert flower.

The Goss Government came to power in 1989 with a policy on women's health that it is said was written by a male party member. Jude Abbs, women's health activist, is credited with having brought women's health to the Queensland branch of the ALP and then into government when she became head of the new Women's Health Unit. From this time on, women's health in Queensland received more stable funding, jointly supplied by the Commonwealth and Queensland under the NWH Program. In the next two years, six new community-based centres were funded from the same source: Townsville in 1990, Rockhampton and Wide Bay in 1991, Logan and Ipswich in 1992 and Gympie and District Women's Health Centre in 1994. Gladstone nurses had campaigned for a centre, which was opened in 1994. In 2011, there are nine women's health centres in

Queensland, all women controlled and community based, except for the Ipswich centre, now called West Moreton Women's Health, which ran into financial difficulties in 2003 and became part of Queensland Health in 2004.

The general situation in South Australia in the key early 1980s was one of strong community and ministerial support for women's health, on one hand, and determined bureaucratic opposition on the other. The story of the closure of Hindmarsh and its reopening as Adelaide Women's Community Health Centre has been discussed. Soon after, Labor replaced the Liberal Government and the new Minister for Health, John Cornwall, was strongly interventionist. He was persuaded to support a social determinants and community-development approach to health and was aware that, despite Australia's relatively good average life expectancy, there were serious inequalities in health outcomes and significant levels of preventable death, disease and injury, especially among low-income groups (Cornwall 1989:157–62). Liz Furler was appointed Women's Adviser on Health at the beginning of 1984, with a brief to increase women's influence in health policy. During his tenure, Cornwall approved funding for three new women's health centres to complement Adelaide Women's Community Health Centre as a State-wide service.

The first was Elizabeth Women's Health Centre (later Northern Women's Primary Health Care Centre), which began providing services in 1983 and officially opened in 1984 after five years of lobbying and preparation by a sponsoring group. In a clear instance of party difference, the centre had been approved by the Labor Government in 1979 but was abandoned by the incoming Liberal Government (Radoslovich 1994:31–7). In the southern part of Adelaide, women mobilised in response to the enormous health and social problems and service gaps that were evident in the area. A formal group was established in 1983 and, supported by the local community health centre, it wrote a submission for a women's health centre. Approval to proceed was announced at the opening of the Elizabeth centre, and Southern Women's Health and Community Centre was officially opened in September, 1984 (Radoslovich 1994:39–44).

Again in 1983, Minister Cornwall gave approval for a steering committee of local women to investigate the feasibility of establishing a centre in the Port Adelaide area. Dale Street Women's Community Health Centre was opened for business the following year. From the beginning, 180 people per month attended group and other sessions and waiting times for appointments with doctors, counsellors and nurses soon extended to several weeks (Radoslovich 1994:45–50).

In keeping with the longstanding bureaucratic preference for government (or health department) control, the SA women's health centres have now lost their independence, although refuges have been allowed to maintain independent management committees. An early amalgamation attempt in 1986–87 by the

Health Commission was staved off by extensive grassroots action (Auer 2003:8). In 1995, however, in a move with the stated aim of achieving 'efficiencies', Adelaide Women's Health Centre was de-incorporated and merged with the Women's and Children's Hospital. A memorandum of understanding was written that outlined the responsibilities of the two agencies and the name, Adelaide Women's, was changed to Women's Health Statewide. The three other women's health centres were amalgamated into the community health services of their regions. In 2004, the Women's and Children's Hospital and Women's Health Statewide were amalgamated to form the Children, Youth and Women's Health Service. According to Jocelyn Auer, a member of the movement from the early days, the SA women's health centres are now clearly part of the health service and can no longer be said to be run 'by women, for women'. They now work for change within the health system (Auer 2003:8, 12).

Various groups interested in setting up a women's health centre formed in Hobart in 1974 but their efforts to get support were unsuccessful and they finally disbanded. In 1984, another group, the Women's Health Foundation, was established. Members were especially concerned that low-income women could not access abortion services because they could not afford to travel to Melbourne. At this time it was estimated that between 75 and 90 per cent of Tasmanian women wanting an abortion were forced to go interstate. Moreover, virtually no counselling services were available in Tasmania. The foundation raised some $33 000 over two years, with which they bought a building at 9 Pearce Street, Hobart. It was renovated and approved as a medical centre; however, medical practitioners willing to do abortions and general practitioners to provide back-up could not be found.

After this setback, it was decided that the house could be leased to the Hobart Women's Health Centre group, to be used as a women's health centre; however, operational funding was not available from the Tasmanian Government. Eventually, 18 months' funding was allocated by the Commonwealth and the centre opened in 1987. A doctor who was able to bill Medicare for consultations was found. Lobbying for expansion continued and, in 1989, in the lead-up to the State election, the Labor Party promised that it would support three women's health centres. Once in government, however, it announced that there was only enough money for one. And so it is that Tasmania, to this day, has one (precariously funded) women's health centre.

After the closure of Collingwood Women's Health Centre in the late 1970s, Victorian activists focused their attention on supporting women to care for their own health and trying to influence mainstream services to be more responsive to women's needs. Information and community education resources were produced, as a variety of health-focused groups began to form, such as an endometriosis self-help group and a DES[4] action group. A Women's Health Resource Collective (later Women's Health Information Resource Collective) was formed in 1982 by a small group of women, some of whom had belonged to the original collective. The group survived on bits and pieces of short-term funding. It focused on information provision, community development, advocacy and lobbying and the development of written health-promotion material. In its first five years, it produced 14 information leaflets and booklets on a range of issues and printed, in total, 95 300 copies. Workers collaborated with other community groups and gave talks and addresses. The centre also operated as a drop-in place (Women's Health Information Resource Collective 1987).

The Ministerial Women's Health Policy Working Party was established in 1985. It reported in 1987, giving rise to a serious struggle that resulted in a period of expansion for Victorian women's health services. The report recommended that at least one women's health service be set up in each of the health regions and that there should be two women's health information services, one of which would focus on the needs of immigrant women. A group called Healthsharing Women was formed, which successfully tendered to run a State-wide information service, opened in 1988. The Women's Health Service for the West, the first regional women's health centre, was initiated by two groups, one a coalition from the northern and the western suburbs and the other the Western Women's Health Network. Under the cost-shared NWH Program, women's health centres were set up in each of the regions between 1989 and 1992, following initiatives by groups of community women, most of which had been mobilised for years.

In 1993, the Women's Health Information Resource Collective and Healthsharing Women amalgamated to form a single State-wide agency. The service changed its name to Women's Health Victoria (WHV) in 1996. It provides health promotion, information and advocacy services, with a focus on informing and influencing health policy and service delivery. Currently there are nine independent regional services and three State-wide services funded under the Victorian Women's Health Program.

The political climate in Western Australia was not strongly conducive to the establishment of separate women's health services, although small windows of political opportunity opened at different times. The network of women's health services that is in place, therefore, testifies to the dedication of grassroots groups and the women in bureaucracies, political parties and other places who support them. Grassroots action continued in the late 1970s and through the 1980s in efforts to get State support for new centres. The establishment of the Goldfields Women's Health Centre resulted from action by community women and nurses over a period of years, for example. Initially, the director of community nursing,

---

4 Diethylstilboestrol, which is discussed in Chapter 4.

Margarita Paul, sent out a questionnaire asking women to identify the services that were important to them. A public meeting was held and the Goldfields Women's Health Care Association formed, followed by fundraising drives and lobbying. A group of volunteers began to provide skeleton services in 1986. The following year, services were expanded, supported by donations and more fundraising. The then Health Minister, Ian Taylor (minister from 1986 to 1988), was sympathetic but the women were required to prove they could run a centre efficiently on a volunteer basis before government funding would be considered. Money for a house was obtained from the Lotteries Commission in 1988 and funds were raised to employ a counsellor. Operational funding was secured from the Health Department in 1989 but had to be supplemented with other grants and community donations.

A similar process took place in the Geraldton area where a group wishing to establish a centre had been organised for several years. A regional planning study had been undertaken and submissions written. Despite supportive government statements, only $5000 had been allocated by 1989, when Labor promised support in its election campaign. Once in government, however, they refused to provide further funding. The centre, initially called the Midwest Women's Health Resource Centre, was eventually funded under the NWH Program in 1991.

Whitfords Women's Health Centre, now Women's Healthworks, was set up under the auspices of the Women's Health Care House in 1989, but the following year it developed its own constitution and became independent. Mirrabooka Multicultural Women's Health Information Centre, now Ishar Multicultural Centre for Women's Health, opened in 1992. Rockingham Women's Health Service was established in 1993, funded by the NWH Program, along with Hedland Well Women's Centre. Gosnells Women's Health Service opened in 1994. By 1997, 11 community-managed women's health centres, metropolitan and regional, were being jointly funded by the Commonwealth and WA governments under the NWH Program (Commonwealth of Australia 1997:26).

Throughout this period, Perth's original women's health centre, Women's Health Care House, continued to operate and expand. At the end of the 1980s, a decision was taken to try to better meet the needs of the significant numbers of clients with alcohol and other drug problems. To this end, Perth Women's Centre was established a block away the following year. In 2005, Women's Health Care House and Perth Women's Centre were amalgamated and now operate as Women's Health Services. The organisation manages numerous community and outreach projects and provides services for more than 45 000 families each year from more than 60 nationalities and from city, rural and remote areas of the State.

In the Australian Capital Territory, efforts to establish a women's health centre go back to 1974 when the first unsuccessful funding submission was made. The ACT Women's Health Network (ACTWHN) established a women's health centre working party in preparation for the NWHP in 1987. The ACT Department of Health suggested a workshop in early 1990 to discuss the implications of the NWHP for local services. The workshop was convened by Dorothy Broom, then Convenor of ACTWHN. There was unanimous agreement that the NWH Program money should be used to establish a women's health centre. The draft recommendations of the meeting were circulated for comment and a special general meeting of the network was called to refine the draft proposals. A subcommittee was formed to progress the decision. The ACT Government and the Commonwealth accepted the recommendations and the Canberra Women's Health Centre, later renamed the Women's Centre for Health Matters, was opened in 1990. Networkers became members at the next ACTWHN meeting and stuck gold stars on their foreheads to celebrate!

The Work of Women's Health Centres

Women's health centres provide a broad range of community-based services. The service mix varies from centre to centre and from time to time, depending on resources and local needs but whatever is offered is highly valued, judging by the queues of women who line up to use them. As well as medical services in some locations, counselling and preventive health advice might be on offer, alongside referral, naturopathic and massage services, for example. Counselling for emotional and mental health issues, sometimes related to abuse and domestic violence, is nearly always in high demand. Centres provide information on countless topics, often in many languages, facilitate the formation of support and self-help groups and hold a variety of workshops and classes in response to changing needs. Most centres provide outreach services. Service provision for individuals and groups involves interaction and cooperation with a wide range of local and State agencies, from individual health professionals to housing departments.

The cluster of services provided is not readily available from primary medical care facilities, such as general practitioners' offices. Moreover, services are provided in a sympathetic manner with time taken to listen, provide information and consider a woman's overall life situation. Waminda Aboriginal Women's Health Centre serves as an example. As well as conventional reproductive health and screening services and childhood health programs, there are domestic violence prevention and support programs, healing camps, grief and loss support systems, social and emotional wellbeing projects and health-promotion activities. Personal growth and empowerment are major goals. This work includes school programs for girls alongside parenting programs and family support workshops for women and their children, involving the development of skills in relation to everyday needs and activities, such as housing, finance, business and IT use. Like other women's health centres, Waminda aims to offer integrated, culturally appropriate, holistic primary health care, with a focus on health promotion and illness prevention.

Political advocacy is a major component of work. Women's health workers write letters and position papers, make submissions to inquiries, and lobby and liaise with governments at all levels, including the local level. They lend their support to other groups, such as unions, during campaigns for equal pay, for example. Typically, a centre will be involved in a number of community-development activities, which can range from sexuality education for young people to the elimination of toxic waste. In facilitating participation in its decision making, a centre contributes to the personal development, health and wellbeing of local women (Broom 1998a:7). The bigger centres undertake research into local needs and conditions and publish and disseminate the findings.

Women's health centres have been able to influence the way things are done in mainstream hospital and medical systems by expanding the scope of debate and developing best-practice models of primary health care, although their influence is less than activists would wish. Centres and the wider movement bring up new issues and suggest new approaches and new ways of working that raise mainstream awareness about what might be involved in women's health care. More opportunities are thereby created for mainstream innovation than would have otherwise been possible (Dwyer 1992a:26–7). Centres influence both by example and through training: staff members are regularly invited to contribute to the education of medical students and centres provide training placements for medical students and students from other disciplines, such as nursing and social work (Broom 1998b:10–11). Information about women's health, both hardcopy and online, finds its way into the nooks and crannies of health systems. It also contributes to the formation of bands of health consumers who expect to be well informed and to participate in decisions about their health and health care. And the day-to-day activities of centres support and reinforce political activism. As Dwyer (1992b:25) has argued, the two arms of the dual strategy reinforce each other: 'the delivery of services legitimates the advocacy and the advocacy disseminates the lessons learned from the people being served and advances their interests.'

Women's health centres are highly valued by the women who use them. Research undertaken in the 1990s by Dorothy Broom probed the reasons. Broom found that many women felt safer in an all-women environment and many were more comfortable with a woman doctor and therefore more willing to discuss problems. Women appreciated the sympathetic hearing they received, the time taken to provide explanations and information and the responsiveness to their health, broadly defined, and their life situations. Women gained empowerment through their participation in groups organised around a range of healing and health-promoting activities, such as education, living skills development, exercise and self-defence. When asked, women wanted other health agencies to replicate features of women's health centres: they wanted more informal environments, more supportive staff, more information and counselling, the availability of more groups, a more holistic approach to health and they wanted more women's health centres, closer to home (Broom 1996, 1998). In summary, the appeal of women's health centres was found to be based in best-practice models of care, including the time taken to deal sympathetically and holistically with complex problems and to provide information. Women felt empowered by their participation in groups and by opportunities made available for health development (Broom 1998b:5).

Refuges, Shelters and Houses

The one women's health issue that the Fraser Commonwealth Government supported was shelter for women escaping domestic violence. At the time, new refuges were being established by churches and welfare-oriented groups, as well as by feminists. In 1975–76, 19 refuges were funded under the Community Health Program and one under the Homeless Persons Assistance Program; however, one year later, there were 40 refuges, with more than 100 in operation by 1979 (Dowse 1984:149–50). As discussed in Chapter 2, in the absence of agreement in the Commonwealth bureaucracy about the appropriate locus of responsibility, refuge funding had been provided through the Community Health Program under the Whitlam Government. The Fraser Government continued to use the same channel but it simultaneously slashed the funding, leaving the Community Health Program to fight for its life (Dowse 1984:151). One result, among others, was reduced refuge funding.

Prime Minister, Malcolm Fraser, seemingly supported refuges: he had personally intervened to ensure that Queensland refuges were funded directly after Premier Bjelke-Petersen refused to pass on Commonwealth money on the grounds that 'Marxist lesbians' were involved in the Brisbane refuge. In 1977, it was decided that the Commonwealth would put refuge financing on a secure basis and the Minister for Social Security, Senator Margaret Guilfoyle, was requested to prepare a submission for the budget that year. The minister was, however, reluctant to take on the new responsibility and the budget approached without a satisfactory proposal. Facing the possibility that funding would cease, the Office of Women's Affairs sent out an alert. Strong community action followed, including a high-profile media campaign. In response, cabinet decided that existing arrangements should continue and that the money allocated would be doubled to $2 million (Sawer 1990:38). At the same time, however, the Commonwealth continued to cut funding for the Community Health Program and called on the States and Territories to take up the slack (McFerran 1990:194). The outcome of this extraordinary situation was that while there was more money for refuges, existing (that is, feminist) refuges, which by this time comprised about one-third of the total, suffered funding cuts. Moreover, newly established refuges received 'only shoestring assistance' (Dowse 1984:151–2).

The entry of private institutions and organisations into the field gave rise to debates and disputes about the legitimacy of 'feminist' refuges. Workers continued to endure poor wages and conditions in feminist establishments, often donating their own money by splitting available salaries among a greater number of workers. Conservative sub-national governments did not support the refuge movement, at least initially, whereas reasonable support, albeit infused with electoral expediency, came from Labor governments. Overall, 'new refuges were set up with ridiculously poor funding and funding for existing refuges stagnated' (McFerran 1990:194).

A funding crisis was created in 1981 when the Commonwealth passed responsibility to the States and Territories for what remained of the Community Health Program, women's health centres, refuges and rape crisis centres. A strong reaction followed from feminist organisations, supported by the National Women's Advisory Council, which issued a media release censuring the Commonwealth for abrogating its responsibility to women and children. A tent embassy was set up outside Parliament House but the decision stood (McFerran 1990:198–9; Sawer 1990:54–5). Refuges limped along on grossly inadequate funding, unable to pay standard wages, until 1984, when a Commonwealth Labor government set up the Women's Emergency Services Program (WESP), which brought with it funding increases. In 1985, WESP, jointly funded by the Commonwealth, States and Territories, was incorporated into SAAP—a move that was initially resisted by feminists on the grounds that refuges were not about homelessness but about domestic violence. The advent of SAAP funding brought a measure of stability, in the form of five-year funding agreements. Perversely, perhaps, the end of the 'annual scramble for bitterly contested money' rendered the refuges invisible in a political sense. No longer forced to draw attention to themselves and to make their arguments public, there was less debate about domestic violence and the homelessness it caused (McFerran 1990:200–2).

The proliferation of refuges did not solve women's emergency accommodation problems. For example, only 19 per cent of women seeking emergency shelter were able to gain a place in Victoria in 1992 (Fredericks 1993). Thus, women from different backgrounds continued to set up new services. For example,

Cawarra Women's Refuge Aboriginal Corporation was established in 1977 and has provided services for Aboriginal and non-Aboriginal women since that time. Wirraway Women's Housing Co-Operative in Moree, New South Wales, was established in the early 1980s to provide Aboriginal women with emergency as well as permanent accommodation. More recently, the Aboriginal Family Violence Prevention and Legal Service Victoria was established to assist people affected by family violence and sexual assault. It has three branches in country Victoria and among its activities are programs for young Koori women. The Yinganeh Aboriginal women's refuge was set up in Lismore, New South Wales, in 2005.

Immigrant women in Victoria set up the feminist Refuge Ethnic Workers Program (REWP) in 1984, which conducted education projects and worked to challenge negative stereotypes, both inside and outside immigrant communities. It adopted a new name and a new mission in 1994 as the Immigrant Women's Domestic Violence Service. Run by a community-based collective, it provides an exceptionally comprehensive range of services. Women of Different Ethnic Backgrounds (WODEB), a subgroup of Women in Health around Melbourne (WHAM), was also formed to explore different ways of dealing with immigrant and refugee health issues. In South Australia, a number of services for women escaping violence were established, including the Non-English Speaking Background Domestic Violence Action Group.

New Anglo-Australian feminist refuges include the Women's Place for homeless or intoxicated women without children, opened in Sydney in 1981 after considerable difficulty finding suitable accommodation. Louisa Lawson House was set up in Sydney in 1982, in response to concerns that women escaping physical and sexual violence were becoming 'mental health statistics' for want of appropriate services (Grahame and Prichard 1996:71). Its founders marched on the Premier's office to demand funding. Coffs Harbour Women's Support Group, formed in 1984, had a turbulent beginning, with serious disagreements in the first year (Grahame and Prichard 1996:34). The Esther Refuge Collective was formed in 1983 to establish a feminist refuge in the Hornsby–Ku-ring-gai area of northern Sydney.

In South Australia, Anne Women's Shelter, Elizabeth, opened in 1978 and Hope Haven Women's Shelter, Adelaide, Port Adelaide Women's Shelter, Port Augusta Women's Shelter and Whyalla Women's Shelter all operated in the 1970s and 1980s. Annie Kenney Young Women's Refuge was set up in Hobart, Matilda Women's Refuge and Woorarra Women's Refuge were established in Melbourne, along with others in country Victoria. In the Australian Capital Territory, the Single Women's Shelter Collective was formed in 1981, in response to problems that emerged when women with different needs were housed in the same place. The group struggled to obtain funding for three years but Toora Single Women's

Shelter, now called Toora Women, opened its doors in August 1983. Demand for services has always been high and, like so many others, it has survived on minimal funding, and, on occasion, even that has been under threat. The organisation has expanded and changed during its 28 years: there are now eight separate Toora services, employing more than 50 women (Rosenman 2003). In Western Australia by 1990, there were eight metropolitan refuges, five country refuges, an immigrant women's service and an Aboriginal women's refuge. One of these, the Patricia Giles Centre, which was opened in 1989 and expanded in 2006, offers programs specifically tailored for Aboriginal women and gay, lesbian, bisexual, transgender, intersex and queer (GLBTIQ) people.

The Women's Health Network in the Northern Territory took the lead in lobbying for a refuge and wrote several unsuccessful funding submissions. Eventually, an application for Commonwealth SAAP funding succeeded and Dawn House, which is about to celebrate its thirtieth birthday, was established.

The remarkable story of how a country refuge, Edith Edwards Women's Centre, in Bourke, New South Wales, was set up is worth recounting in detail because it illustrates the extraordinary efforts women undertook to set up basic services and demonstrates that women from different cultural backgrounds can work together successfully. Its establishment took a series of community meetings, stretching over a decade, and dedicated collaborative action by Aboriginal women, non-Aboriginal women and other members of the Bourke community. In response to high rates of violence, the first public meeting was held in the early 1980s, followed by the formation of a committee, a succession of further meetings and several unsuccessful funding submissions. In 1987–88, the District Manager of the then Department of Youth and Community Services supported the committee, making strong representations to her department and documenting the need for a facility in this isolated town. Her efforts also failed but the committee persevered.

In the meantime, Mygunyah Aboriginal Corporation, formed by Dubbo women, had obtained funding for a number of domestic violence workers to be located in western towns. The Commonwealth Department of Family and Community Services proposed that a support worker be provided through Mygunyah. Bourke women protested strongly because women and children would need to be transported to the nearest refuge in Parkes, about 500 km away. A support worker nevertheless arrived.

The Bourke committee continued to agitate for separate funding. It was assisted by a nun from Cobar who had helped set up another country refuge. In 1991, another public meeting was held. The result was an offer from the Historical Buildings Cooperative of a heritage-listed 'Grand Mansion' with a large garden in the centre of town, on condition that the group take responsibility for maintenance. An added attraction was that it was only half a block from the police station. The group became incorporated, applied for charitable status and decided to wait no longer for government funding.

A mammoth community fundraising effort ensued. The solicitor employed by the Aboriginal Legal Service cooked curries to sell in the main street, helped by others making salads and rice. A radio auction was organised, with donated goods and services from surrounding towns. There were cake stalls, bingo games and the like, a small bequest and a local businessman who, facing a court appearance, donated $2000 to show he was of good character. The council agreed to waive water, sewerage and land rates. During the preparatory phase, informal community consultations were held, which included talking to older women about expectations, needs and concerns. Given that renovations, building maintenance and insurance had to be paid for, the committee was fortunate in finding a qualified, highly respected Aboriginal woman who agreed to live in, rent free, as unpaid manager.

The refuge opened on International Women's Day, 1992. The first clients had arrived two weeks beforehand and in the first month 100 bed nights were occupied. Donations from religious organisations allowed the employment of two casual employees; otherwise all work was voluntary. Fundraising continued: donations included half a sheep a week from a fundamentalist Christian community and a towel service supplied by the Country Women's Association. Aboriginal and non-Aboriginal women worked together and volunteers were included in decision-making processes, fostering feelings of ownership. By 1992, the refuge was providing a 24-hour, seven-day-a-week service without public financial support. In 2011, Edith Edwards Women's Centre is a publicly funded, community-controlled service, with the capacity to house three families. Additional accommodation options are available in private homes, if needed (Alvares 1992; Personal communication with refuge staff).

A variety of other services to support women experiencing domestic violence has been set up over the years. To give just a few examples, the NSW Women's Refuge Resource Centre has operated since 1986 as a referral, information and awareness-raising service. In Queensland, a State-wide domestic violence service offered counselling, community education and produced resources until 2002, after which it became an advocacy and outreach service. A domestic violence crisis service was set up in the Australian Capital Territory in 1988 to provide crisis intervention at the scene of the incident alongside the police and a 24-hour, seven-day-a-week crisis telephone service. Aboriginal women have devised various projects, using art and storytelling traditions for therapeutic purposes. Community arts projects are also used in multicultural settings (Cazalet and Lane 2000). In Townsville, in the late 1990s, a women's collective established a community garden in the grounds of the North Queensland Combined Women's

Services Centre, as a symbolic project to work for peace and against violence (Lynn and Perkins 2000). Another creative project is the collection of stories by workers in a north Queensland women's shelter, published as *Dragonfly Whispers* (Sera Women's Shelter et al. 2006).

Like women's health centres, refuges, shelters and houses operate with dual aims: they try to meet the immediate support and accommodation needs of women and children escaping violence while engaging in political action. Intensive case-management services for diverse groups of women and children are provided and some agencies have special programs for children. Refuges advocate on behalf of clients, produce information and research and conduct community education, aiming to generate awareness of domestic violence and promote the rights of women who have suffered from it. Training packages are developed for relevant professionals, along with a full range of information production and dissemination activities.

Sexual Assault Services

Despite campaigns against sexual violence in the 1980s and 1990s, the issue has been difficult to keep on political agendas. A couple of well-reported pronouncements helped the cause. In South Australia, Supreme Court Judge Justice Bollen said in 1993 that a husband may use 'a measure of rougher than usual handling' to persuade a wife to consent to sex. In the same year, Justice Bland told a Victorian County Court in a rape case that 'no often subsequently means yes'. Such statements prompted public debate and intensified feminist campaigns.

As with domestic violence, in relation to rape and sexual assault the importance of considering cultural factors gradually became more widely recognised. In communities where shame was attached to victims and their families, sexual crimes were rarely discussed (Yarrow Place web site). Despite the establishment of services such as the Migrant Women against Incest Network in New South Wales in 1986, immigrant and refugee women usually maintained silence about sexual assault (Jung 2003). Regardless of these barriers, sexual assault became a major issue in many multipurpose centres set up by immigrant women.

As far as I have been able to discover, only a few sexual assault services along white feminist lines have been established by Aboriginal women.[5] One such is the Yorgam Aboriginal Corporation, set up in 1993 in East Perth to overcome the

---

5   Aboriginal women have their own ways of meeting community needs.

problem that available services were inappropriate. Yorgam supports spiritual, physical, emotional and mental health needs and provides a range of counselling services to address violence and sexual abuse affecting Aboriginal people.

Anglo-Australian women set up many new services. In New South Wales, the Dympna House incest service secured funding for the Dympna Accommodation Program in 1986, which was incorporated as the Stepping Out Housing Program in 1987. Dympna staff recognised that clients who were homeless would benefit from more stability in their lives. The Stepping Out Housing Program provides supported accommodation for women (with or without dependent children) who have experienced childhood sexual abuse. Many such women fled to the streets at a young age. Another New South Wales service is the Southwest Women's Child Sexual Assault Resource Centre, set up by women with CEP funding in 1985. Later called Rosebank, the service struggled to locate appropriate accommodation but, in 2006, premises were secured until 2011.

Women's House, Brisbane, which began as a rape crisis centre in 1975, had to wait until 1983 to receive temporary funding and until 1991 to obtain secure funding. The following year, it added the word 'incest' to its title, to better acknowledge the scale of sexual violence, becoming the Brisbane Rape and Incest Survivors Support Centre. A multipurpose women's centre was established in Cairns in 1986, providing a sexual assault crisis service. Similar services have been established on the Gold Coast and the Sunshine Coast.

In South Australia, the feminist Adelaide Rape Crisis Centre was still struggling financially in the 1980s, although it received some government funding. In 1993, the Government decided to amalgamate the service with the sexual assault service run by Queen Elizabeth Hospital. Feminists campaigned against the 'amalgamation', which meant disestablishment of the management collective, but the merger went ahead. The service, called Yarrow Place, has a strong preventive focus. It challenges attitudes and beliefs and works towards 'a society free of sexual violence'. Two Aboriginal health workers are employed.

The Women Against Rape group formed in Tasmania in the 1970s and worked towards law reform but was hampered by internal divisions. Roughly, one group of professional women favoured workers with professional qualifications while another thought that experience was the most important qualification and that cooperation with government would lead to cooption. Another issue was whether the service would participate in police training. Complicating matters was the position taken by male gynaecologists, who wanted a hospital-based, medically oriented service. In the event, women were able to cooperate sufficiently to set up a service in 1986.

As mentioned in the previous chapter, the publicly funded Sexual Assault Centre was established at the Queen Victoria Medical Centre, Melbourne, in 1977. The centre developed within a feminist framework and part of its early work was to undertake community and professional education. In 1982, the Cain State Labor Government was elected on a promise to establish a sexual assault service in each of the State's health regions. By 1985, six Centres Against Sexual Assault (CASA) had been put in place. In response to the recommendations of the inquiry into women's health, which reported in 1986 (of which more below), another seven centres were established by the end of the 1980s, followed by two more in 1992 and 1995 respectively, completing a network of 15 services. The centres have a variety of management models. Although government controlled and funded, some are community based and some have mixed boards, which include hospital administrators and community members—a structure designed to facilitate community input and accountability. According to Hewitt and Worth (n.d.), it is something of an open question whether CASA are an expression of the feminist struggle against patriarchy or 'whether they had been co-opted to create a well serviced class of victims'.

Western Australia's original Sexual Assault Resource Centre (SARC) was relocated in a house close to the King Edward Memorial Hospital in 1985. The aim was to provide a confidential, non-hospital environment, with hospital backup nearby. Workers enjoyed a considerable degree of autonomy, were organised as a collective and able to operate from a feminist perspective, although tensions existed 'vis-a-vis the bureaucracy of a large teaching hospital' (Farr 1987). A number of regional services also operate in Western Australia, including Waratah Support Centre, in Bunbury, which is a combined sexual assault and domestic violence service, set up in 1988. It runs the Mooditj Healing Program, which originally provided healing services for Aboriginal women and children but now also supports Aboriginal men. The Eastern Goldfields Sexual Assault Resource Centre is a community-based, government-funded centre, with a voluntary board of management, established in 1993 as part of the NWH Program. New sexual assault resource centres were set up in Port Hedland and Albany using NWH Program money.

In the Northern Territory, a group of women volunteers who saw an urgent need for a feminist service set up the Darwin Counselling Group in 1985 to provide support for women and children who had experienced sexual assault. The women lobbied for funding and, after two years, were successful. Ruby Gaea was opened in 1987 and is still managed by a collective today. Decision making is done on the basis of consensus and women from a variety of ethnicities have served on the collective.

In summary, what has emerged after almost 40 years is a variegated patchwork of government and non-governmental sexual assault services across the States and Territories. All provide services as well as engaging in advocacy and other political activities. Preventive programs are devised to challenge attitudes and beliefs, along with training programs for police, lawyers, doctors, nurses, social workers, youth workers and others. Two services, the NSW Rape Crisis Service and the Canberra Rape Crisis Service, have a continuous history back to the 1970s. Both provide 24-hour, seven-day-a-week telephone or online access to experienced counsellors. In Victoria, the services can be described as 'arm's-length' government services, as each of the 16 CASA has its own community-based board and has been heavily influenced by feminist principles. In Queensland there are 16 services, all of them non-governmental organisations (NGOs). In Tasmania there are three services, one in each of the health regions, and all three are NGOs. All States and Territories provide 24-hour services but not all provide access to specialist counsellors. In some States, after-hours calls are referred to nurses or mental health workers. In other locations, only recent assaults are dealt with at the time of a call, with less recent assaults referred to daytime services.

Direct Activism in Relation to Sexual Violence

Following Italy and the United Kingdom, in Australia the first 'Reclaim the Night' marches were organised in 1978. The aim is to draw attention to sexual violence against women and to protest against the virtual curfew imposed on women because walking on the streets at night can be dangerous.

Direct action has included drawing attention to rape during war. One of the most publicised activities of the early 1980s was women marching on Anzac Day in memory of women who were raped in war. The Sydney Women Against Rape Collective was formed in 1980. In 1981, approximately 300 women joined the end of the Anzac Day march in Canberra, resulting in 65 arrests. The magistrate who heard the case used the language of terrorism and mutiny and sentenced three women to a month in jail for coming within 400 m of the march (Elder 2007:251). The Rape Action Group for Every Woman, established in Perth, was involved in Anzac Day activism in 1983, which resulted in 168 women being arrested when they marched, after having been refused a permit. The emphasis was, nevertheless, on non-violent protest (Grahame and Prichard 1996:111). Reclaim the Night marches are held annually in cities around Australia, as they are overseas. These attempts to decentre the dominant narrative of military heroism were met with outrage in many sections of society and they also sparked controversy and debate within the women's movement about appropriate strategy (Howe 1984:22).

In recent years, Reclaim the Night activism has been partly overshadowed by the more male-oriented White Ribbon Campaign. Initiated by a small group of Canadian men in the early 1990s, it was a response to the massacre of 14 young women in Montreal. The United Nations followed up in 1999, declaring 25 November the International Day for the Elimination of Violence against Women, to be symbolised by the White Ribbon. Generally led by prominent men acting as White Ribbon Ambassadors, the international campaign asks men and boys to speak out and take an oath, swearing never to commit, excuse or remain silent about violence against women.

Conclusion

Members of the women's health movement from a variety of backgrounds worked tirelessly to build an institutional infrastructure that would provide urgently needed services, giving generously of their time and energy and often their own money. Most of the services that were set up are not available elsewhere and are highly valued and strongly sought. The work of the movement has given rise to significant opinion shifts: taboo subjects that were not spoken about in public are now inscribed in government policies and many people now consider that access to appropriate services is a basic right. Moreover, although considered highly unconventional in the early years, separate women's health services now enjoy a level of legitimacy in most jurisdictions.

The network of centres and services across the country provides an institutional base for the movement from which political action in all its forms can more readily be undertaken. Since the 1980s, those women working in women's centres and services, both government and non-government, have constituted a core network of women's health advocates. Surrounded by a growing constellation of funded and unfunded advocacy groups—some tiny, some large—a strong foundation is in place for continuing work.

In keeping with these developments, advocacy work took on a steadier, more predictable character from the 1980s onwards. After the heady days of the 1970s, when direct action was common, new institutional structures, set up in response to the earlier activism, created opportunities for new ways of working. A wider range of avenues through which governments might be approached and policy might be influenced was put in place. These included the channels opened through women's health policy machinery in all jurisdictions and the extensive consultation processes that formed an important part of government inquiries into women's health and aspects of women's health in the 1980s. Inquiries, task forces and advisory bodies created representative roles and movement members were able to serve in the new positions and present a feminist perspective.

The possibility of working effectively through institutionalised structures is, however, strongly influenced by the political orientation of the government in power. Governments with no interest in women's health have held power both nationally and sub-nationally at different times. The commitment and perseverance of movement members has been such, however, that advantage has been taken of political opportunities as they became available. In some cases, such as when Brisbane activists devised a means of having Commonwealth money for their centre channelled through national and State community health associations, women opened up opportunities for themselves. The institutional base that the movement has built for itself is small but strong.

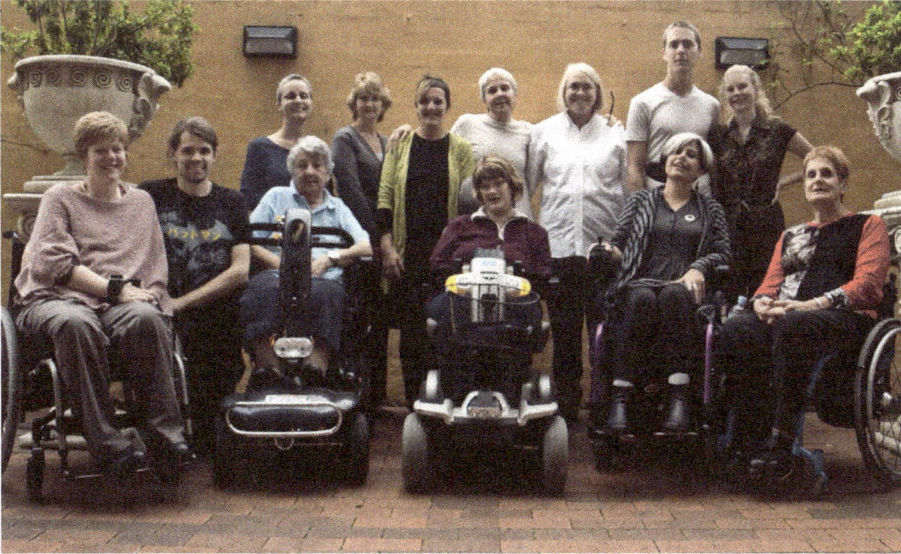

Women with Disabilities Australia (WWDA) Management Committee and staff, Hobart, 2010. Executive Director, Carolyn Frohmader, centre back; Convenor of WWDACT, Sue Salthouse, far right.

Photo: Women with Disabilities Australia

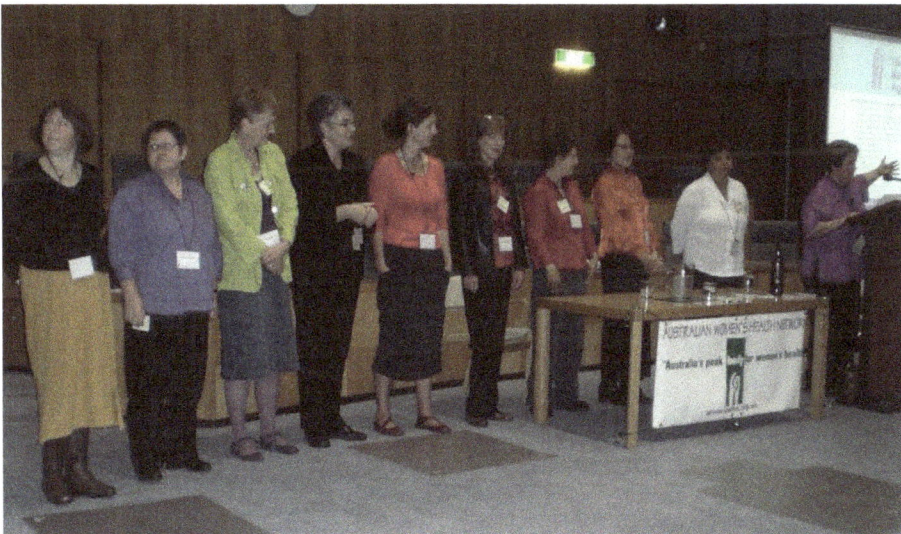

Members of the AWHN management committee at the Women's Health Summit held at Parliament House, Canberra in 2007 to draw attention to the need for a review and update of the National Women's Health Policy. From left: Vicki Lambert (WA), Denele Crozier (NSW), Cobi van der Es (Qld), Marilyn Beaumont (Vic), Marian Hale (Tas), Morven Andrews (Tas), Tracey Wing (Tas), Gwen Gray (ACT) Dot Henry (WA) and Celia Karfpen (SA).

Photo: Gill Wann

123

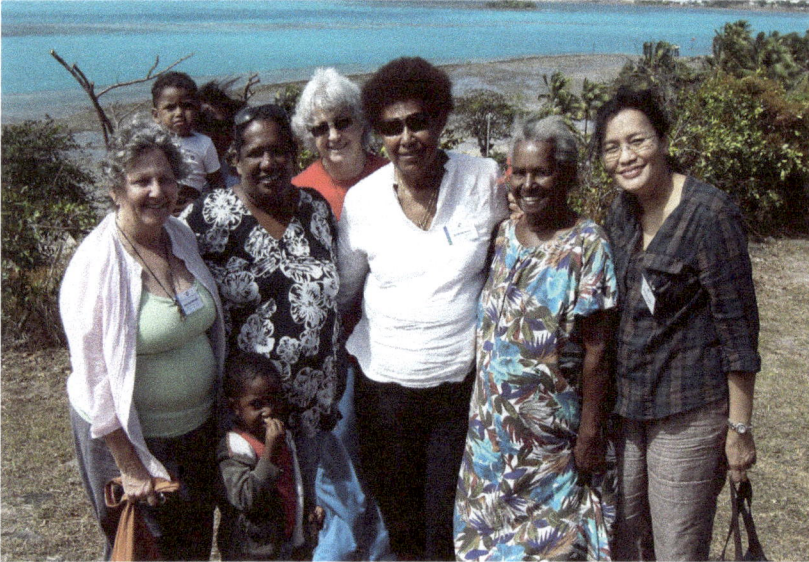

Members of the Queensland Women's Health Network voluntary management committee facilitate Women's Health Forums in the Torres Strait Islands, 2010. Pictured: Dr Betty McLellan, Chair of Queensland Women's Health Network (centre), with local women and children on Hammond Island.

Photo: Queensland Women's Health Network

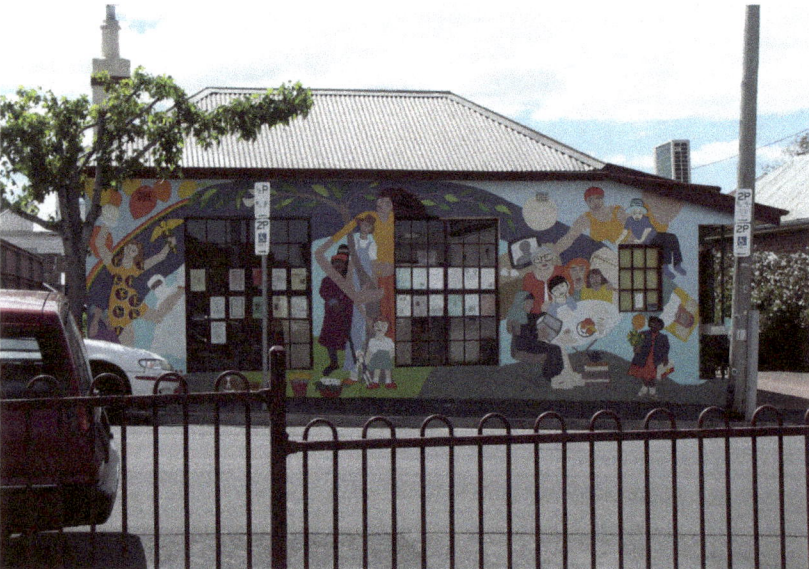

Hobart Women's Health Centre.

Photo: Tracey Wing

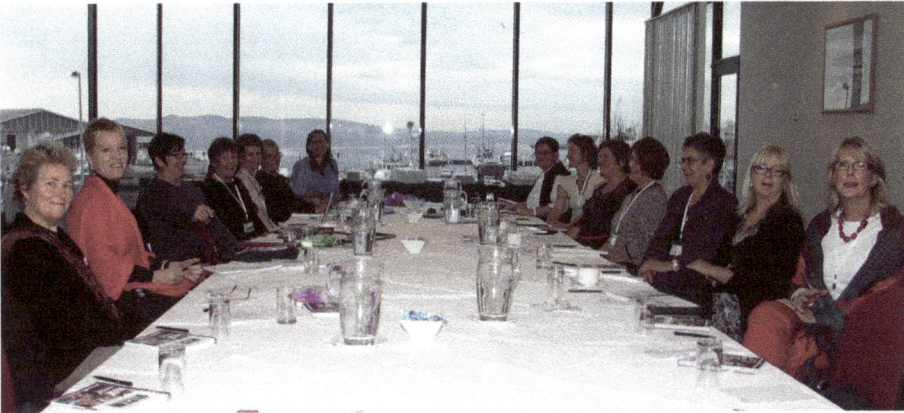

Unaccustomed to gathering in salubrious surroundings: the AWHN management committee plans the Sixth AWHN National Women's Health Conference, Hobart, 2008. From left: Mandy Stringer, Megan Howitt, Kelly Bannister, Cathy Crawford, Maree Hawken, Annie Flint, Marian Edmondson, Daniel Crozier, Patti Kinnersley, Celia Karpfen, Gwen Gray, Marilyn Beaumont, Cheryl Barker, Susie Reid.

Photo: Tracey Wing

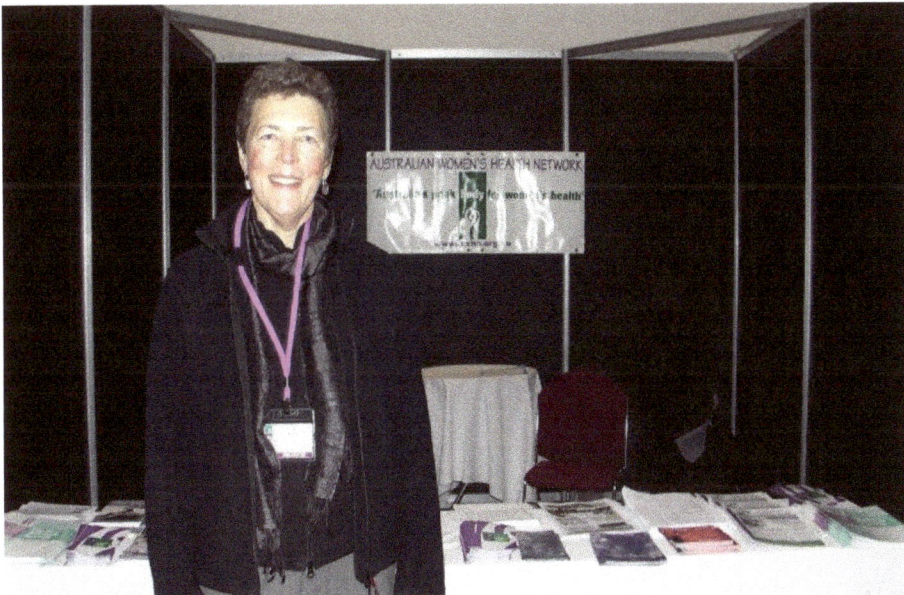

Dorothy Broom, inaugural convener of the ACT Women's Health Network, who has written extensively on the Australian Movement, in front of the AWHN stand at the Sixth National Women's Health Conference. Dorothy had attended all six national conferences, 1975-2010.

Photo: Tracey Wing

4. Group Proliferation and Formal Networks

> There are hundreds of community-based groups of women organised around particular health issues. (Dwyer 1992b:211)

Like the women's movement, which has been described as 'broad-based' and 'somewhat protean', 'loosely made up of many disparate parts' (Dowse 1988:207), the women's health movement has always encompassed groups with different views and priorities. From the 1980s onwards, however, it became even more diverse as groups proliferated and the movement took on the appearance of a variegated array of assemblages, some of them tiny. Most of the new health groups were concerned with specific issues, such as maternity services or breast cancer treatment, but some focused on the health of particular groups, such as women with disabilities or sex workers. Immigrant and refugee women continued to set up their own associations and services, as did Aboriginal women. Not all of the new groups were feminist but most undertook advocacy, provided support and facilitated information sharing and self-help. As new interests and needs emerged, existing centres and services modified their activities in response. In the academy, the proliferation of groups was reflected in feminist theory building, where attention moved from a focus on similarities to the importance of difference and different experiences, whereupon the notion of a 'variety of feminisms' gained currency.

In the 1980s, women in the movement turned their minds to the problem of how to improve the effectiveness of political action. One response was the formation of generalist networks and associations that were established in most jurisdictions, along with a national peak body: the Australian Women's Health Network (AWHN). Specialist associations and peak bodies were also set up in the refuge and sexual assault sectors. Over time, most of the generalist State and Territory networks have been replaced with associations of service providers but AWHN and the Queensland Women's Health Network (QWHN) continue.

Group proliferation can be seen as both a strength and a weakness. The formation of multiple organisations is one of the criteria that has been used to assess the strength of women's movements: the more organisations and the more members, the stronger is the movement (Weldon 2002:80). The creation of so many groups demonstrates the importance that women attach to health and it facilitates the articulation of a much broader range of issues. On the other hand, movement members often no longer know each other, even at the local level. The capacity of the movement to speak with a single voice is reduced. The list below and the following survey of new groups are far from exhaustive.

Selected Specialist Women's Health Groups Formed from the 1970s Onwards

- ACT Incest Centre
- AIDS Council of New South Wales
- Australian Lesbian Medical Association
- Australian Women's Health Nurse Practitioners Association
- Australian Women's Health Nurses Association
- Bonnie Babes Foundation
- Breast Cancer Network of Australia
- Centre for Women's Action on Eating Issues
- Coalition against Depo-Provera
- Coalition of Activist Lesbians
- Collective of Australian Prostitutes
- Continence and Women's Health Physiotherapy
- Council for the Single Mother and Her Child
- DES Action
- Eating Disorders Foundation of Victoria
- Eating Issues Centre
- Endometriosis Association of Victoria
- Female Doctors Group (Gender and Medicine)
- Feminist Therapists Group
- Girl2girl
- Incest Survivors' Association of Western Australia
- Jean Hailes Foundation
- Medea
- Migrant Women against Incest Network
- National Breast Cancer Foundation
- National Council for the Single Mother and Her Child
- National Network against Trafficking in Women
- National Rural Female GP Network Steering Committee
- National Rural Women's Coalition
- Older Women's Network
- Older Women's Network of New South Wales
- Older Women's Wellness Forum
- Pelvic Instability Association of Victoria

- Pink Links
- Polycystic Ovarian Syndrome Alliance
- Polycystic Ovarian Syndrome Association of Australia
- Positive Women
- Post and Antenatal Depression Association
- Post and Antenatal Support and Information Group
- Postnatal Depression Support Association
- Project Respect
- Project without a Name
- Real Rape Law Coalition
- RSI Group Canberra
- Scarlet Alliance
- SIDS Council of Australia
- Stillbirth and Neonatal Death Support
- Sydney Incest Survivors Collective
- Tenosynovitis Association
- Victorian Women with Disabilities Network
- Women against Incest
- Women and Addiction Group
- Women with Disabilities ACT
- Women with Disabilities Australia
- Women's Addiction and Recovery Service
- Women's Healing Centre
- Women's Incest Survivors Network
- Women's RSI Support Team

A Proliferation of Groups

Specialist and single-issue women's health groups had already begun to emerge in the 1970s. One of the early specific concerns was use of the drug diethylstilboestrol (DES). DES Action was initiated by the Union of Australian Women in 1979 as a support and advocacy group for women exposed to synthetic hormones, which can have cancerous and other adverse reproductive side effects for mothers and daughters and possibly sons. Other groups followed in different parts of the country. Initially, pharmaceutical companies, health authorities, doctors and gynaecologists denied that the drug had been used in Australia but, in 1983, after a long campaign, a DES clinic was opened at the Royal Women's

Hospital, Melbourne. Its existence, however, was not publicised and neither doctors nor the Victorian Government knew of its existence. It was eventually privatised (DES Action Australia web site). A coalition against another drug, Depo-Provera, was arranged in Victoria in 1987, after a 10-year campaign by a number of organisations (National Women's Health Centres Newsletter 1988).

Groups began to form around women's mental health issues from the late 1970s onwards, partly in response to reluctance in the mainstream movement to address serious mental health issues. The Feminist Therapists Group began in Adelaide in 1981 to provide mental health care and facilitate the formation of support groups. The Project without a Name was set up in Sydney in 1982, with mental health among its several concerns. The Leichhardt Women's Community Health Centre (LWCHC) collaborated with feminist therapists and others to establish Louisa Lawson House, which was opened in 1983, first to provide support for women in severe emotional crisis and, later, when more public funding became available, to provide emergency accommodation. In 1985, funding was received to operate a women's mental health and therapy centre, including provision of counselling services and group programs. Later, a minor tranquilliser clinic was established to offer education and mental illness prevention programs. Obtaining funding was always a struggle (Shaw and Tilden 1990:94–5).

Meg Smith, one of the original workers at LWCHC, set up a mood-disorder support group in 1982, which grew rapidly. Many similar self-help and support groups were formed, some of which also undertook advocacy, concerned about the poor state of mental health services and the shortcomings of mental health legislation. Other issues were discrimination against people with mental illness and lack of rehabilitation services for people in the recovery stages (Smith n.d.). In the Australian Capital Territory, a group of friends who had experienced mental illness themselves formed a collective in 1984 and opened Medea in 1986 when funding was obtained. Medea was a holistic alternative to the limited mental illness management options that existed in the Territory at the time. Workshops, open to any member of the community, were held three days a week on issues such as anger release, unresolved childhood issues, child sexual abuse, resolving conflict and the like (Australian Women's Health Network 1988:2–4).

Feminists brought incest out of the shadows and publicly identified it as a major, long-term women's health issue. Women against Incest was formed in Sydney in 1983, and worked to attract funding for a community-based centre. Dympna House, Australia's first feminist incest facility, was opened a year later, to undertake counselling, research, training, community education and accommodation provision. Its priorities were the protection of children, the empowerment of women and girls and the creation of a referral network for offenders. Women against Incest continued to work with Dympna House as a policy advice and advocacy group. Originating at Women's Health Care House,

Perth, the Incest Survivors Association of Western Australia was incorporated in 1984. It deals specifically with child sexual abuse and post-traumatic stress disorder (PTSD) in later life, and produced a parenting manual in 2007. The Migrant Women against Incest Network was established in 1986, which broke new ground by conducting public awareness and education programs around this previously taboo issue (Jung 2003:111). The Women's Incest Survivors Network Incorporated (WISN), which still operates, was formed in Sydney in 1992 after the First National Confest for women survivors of incest and child sexual abuse, which was organised by the Sydney Incest Survivors Collective (Martin 2000). Women in the Australian Capital Territory set up an incest centre in the 1990s but it was forced to close when funding was withdrawn by a Liberal Party government.

Recognised as a major women's health issue in the 1980s, eating disorders became a focus for program development work and research. A variety of community-based associations and foundations was established to support sufferers and undertake advocacy. Most were not women specific, which is perhaps surprising given that women are the main sufferers. Only about 10 per cent of the young adults diagnosed are males (Eating Disorders Foundation of Victoria web site). The new organisations provide services for women, of course, and there are one or two that are exclusively for women. Brisbane feminists set up the Centre for Women's Action on Eating Issues in the 1990s, changing its name to the Eating Issues Centre in 2009. It provides services for women on Tuesdays and Thursdays and for men, women, transgender and intersex people during the rest of the week. The centre takes a holistic view and uses the term 'eating issues' in preference to 'eating disorders' to denote a social view rather than a medical, individual pathology perspective (Isis web site).

A number of specialist groups formed around issues related to pregnancy in addition to maternity care reform and pro-choice groups. Postnatal depression (PND), trauma and grief after miscarriage, stillbirth and neonatal death emerged as important women's health issues from the 1980s onwards. The Post and Antenatal Depression Association (PANDA) is a Victorian community-based, self-help organisation formed to provide support, including telephone support, information and referral services, to women and their families. An average of 200 calls per month is received through the helpline. PANDA trains volunteers, undertakes advocacy, supports the establishment of new support groups and offers information, education and training seminars for professionals and community groups. In 2003, it established a network of postnatal depression group facilitators to bring health professionals and facilitators together. In the Australian Capital Territory, the Post and Antenatal Depression Support and Information group (PANDSI) and, in Perth, the Postnatal Depression Support Association (PNDSA) provide a similar set of services. Groups that formed in the 1980s around miscarriage, stillbirth and neonatal death include Stillbirth and Neonatal Death Support (SANDS Australia), which has branches in several jurisdictions, and the National Sudden Infant Death Syndrome (SIDS) Council of Australia, with branches in all jurisdictions and the Hunter region of New South Wales. The Bonnie Babes Foundation, established in 1994, provides a range of services, including counselling, in cases of infertility, miscarriage, stillbirth, pregnancy loss, neonatal loss and premature birth.

Groups also sprang up around the 'new' malady repetitive strain injury (RSI) in the 1970s and 1980s. The problem was new only in the sense of having been recently brought to public attention: reports of its occurrence had appeared in journals for 100 years. The Workers Health Centre in Lidcombe, Sydney, ran support groups from 1979 onwards. Victorian women set up the Women's Repetitive Injury Support Team (WRIST) in 1982. In the same year, Adelaide women set up RSI Campaign and in 1984 the Tenosynovitis Association was formed in Sydney and the RSI Support Group in Canberra. Most groups provided information in a number of languages. Doctors at Adelaide Women's Community Health Centre discovered that women prefer support groups rather than individual counselling because it reassures them to know they are not alone. Moreover, groups were found to be an efficient way of disseminating information (Brown et al. 1986).

The advent of HIV/AIDS was the stimulus for the formation of yet another set of issue-specific groups when women felt that their concerns were not being fully recognised. By 1993, there were groups in most major cities providing support and information and conducting advocacy. Positive Women was established in Victoria in 1988, for example. The organisation obtained funding to develop a resource kit for women with HIV/AIDS and for service providers. It was also funded to facilitate support group formation and to develop a sense of community. Women had expressed a strong need to meet other HIV/AIDS-positive women to break down the sense of isolation they felt. To help meet these needs, a book and a video were produced.

There is a women's health sub-movement around alcohol and other drugs but it has always been small. Most community-based associations and public agencies are mixed-sex services, and, in the early days, in particular, the focus was on the needs of men. High relapse rates were attributed to the inability of services to meet women's needs. In 1989, an Australia-wide survey showed that there were no arrangements in place in 44 per cent of agencies to meet the needs of women with children. There were even fewer services for women with special needs, such as migrant women, Aboriginal women and lesbians (Crawford and Elliott 1994:143–53). The Royal Women's Hospital, Melbourne, however, does provide a voluntary, State-wide women's alcohol and drug service for pregnant women with ongoing drug and alcohol issues, along with professional support and education programs.

Otherwise, nearly all women-specific drug and alcohol programs originated in women's health centres. Most of the larger women's health centres, such as Leichhardt, employ drug and alcohol workers. The Women and Addiction Group associated with the Leichhardt centre was formed in 1981. Women's Health and Family Services (formerly Women's Health Care House), Perth, offers a comprehensive set of services for women and those living with women who are experiencing drug and alcohol problems. As well as a general program, separate services have been fashioned for immigrant and refugee women, and for pregnant and parenting women and their families, and the Singing Up Project has been created for Aboriginal women and their families.

ACT initiatives include the establishment in 1985 of the feminist Women's Addiction Recovery Service (WARS) by the Toora Single Wimmin's collective. WARS was a community-based information, referral, education, training and counselling service for women and children; however, the service had only one paid worker and so could not provide effective support for more than a few individual clients. It therefore set about developing a broader approach, which included a critique of existing services. It attempted to counter negative attitudes towards drug-dependent women, redefined women's dependence and developed new models to promote positive change. Experience showed that it is impossible to separate women's experience of drug dependence from the conditions of their everyday lives, including past and present abuse, levels of self-esteem and motherhood roles (Morgain 1994). Focusing on both licit (pharmaceuticals, alcohol) and illicit drugs, a policy of resourcing communities to respond to their own needs and experiences was developed.

The ACT Women's Health Network, of which more below, established a longstanding working group on alcohol and other drugs. One issue of concern was the provision of safe injecting equipment for the local remand centre. It successfully lobbied for a halfway house, opened in 1994, where women recovering from addiction could be with their children.

The availability of information about breast cancer and its treatment became a concern in the 1980s when survivors began to form support, advocacy and exercise groups around the country. The Breast Cancer Network of Australia (BCNA) was established in 1998, after public meetings in each State and Territory had brought women together to discuss their concerns. The network is supported by well-known people such as Olympian Raelene Boyle, a breast cancer survivor, and by donors with significant capacity, such as Baker's Delight. After only two years, the organisation had 5100 members. At the time of writing, BCNA has

33 000 individual members and 200 member groups. It aims to ensure that all women diagnosed with breast cancer receive the best information, treatment, care and support available. In the first decade, it conducted public awareness campaigns, such as setting up (pink) 'Fields of Women' in various locations, and lobbied extensively on breast cancer treatment issues. It has established a free telephone information service, produces brochures and publishes a newsletter four times a year (Breast Cancer Network of Australia web site). The non-profit National Breast Cancer Foundation, which gathers support from both the corporate and the community sectors, was formed in 1994 to raise money for breast cancer research. In the Australian Capital Territory, Pink Links has been formed as a support group for younger women with breast cancer. These groups have lobbied successfully for improvements in treatment, gaining, among other things, the provision of more information, more supportive care and, in 2001, the establishment of a lymphoedema research network (Redman et al. 2003).

New groups continued to form around violence against women, especially in response to notorious statements by members of the judiciary, mentioned above. For example, the Justice for Women Action Collective was formed at Melbourne University in response to comments by Justices Bollen and Bland in 1993. About the same time, the Victorian Police Service conducted a sexual assault phone in, called Operation Pegasus, which met with an overwhelming response. Ten extra phone lines had to be installed to cope with calls and the police who took the calls are reported to have wept openly. Another Victorian group, the Real Rape Law Coalition, was active in the 1990s, along with the Brisbane Rape Crisis Centre, which partnered with the Women's Legal Service, the Domestic Violence Resource Centre and the Brisbane Women's Health Centre to produce a critique of Queensland's Criminal Code, entitled *Rougher Than Usual Handling*: *Women in the criminal justice system* (Fredericks 1993).

A variety of other issue-specific groups, too numerous to list, includes the Women's Healing Centre, formed in Sydney in the early 1980s, which, like dozens of others, was concerned with promoting alternative therapies, including relaxation, meditation, acupuncture and herbal remedies. Menopause-awareness groups sprang up in many places and the self-help Endometriosis Association was formed in Victoria in 1984, following calls to the Women's Health Resource Collective from more than 200 women seeking information. The Polycystic Ovary Association of Australia began in 1998 as an information-dissemination, awareness-raising and support group. In 2008 it established an alliance with the Jean Hailes Foundation and the Robinson Institute and in 2009 received Commonwealth funding support. The alliance lobbied for the development of a set of evidence-based guidelines for the assessment and management of polycystic ovarian syndrome, which was released in 2011. The Pelvic Instability Association was formed in Victoria in 2003. The Australian Physiotherapy

Association set up a subgroup, Continence and Women's Health Physio, which provides information and resources about back and pelvic-floor health during pregnancy. A national e-newsletter is produced four times a year and one of the aims is to provide resources for rural and remote-area physiotherapists who do not have access to specialist services (Australian Physiotherapy Association web site).

As well as forming around specific health issues, women organised to promote the health of particular groups. The need for a specific focus on women prompted the formation of Women with Disabilities Australia (WWDA) as a national peak body in 1995. Founding women felt that their issues were not getting a full hearing either in the disability sector or in the women's health movement. The organisation evolved from a women's network within Disabled Peoples International Australia (DPIA), where it had operated as an unfunded subgroup for some years. WWDA is managed by women with disabilities and has a strong human rights focus. A large part of its work concentrates on health issues, including activism around enforced sterilisation, the facilitation of access to appropriate hospital and medical services and violence and sexual assault issues. Affiliated groups include the Victorian Women with Disabilities Network and an ACT group formed in 1995. Women with Disabilities ACT (WWDACT) is a feminist collective that undertakes systematic advocacy on the impact of disability across all areas. It was funded by Disability ACT in 2011, allowing it to employ two part-time workers who are co-located with the local women's health centre, the Women's Centre for Health Matters.

Health is a priority for many same-sex-attracted women who have experienced having their sexuality overlooked in medical encounters. Homophobia, social isolation and discrimination often lead to mental and physical health conditions, which can result in other problems, such as substance misuse.[1] Lesbians might also have special needs, such as those arising from a disability, for example (Women's Health in the North 2009:6). While some Australian lesbians thought that the women's health movement was not fully cognisant of their issues, they have, on the whole, been far less critical of it than their North American sisters, probably because so many have been involved as members. Sylvia Azzopardi (quoted in Robertson n.d.:Ch. 19) notes the importance of this contribution, which resulted in many women's health centres developing specialised services.

As well as working with multipurpose women's health groups, lesbians have also formed separate groups. In 1999, the Australian Lesbian Medical Association (ALMA) was founded to offer support and mentoring for lesbian doctors, medical students and their partners. It funds lesbian health research, lobbies to have lesbian health included in medical curricula and fosters links with like-

---

1 For an excellent review of health problems faced by sexual-minority women, see McNair (2003, 2009).

minded organisations. The voluntary committee runs an annual conference and produces a newsletter. The Coalition of Activist Lesbians (COAL)[2] is an advocacy and lobbying association formed in 1994 to campaign for an end to discrimination. It produced a major paper on lesbian health issues in 1997 (Myers and Lavender 1997) along with research papers on violence against lesbians, 'lesbophobia' and lesbian domestic violence. Girl2girl is a web site providing information for lesbians about safe sex and sexually transmitted infections. The AIDS Council of New South Wales (ACON) is a community-based Sydney group with 150 staff members and 700 volunteers that operates extensive programs to promote the health and wellbeing of the gay, lesbian, bisexual and transgender (GLBT) community and men and women with HIV. In Victoria, action by the gay and lesbian communities led to the introduction of the Gay and Lesbian Health Action Plan, announced by the Minister for Health in 2003. As part of the plan, a health resource unit was established for gay, lesbian, bisexual, transgender and intersex Victorians, which is jointly managed by the Australian Research Centre in Sex, Health and Society, the Victorian AIDS Council/Gay Men's Health Centre and Women's Health Victoria (WHV).

Many generalist women's groups see health as one of their major concerns. Said to be the first of its kind in the world, the Council for the Single Mother and Her Child was formed in 1969 by a group of Victorian single and relinquishing mothers who had experienced prejudice and discrimination. From the beginning, the group worked within a self-help framework and its twin objectives were to support single mothers and at the same time work for social change and legal reform. The council aims to change practices and laws that have an adverse effect on women's health. Early concerns were social and institutional pressures to relinquish babies for adoption, refusal of the right for mothers to see babies prior to adoption and adoption processes that were shrouded in secrecy. There was no reliable income support for single mothers at the time and such special benefits as might be available were discretionary. 'Illegitimate' children and their mothers were stigmatised and legally discriminated against in a variety of ways. Similar organisations were set up in other States soon afterwards and the National Council was established in 1973. The organisation has successfully fought for and achieved a range of important reforms.

Health is a central concern for many immigrant women's organisations such as the Association of Non-English Speaking Background (NESB)[3] Women of Queensland, formed in the early 1990s as a lobby group. The YWCA has advocated and worked for women's health on its own and in collaboration

---

2   There is a group with the same name in the United States.
3   'Non-English-speaking background', a term that appeared to be widely accepted in the 1980s and 1990s, has largely fallen into disuse. It is sometimes replaced with 'culturally and linguistically diverse' (CALD), or, more simply, immigrant and refugee women.

with women's health groups over many years. Older Women's Network (OWN) groups have been established across Australia, including an Australian peak body, beginning with a group formed in New South Wales in 1985. Health has always been a major issue for OWN members. Betty Johnson, the first Convenor of OWN Australia, who regularly collaborates with AWHN and other women's groups, was appointed an Officer of the General Division of the Order of Australia for her advocacy on aged care and health care. She serves on numerous health committees in New South Wales.

OWN has developed a positive approach to older women's wellbeing, based on the social perspective. Women are encouraged to define their own needs and to design and implement programs that will meet those needs. With public funding support from health departments, local councils and other places, OWN New South Wales supports groups that wish to establish wellness centres. The Older Women's Wellness Forum in 1999 resulted from collaboration between OWN New South Wales, the Benevolent Society and the Departments of Health, Women, Sport and Recreation and Ageing and Disability. There are currently 14 regional groups in New South Wales, which aim to provide an inclusive, welcoming, drop-in environment for women from a diversity of cultures. At the time of writing, there are OWN Wellness Centres in The Rocks, Bankstown, Chatswood, Sutherland and in Coniston, in the Illawarra area.

Health is a major concern for women living in rural and remote areas where all services are in short supply. Some areas have access only to the Royal Flying Doctor Service and perhaps a clinic staffed by a remote-area nurse and an occasional doctor on a flying visit. Such circumstances reduce the likelihood of regular screening, for example, so it is not surprising that women in the bush have higher morbidity rates from cervical cancer. Domestic violence is a serious concern, partly because support services are few and partly because disclosure can create socially difficult situations. Problems of isolation from family and friends can be exacerbated because rural and remote mental health services are under resourced (National Rural Women's Coalition 2008; Whittle and Williams 2001).

A number of organisations have been established to promote rural health. While only a few are women specific, all have women members. The National Rural Health Alliance is a mixed-sex, Commonwealth-funded coalition, with 27 member organisations. It was set up in the early 1990s as an advocacy and information-providing agency. The Rural Doctors Association of Australia was formed in 1991 and has a women's special-interest group, the Female Doctors Group (Gender and Medicine), which keeps the organisation abreast of current research. In 1992, a group of rural women in Victoria met to discuss the possibility of a State-wide organisation, which resulted in the formation of Australian Women in Agriculture the following year. The National Rural

Women's Coalition, whose member organisations are mostly mixed-sex groups, is one of the six national women's alliances funded by the Department of Families, Housing, Community Services and Indigenous Affairs (FaHCSIA). It currently focuses on women's health issues, including family violence. On the basis of extensive consultations, it produced a report on rural health infrastructure in 2008. The National Rural Female GP Network Steering Committee has also been formed for the purpose of encouraging other organisations to value and support female general practitioners.

Women set up groups in the 1980s to agitate for the rights, including the health rights, of sex workers, with policy reform as a major goal. The Collective of Australian Prostitutes was formed in Sydney in 1983, concerned with legal rights, policing and health issues. In 1989, Scarlet Alliance was established as the national body for State and Territory sex-worker associations with the aim of achieving optimal OHS and legislative provisions (Scarlet Alliance web site). One of the key aims of sex-worker organisations is to develop effective responses to HIV. In 1998, a non-profit community-based organisation, Project Respect, was formed to support women in the sex industry, including women trafficked to Australia, and to prevent exploitation and enslavement. The organisation conducts outreach support and advocacy work in relation to law and policy reform. The National Network against Trafficking in Women has also been formed.

Unlike their Canadian counterparts, Australian nursing organisations have not mobilised strongly around access and equity issues in health, although a couple of 'Keep Medicare Healthy' campaigns were run in the 1980s. Nurses have, however, been active in relation to industrial issues, including remuneration, occupational health and conditions of work. From the 1970s onwards, several groups promoted the transfer of nursing education to the tertiary sector. An extended strike over inadequate staffing levels and pay was staged by Victorian nurses in 1986, following direct action in other jurisdictions (Ross 1987). OHS issues have been a major concern for the Australian Nurses Federation (ANF). The Australian Women's Health Nurse Practitioner Association was formed in 1988, first in New South Wales, where the first women's health nurse practitioners were trained. Its name was changed to the Australian Women's Health Nurse Association in 1999—a peak body for women's health nurses throughout Australia. The Community Health Nurses Association was formed in Victoria and groups have been active on environmental health issues. A 'lead in the soil' campaign, for example, was conducted in Port Pirie, South Australia, a lead-smelting town where, among other problems, citizens had high blood-lead levels.

A different type of women's health organisation is the non-profit Jean Hailes Foundation, established in Victoria in 1992, in honour of the female doctor after whom it is named. The foundation is Commonwealth funded and focuses on research and education. Meanwhile, partly in response to the fragmentation that came with the movement's expansion, women decided to established specialist advocacy groups, generally called networks, in the mid-1980s.

Generalist Women's Health Networks

Networking is a way of working that has been used extensively by women's groups in Australia and overseas. It has been found to be an effective way of problem solving, exchanging views and information, building confidence, morale and professionalism, sharing resources and improving skills. Networks are also used to increase visibility, to access sponsors and mentors, to build alliances with like-minded organisations and engage in collaborative projects (Townsend 1994:12–13).

In the 1980s and 1990s, the women's health movement established formal networks with the aims of strengthening capacity and creating advocacy arms that were independent of funded centres and services. During unfavourable political times, established agencies were in danger of becoming 'activists on a leash'. In Victoria under the Kennett Government, for example, the threat of being de-funded had a 'gagging effect' on women's health services and tended to subdue criticism of policy changes that were detrimental to the community sector (Horsley 1994:10). Independent networks, it was therefore thought, would allow women to speak out strongly. Moreover, women's voices would be more unified and advocacy work could be planned. Intelligence about community perspectives was to be gained through the centres and services that are in daily contact with clients and other community agencies. At its best, this set of arrangements would work as a type of standing consultation process, which, under the right conditions, could feed ideas into policy on a regular basis. In addition to service providers, networks were open to all women who agreed with the aims and objectives.

Establishing a National Women's Health Network

In the wake of momentum generated by the successful 1985 Adelaide women's health conference and the subsequent announcement by the Prime Minister that a national women's health policy would be developed, the Australian

Women's Health Network (AWHN)[4] was formed by women attending the inaugural Community Health Association Conference in September 1986. About 50 women from different States and Territories, mindful of the need for a feminist perspective to be represented in general health policy debates, agreed to form a national network. The new association was announced at the final conference plenary session, attended by Commonwealth Health Minister, Neal Blewett, and was greeted with a spontaneous ovation. Yoland Wadsworth, a sociologist, was the first convenor. Immediate expressions of interest and offers of assistance came from officers of the Commonwealth Health Department (Abbs 1994; National Women's Health Centres Newsletter 1987a).

Jude Abbs, long-standing women's health activist, became interim national convener in 1987. She and the State and Territory representatives of the new organisation generated interest across the country, assisted by a Commonwealth Women's Health Development Program Grant. A funding submission for a secretariat was written to the Commonwealth setting out the long-term goals, proposed activities and a provisional organisational structure (Abbs 1987). Links were established with the Consumers Health Forum and maintained with the Australian Community Health Association. AWHN gained a place on the newly formed Australian Health Ministers Advisory Council (AHMAC) Subcommittee on Women and Health, a position that served the movement well (Abbs 1994:4– 5). It allowed women's views to be fed into policy processes while facilitating the dissemination of information about policy developments within government to the wider movement.

The first national meeting of AWHN was funded by the Commonwealth Department of Health and took place in the Board Room of the Royal Women's Hospital, Melbourne, in October 1987. Women worked strenuously for two days to develop a set of aims and objectives and work out a structure. It was decided the organisation would be feminist, with as broad a base as possible. The main purpose was 'to present a well-articulated set of demands to Commonwealth and State Governments' (Donovan 1987:9). Liza Newby, who headed the consultation team for the first NWHP, attended, outlining the main issues that would be canvassed in a forthcoming discussion paper. Participants reported on the state of play in each jurisdiction, which varied considerably from place to place. At the time, it was expected that AWHN would soon receive funding. The plan was to become incorporated and 'advertise for a national coordinator as soon as possible' (Donovan 1987:9). In the event, AWHN was to wait 25 years for the funds to employ a coordinator.

At the same time, enthusiasm for connection prompted women's health centres to produce a newsletter—a process assisted by Senator Patricia Giles, Labor

---

4   It was at first called the National Women's Health Association; the name was not settled for a year.

Senator for Western Australia, a founder of WEL and women's health activist. 'At last! A thousand welcomes, sisters; we've needed you so much', wrote the Hunter Region Working Women's Centre in a letter to the editor of the first issue. Issue 2 came out in October and flagged that the newsletter might become a vehicle for the distribution of information from AWHN, as the network became further established (National Women's Health Centres Newsletter 1987b). And so it was. The decision was taken to rename the newsletter and to make its receipt an AWHN membership benefit. Issue 4, produced in April 1988, became the first *Australian Women's Health Network Newsletter*. Two further newsletters were produced before production ceased in early 1989. The 1987 funding application had not succeeded. AWHN continued to participate in the work of the AHMAC Subcommittee on Women and Health and that of the Consumers Health Forum but, by 1990, it had not been incorporated, it no longer communicated with members and was effectively in recess.

Three years later, ACTWHN, whose financial management system consisted of collecting money in a polystyrene cup to cover meeting expenses, held a women's health festival outside Old Parliament House. The festival, organised by a committee led by Jenny Lyons, made a profit! With a few hundred dollars to spend, members decided to pay someone to write a funding application for AWHN. At the time, Leanne Webster, the first coordinator of the Canberra Women's Health Centre, was on maternity leave and was available to do the work. The 1993 application to the Commonwealth Department of Health was successful and AWHN received seed funding of $61 180.

The Interim Steering Committee of ACTWHN members—Convenor, Manoa Renwick, Dorothy Broom, Jenny Lyons and Gwen Gray—was formed. A project officer, Julie McCarron Benson, was employed and the first (and so far the only) AWHN office was established in Kingston, ACT, complete with office equipment, including a computer and a photocopier. A teleconference of State network representatives was called and arrangements made for a two-day face-to-face meeting in February 1994. Representatives from all jurisdictions attended, the aims and objectives were clarified and the structure and constitution agreed. AWHN was incorporated in the Australian Capital Territory on 3 March 1994. During the funded 12 months, strong communication channels were established across the country, not only with AWHN members but also with like-minded organisations. The 1994 submission for continued funding, however, was not successful. The photocopier was sold, the national office disbanded and newsletter production once again ceased.

During the years until the end of 1998, the position of convenor remained in the Australian Capital Territory, with Gwen Gray filling the position. AWHN worked closely with QWHN members, especially with Carol Low and Marybeth Sarran, who took the role of secretary for several years. These were frustrating years of repeated, unsuccessful funding submissions. Communicating with members was difficult, with fax the main method. Telephone calls and teleconferences were expensive and mostly outside the capacity of the tiny budget. Non-governmental sources of funding, such as foundations, were explored without success. In 1994, AWHN was told that the Commonwealth Department of Health would no longer provide operational funding. Henceforth, one-off project grants would be all that were available—a development influenced by encroaching neo-liberal ideas. A funding application was made to the National Agenda for Women Grants Program in 1995, but it, too, failed. In 1996, however, AWHN was chosen by the Office of the Status of Women (OSW) to be one of four national organisations to be assisted by a consultancy firm to develop strategic and business plans. The plans were duly developed but could not be used effectively by an organisation that could scarcely afford a teleconference.

Undaunted, the 1996 AWHN AGM agreed that efforts to gain funding should be the top priority in the next year. At the time, the network was fortunate to have Carolyn Frohmader[5] to assist with submission writing and other AWHN work. An unsuccessful application was made to the Rural Health Education Support and Training Grants Program 'to improve access to women's health information, education, training and support in rural and remote areas'. In early 1997, office-holders met once more with officials in the Commonwealth Department of Health and Family Services to consider possibilities. Extensive discussions took place about an expanded role for AWHN, the outcome of which was another major funding submission. After a protracted process, that application, too, was eventually rejected.[6] In June 1997, a repeat application to OSW for operational funding resulted in a grant of $25 000. The organisation was able to develop a web site, arrange for information and membership pamphlets to be printed, pay for a post office box, hold teleconferences and continue to research and write submissions to a range of grant programs and funding bodies. A third submission to OSW for the 1998–99 year was turned down.

At the end of 1998, Helen Keleher was elected convenor and the centre of gravity shifted to Victoria until 2005. During that period, the enormous job of organising two successful national women's health conferences, one in Adelaide and the other in Melbourne, was undertaken. Small profits from the conferences allowed the web site to be upgraded and maintained and regular newsletters produced. In 1995, the position of convenor moved to South Australia under Anne-Marie Hayes and, subsequently, Celia Karpfen. As the costs of communication fell, it became possible to hold regular teleconferences and was easier to have office-

---

5   Carolyn Frohmader has been Executive Director of Women with Disabilities Australia (WWDA) since the second half of the 1990s.
6   Rumours had it that when the proposal came to the notice of staff in the office of the Minister for Health, it was swiftly conveyed to the 'no' tray.

bearers located far from each other. In 2008, the position of convenor moved back to the Australian Capital Territory, with the convenor, program convenor, secretary and treasurer of the 2010 Sixth AWHN National Women's Health Conference Organising Committee all living in different States.

Since incorporation in 1994, AWHN has financed operations from membership fees, small conference profits and a handful of small project grants. It has responded to relevant political issues as they emerge, as resources allow. It has participated in 'Defend Medicare' and right-to-choose/reproductive rights campaigns. In 2002, it was one of seven original members of the National Medicare Alliance—a group that met frequently by teleconference and lobbied to try to persuade the Commonwealth to preserve the universality of Medicare, on the grounds that universal access to hospital and medical services is essential for women's health. It is a member of the Australian Health Care Reform Alliance, formed in 2003, a coalition of some 53 health organisations and associations advocating structural health reform.

AWHN has written submissions to government commissions and inquiries. It has written letters and otherwise lobbied on a range of issues, providing support for State women's health services when they seemed to be under threat. It was instrumental in warding off a Commonwealth attempt to discontinue its funding for women's health centres through the Public Health Funding Outcome Agreements (PHOFAs) in 2004. It campaigned for an update of the first NWHP from 1995 onwards and influenced the Labor Party's commitment to develop a second national women's health policy, launched in 2010. It has increased its membership, communicates with them weekly, maintains a web site and produces regular newsletters. Successful national women's health conferences have been staged every five years since 1995, when the Third National Women's Conference was organised jointly by ACTWHN and WEL ACT. Generous Commonwealth subsidisation facilitated the participation of more than 160 Aboriginal women in the 1995 conference, which laid the foundation for the later development of an Aboriginal women's subgroup, the AWHN Talking Circle, of which more below.

Between 2007 and 2011, efforts to secure operational funding were stepped up. The matter was discussed with relevant departmental officers and ministerial staff. Applications were written variously to the Women's Development Grants Program of the Commonwealth Office for Women, the Department of Health and Ageing and to the office of Health Minister, Nicola Roxon. AWHN's submission to the new NWHP stressed the need for funding support if the organisation was to be able to represent its membership and provide good policy advice to the Commonwealth. In 2009, on the basis that it was already an alliance with 64 organisational members at that time, AWHN applied to become one of the six National Women's Alliances funded by FaHCSIA. In a review of the alliances the previous year, there had been strong support for a national alliance focusing on women's health. That application was also unsuccessful. Quite unexpectedly, however, in September 2011, Minister Roxon endorsed a proposal that AWHN had put to her office several months earlier and the organisation received secretariat funding for 2011-2012 from the Community Sector Support Scheme. At the time of writing, negotiations are taking place about the details of the contract with officers from the Department of Health and Ageing.

State and Territory Networks

The first general State and Territory-based networks were formed in the mid-1980s, as branches of the newly formed national network. Formal networks operated in every State and Territory by 1988, most focusing on lobbying for the development of sub-national women's health policies and plans and the establishment of more women's health services, especially women's health centres. The Victorian network held bimonthly meetings and produced a bimonthly newsletter, named *Hot Goss*, while the New South Wales network aimed to link a large number of informal networks that had already been established (Community Development in Health 1988:3–12). Several of the early sub-national networks did not survive as the level of voluntary contribution needed to keep them going was too heavy. Others fell into abeyance and were revived from time to time.

Among the earliest and most active was the ACTWHN, which began with informal meetings, followed by the establishment of a formal network in 1986, at much the same time that AWHN was formed. It held well-attended monthly meetings and carried out advocacy work for more than a decade. At the height of its strength in the early 1990s, a number of standing working groups managed their own meetings and their own agendas. The working parties included those on reproductive technology, the health centre working party, alcohol and drugs, information and resources, alternative therapies, the national women's health policy, assertiveness/self-esteem and a party working party (planning an end-of-year celebration).

In 1991 and 1992, ACTWHN members, especially Dorothy Broom and the staff of the Canberra Women's Health Centre, which was still only in the planning stages, were distracted by a challenge to the legality of the centre. Indeed, the case, which was 'full of outrages, ironies and contradictions' (Broom 1992:62), challenged the legality of all separate women's health centres, including those being established under the NWH Program. Three men, led by a Canberra doctor, claimed that the centre breached the *Sex Discrimination Act* because it excluded men from taxpayer-funded services. The case involved much that was abhorrent. During the hearings, women were asked to provide evidence that the women's health movement was not 'special pleading by a lunatic fringe' and that women's needs were real rather than merely perceived by women themselves. The reality and integrity of the claims that the women's health movement had made over the previous 20 years were 'distorted, demeaned and discarded' (Broom 1992:63–4). In the event, the President of the Human Rights and Equal Opportunity Commission, Sir Roland Wilson, decided that it is not unlawful under the provisions of the Act to ensure that persons of a particular sex have equal opportunities with other persons. He argued that because women are disadvantaged, measures that promote equal opportunity between women and men in the health field are lawful. Mounting a defence, however, which included a not inconsiderable nationwide fundraising effort, was extremely stressful and time consuming for the women involved.

Reviewing operations in May 1994, a meeting of ACTWHN listed among its achievements the establishment of the Canberra Women's Health Centre, a birthing centre and a halfway house for women with alcohol and other drug problems. It had organised the incorporation of AWHN, provided support for key defendants in the Canberra Women's Health Centre case, contributed to surrogacy legislation, influenced alcohol and drug policy and participated in the consultation processes for the NWHP. It had lobbied for the establishment of an abortion service, which was opened the same year by Sexual Health and Family Planning ACT, and lobbied against the Hawke Government's 'New Federalism'. As mentioned, it had jointly with ACTWEL organised the 1995 AWHN National Women's Health Conference. This event was so popular that women had to be turned away after 760 registrations were received because of the capacity of the venue.

The AWHN Top End Branch, NT, was established in 1987, at the prompting of Pip Duncan, a member of the Central Australian Aboriginal Congress (CAAC) who had heard about AWHN. At first energy was low because women were already overwhelmed with meetings in a small jurisdiction (the saying was that the same five women often attended the same five meetings). Enthusiasm was stimulated, however, by the news that there was to be a national women's health policy, and regular monthly meetings soon became the pattern. The first major project was to plan a women's health conference. An Alice Springs branch was formed and the two groups kept in touch by exchanging minutes of meetings. Both supported the establishment of the Alukura Birthing Centre (Australian Women's Health Network 1988:8–9). In April 1989, the first AWHN women's health conference was held in Darwin and was well attended by both Aboriginal and non-Aboriginal women.

The Queensland Women's Health Network (QWHN), the most enduring of the sub-national bodies, was formed at a public meeting in 1986, after which volunteers worked at home to progress establishment. A State-wide survey led to a publication, *The Health Needs of Queensland Women*. Without funds, the network went into abeyance but was revived when the State Government changed and the NWHP was launched in 1989. Funding submissions were written and the first grant of $21 000 was received from Queensland Health in 1993 (QWHN 1995).

Once funded, the network was able to produce communication bulletins, organise planning days and teleconferences, link groups in Brisbane with regional centres, gather and disseminate information and increase its membership. The management group met monthly by teleconference and a members' gathering was held every three months (QWHN 1995). The network carried out advocacy in relation to the implementation of the NWH Program in Queensland and, later, worked with Queensland Health's Women's Health Policy Unit. A longstanding tradition is the organisation of regional women's health forums (QWHN 2003). A linked rural women's health network operated for a time, as did local network groups that worked with regional health authorities.

Queensland is currently the only jurisdiction with both a formal Women's Health Network and a providers' alliance. In 2009, when funding insecurity was restricting the work of women's health centres, the coordinators gathered in Gladstone to share ideas and discuss strategies. From the meeting, the Women's Health Services Alliance was formed. QWHN provides secretariat services, acts as a contact point, assists with communication and correspondence and provides a direct link with AWHN (QWHN 2009:7).

The South Australian Women's Health Network was formed in the mid-1980s and survived into the 1990s. It received funding support for two years from the NWH Program, which enabled it to employ a part-time worker, and was responsible, with Adelaide Women's Community Health Centre, for the newsletter *Stating Women's Health*. Country women's health service providers joined, along with women from the community health movement. Members served on a number of key women's health committees. An application to the South Australian Government for funding for a permanent part-time executive officer, which had been promised at one time, was unsuccessful.

After a recess, a women's health network was re-established in Tasmania in the mid-1990s and a branch was formed in the north of the State in 1997. A web site was developed that carried a comprehensive range of health information for clients and providers. The Women's Health Forum was staged in Launceston in 2002, along with a hysterectomy awareness forum. In the same year, a domestic violence symposium was organised in Hobart. Neither branch, however, has met since 2006. The Independent Women's Organisations of Tasmania (IWOT), which represented women's services, including shelters, support and information services, was a peak body formed by the Hobart Women's Health Centre and others, to provide a stronger voice when negotiating with government. It, too, lost momentum and has not met since 2006; however, the Women's Emergency Service Providers (WESP) group continues to meet.

Several network groups were formed in Victoria at different times, including Women in Health around Melbourne (WHAM) and the Women's Services Coalition, developed with the assistance of the Victorian Council of Social Services in 1991. The coalition's membership included refuges, housing services, domestic violence and rape crisis centres, drug and alcohol and women's information services. It was disbanded because the broad-based membership could not agree on principles and objectives. According to one participant, a 'heavy, restrictive feminism' was embraced by some members but not others.

After a period of dormancy, the Victorian network reactivated in 1998 in response to interest from women who were not service providers but wanted to participate in the movement. It was incorporated the following year. It aimed to enhance communication about women's health, create a coalition of like-minded organisations, provide a forum for debate and consultation and undertake advocacy. It organised forums on the Victorian Women's Health Plan, women's access to reproductive information and services and a rural forum. After a couple of years, energy fell and the network again ceased to meet; however, women's health services and agencies are networked with each other through the Women's Health Association of Victoria (WHAV), the peak body, which has nine regional and two State-wide member services. WHAV now encourages organisations with compatible goals to join as associate members. It is a central point of contact for policy consultations.

Network organisation has an uneven history of recess and revival in Western Australia as well. The Australian Women's Health Network (WA) was revived in Perth in 1992 in response to threats to women's health centres. At the time, the centres, most of which were newly established, had had their counselling positions abolished. The network made public statements and organised a media campaign. At its peak, it had a membership of approximately 180 women, many of whom had worked in women's health centres, plus miscellaneous supporters, including women from environmental and consumer groups. There have also been various manifestations of a peak service provider body, including the WA Women's Health Organisation (WAWHO), which operated from 1998 until 2003. At the time of writing, however, only the managers of the women's health centres meet regularly.

In New South Wales, the original network did not survive, which is partly explained by the prior formation of a strong service providers' network. In 1981, when the Commonwealth was handing responsibility for the Community

Health Program back to the States and Territories, the Women's Health and Information Resource and Crisis Centres Association (WHIRCCA) was formed.[7] It aimed to support centres, create regular connections between them and to advocate and lobby on behalf of communities trying to establish new centres. The association met quarterly and developed a list of some 26 policy guidelines, major and minor, in the early 1980s, which included establishment of a women's health service for each administrative region of NSW Health. Another priority was the provision of broad preventive health care for the most economically disadvantaged women. In the first half of the 1980s, it engaged in regular consultative meetings with NSW Health.

Partial success came in 1985 when three new centres in the western suburbs of Sydney—Blacktown, Penrith and Campbelltown—were opened, along with others in rural areas. Funding, however, has always been seen as inadequate. In 2000, WHIRCCA changed its name to Women's Health NSW and now represents 23 centres across the State. It assists members where appropriate, undertakes advocacy and policy development work, develops training modules and other resources, gathers and disseminates information, assists with infrastructure and standards, organises State-wide meetings three times a year, provides facilitation and mediation services and participates in the work of AWHN. The management board is elected and is representative of the different services and regions (Women's Health NSW web site).

The AWHN Aboriginal Women's Talking Circle

The major recommendations formulated by the Aboriginal contingent at the Third National Conference and endorsed by the full conference were the establishment of a National Indigenous Women's Coalition, the staging of an Indigenous women's health conference and the development of a national Aboriginal and Torres Strait Islander Women's Health Policy. Within its limited resources, AWHN attempted to further the recommendations. In 1997 the organisation wrote to the Council for Aboriginal Reconciliation, informing it of the resolutions. AWHN's proposal was endorsed by the council and discussed in its 1997 report (Australian Institute for Women's Research and Policy 1997:20). Subsequently, a delegation from AWHN attended a meeting with the then head of OSW, Pru Goward, to discuss the proposals, but Commonwealth support was not secured.

---

7   The original name of the association appears to have been Women's Health and Information and Rape Crisis Centres Association; however, Rape Crisis Centres resigned in 1985 when WHIRCCA agreed to be part of a government working party to develop service guidelines for NGOs.

In 2004, an Aboriginal woman from Perth, Dot Henry, joined the AWHN committee. As one of AWHN's representatives on Womenspeak,[8] Henry was able to use that forum to draw attention to Aboriginal women's health problems. AWHN obtained funding from the Office of Aboriginal and Torres Strait Islander Health (OATSIH) in 1997 to bring Aboriginal women from each State and Territory to Canberra for a national summit staged in September, of which more below. The Aboriginal women met the day before, developed an initial position paper and decided to form an Aboriginal women's talking circle as a subgroup of AWHN. A further grant was obtained from Womenspeak in 2008, which enabled the group to meet again, in Adelaide in 2009. At approximately the same time, AWHN obtained a grant from the Women's Development Program of FaHCSIA to manage a consultation process with Aboriginal women and write a submission to the proposed new NWHP. The contract also required the development of an Aboriginal women's health strategy and the strengthening of the Talking Circle. A working group to oversee the project was formed at the Adelaide meeting.

Sandra Angus took leave from her position at Queensland Health to become the project officer and undertake the consultations, which were held in every jurisdiction. Unfortunately, time constraints prevented consultation with women living in the Torres Strait Islands.[9] The Talking Circle Working Group met regularly by teleconference to steer the project and to comment on various drafts of the submission, which was written by Sandra Angus and delivered to the Commonwealth Department of Health and Ageing in September 2009. The working group continued to meet by teleconference, with one face-to-face meeting, to work on an Aboriginal women's health strategy. The writing process was ably assisted by Dr Bronwyn Fredericks and Dr Karen Adams, and the strategy was launched at the Sixth AWHN National Women's Health Conference in 2010. It received considerable press attention. At the time of writing, advocacy is continuing to try to progress implementation of the recommendations but the political response is disappointing.

---

8   WomenSpeak was one of four National Women's Alliances that were funded by the Commonwealth Office for Women to undertake consultations on issues affecting women. The alliances were introduced by the Howard Government and replaced the Hawke Government's National Women's Non-Government Organisations' Funding Program, under which operational funding had been made available to a number of women's NGOs. In 2009, the number of alliances was expanded to six.
9   Such work requires a long lead time, as women are scattered and transport between islands is often infrequent.

Domestic Violence and Sexual Assault Networks

A variety of networks and coalitions has been set up in the domestic violence and sexual assault sectors. As the number of refuges increased in New South Wales, the need for unified action led to the formation of a State-wide organisation in 1979. The feminist Women's Refuge Movement Resource Centre, established in 1986, is the central contact for the movement in the State, where there are currently 57 member refuges. It aims to promote community awareness and provides information, resources and advocacy. A longstanding commitment to facilitating participation in decision making is maintained, and, to this end, regional and State conferences where major policy decisions are made are held quarterly. The NSW Women's Refuge Working Party is a smaller management body with authority to make decisions between conferences, in line with endorsed policies and philosophies. Within the movement, Koori, immigrant and lesbian women have formed their own support groups and there is also a child-support group. The Stop Violence against Women Network has also been established in New South Wales.

The incorporated Coalition of Women's Domestic Violence Services was established in South Australia in 2003. It works to raise the profile of violence against women and children in the public domain and to broaden the focus of discussion. It has explored the possibility of coordinated relationships with sexual assault and women's health services and, to this end, has developed a multi-agency working party. It produces policy documents, collects and analyses statistics, collaborates in awareness campaigns and writes submissions to inquiries and consultations, drawing attention to a range of unmet needs, particularly the health problems of children who have experienced violent situations. Among such children, PTSD, developmental delays and behavioural problems are more common.

A women's refuge group was established and incorporated in Western Australia in 1977. Now called the Women's Council for Domestic and Family Violence Services (WA), it is a peak organisation that operates within a feminist framework, representing 54 refuges and other domestic and family violence services. It makes referrals and carries out a range of capacity-development, representation, advocacy, information dissemination, community education, research and training functions. In 2009, it conducted a State-wide survey of services, which found unacceptably low pay levels for workers and disparities between services. It found that the non-governmental not-for-profit community sector is underpaid by up to 30 per cent, compared with other sectors in the State, creating serious staff and recruiting problems (Hartwig 2009).

Nationally, the Women's Emergency Services Network (WESNET) was established in 1992, as a peak advocacy body for SAAP-funded women's services. The impetus for action was an identified need to bring representatives from all jurisdictions together to address issues of common concern. Members at early meetings unanimously agreed that the advancement and recognition of the essential nature of the work required better organisation at the national level. Funding was obtained to employ a consultant to develop a national structure and gather information for incorporation. The first National Joint Forum of SAAP-funded organisations was held in Canberra in 1994 (Townsend 1994:9–11).

WESNET works within a feminist framework and recognises that women's and children's experiences are shaped by their ethnicity, ability, age, sexuality and class. It collaborates with member organisations to identify unmet needs and emerging issues. Like other peak groups, it provides policy advice and lobbies for legislative and program reform. At the time of writing, WESNET has almost 400 members across the country. It has developed a comprehensive domestic violence policy, which includes recommendations for law reform. Changes proposed include the strengthening of mechanisms to remove a violent partner from the family home and the training, including cross-cultural training, of police, court staff, legal representatives and magistrates. The full provision of interpretative services, the compilation of comprehensive statistics in relation to sole-occupancy and exclusion orders and the development of model domestic violence and related legislation through Commonwealth, State, Territory and community-sector collaboration are all objectives. WESNET facilitates national debate, stages national conferences and sector forums and lobbies on all relevant issues (WESNET web site).

The Victorian Centres against Sexual Assault Forum was formally established in 1992 and was incorporated in 1994. It is a peak body for 15 sexual assault services in the State and is committed to addressing all inequalities that result from sexual violence against women, children and men. It takes the view that the occurrence, consequences and elimination of sexual violence should be the responsibility of the whole community and all tiers of government.

The National Association of Services against Sexual Violence (NASASV) has been established nationally to facilitate information exchange, undertake policy and advocacy work and promote the development of a national response to sexual violence within a feminist framework. It aims to challenge and change the attitudes that underpin the perpetuation of sexual violence and, eventually, to see it eliminated. An initial meeting was held in Sydney in 1989, attended by representatives from all States and the Australian Capital Territory. The association was incorporated in 1997 with assistance from the Office of the Status of Women but has no secure funding. NASASV coordinates information, skills and resource sharing between services, lobbies and negotiates with governments, provides policy advice, promotes community awareness, undertakes research, promotes quality training and skills development, monitors innovative service models and organises national meetings, conferences and seminars. In 2002, it released a major report, *Cultural diversity and services against sexual violence* (Weeks 2002). The *National Standards of Practice Manual* has been produced and work on the development of a national data set has been undertaken. In 2009, *Framing best practice: national standards for the primary prevention of sexual assault through education* was produced by a small research team in partnership with other groups, including the Commonwealth and VicHealth.

Conclusion

The Australian women's health movement expanded and grew more diverse as groups multiplied from the early 1980s onwards. A decade later, there were literally 'hundreds of community-based groups of women organised around particular health issues' (Dwyer 1992:211). A panoply of networks and associations was established that facilitated the articulation of women's health issues despite the restrictions imposed by unfunded operation in most cases. The movement established a number of formal networks over the years but public funding to support them was difficult to obtain and many fell into abeyance or were dissolved. Clearly, the movement does not have the political clout that other health provider groups enjoy.

It was thought in the 1980s that the political arms of the movement—the State, Territory and national networks—needed to be one step removed from funded services in order to protect funding and independence. And certainly there have been unfavourable political times when this consideration was important. In 2011, however, most service-provider organisations are independent but part of the institutional apparatus. They work constructively with governments, pressing strongly for the sector's interests and for changes that will improve the conditions of women's lives. In most cases, they refrain from public criticism of the government in power. This way of working demonstrates the significant level of legitimacy that the movement has gained at the State and Territory level.

Growth and diversification within the movement seem to have had both costs and benefits. Expansion is generally considered to be a sign of strength and it certainly facilitated the public discussion of a broader range of women's health issues. In addition, it facilitated the generation and sharing of more and more detailed health information. The capacity of the movement to lobby on specific issues was increased and its ability to provide support to women was enhanced. Self-help groups make a vital contribution to women's health.

But proliferation has contributed to a fragmentation of the movement, at least since the very early days. As time passed, groups developed considerable expertise in their own areas and tended to undertake advocacy separately. More opportunities to address and articulate a wider range of issues have thus been offset by an increasing lack of cohesion, undermining the extent to which the movement can be seen, or can see itself, as a coherent entity. We will see in Chapter 6, for example, that the maternity-care reform movement has tended to work separately from other movement groups. In some areas, fragmentation can be a very real problem. Multiple groups lobby on specific disability issues, for example, and provide valuable support and information to their own client groups. It can be, however, that no group is working at the level of the broad picture where it is necessary to advocate for the general rights of all people with disabilities.[10]

Other processes were at work at the same time that groups were proliferating. Neo-liberalism and managerialism were gaining strength and these ideas influenced the way governments responded to community organisations. Many women who had previously worked at the grassroots level were taking paid positions in the newly created services, in the bureaucracy and in other places. According to Carmody (1990:307), these changes resulted in fewer opportunities for advocacy and collective action and a diminution in the quality of feminist political analysis, all of which was exacerbated by the demands of service provision in poorly funded services. Compared with the 1970s, feminists were becoming separated from each other in different spheres of activity, she argues.

Clearly, many forces were important in changing the way the 1970s women's health movement operated, including changing political opportunity structures. Fragmentation seems to be an unavoidable consequence of expansion, which as we have seen brought benefits as well. While it is hard to isolate the impact of each of the impinging forces, the evidence suggests that the movement has been able to make progress towards its goals, no matter what the changes, when governments sympathetic to its objectives have held power.

---

10   I owe this insight to Sue Salthouse, Convenor of WWDACT.

5. Working Together for Health

> So much of what affects women also affects children and men, so many
> agencies have responsibilities…and our agenda is so large, that we need
> to work with and through others as much as possible. (Dwyer 1992a:25)

The value of a collaborative approach to health care, pioneered in the community sector,[1] is now widely accepted among public health experts. Collaboration between team members and with outside services and agencies is considered a foundational element of effective, comprehensive primary health care. Collaborative ventures are undertaken between governments and non-governmental agencies and between agencies in the health sector itself. Health workers collaborate with local governments and social and community services, including housing, income security, child services and services responsible for safety from violence (Keleher 2001:59). Partnerships between government, non-governmental agencies and communities are now considered indispensable when addressing health promotion. Community-based partnerships are a means through which local needs and capacities can be evaluated and appropriate projects and programs designed. National, State and Territory partnerships of various kinds are being put together in most jurisdictions.

Collaboration is an essential element of everyday work in women's health centres and services. Within a few months of opening in 1975, Liverpool Women's Health Centre was already working with local agencies. Referrals were coming in from local doctors, invitations to speak to local groups and organisations had been received and liaison with local agencies and government departments was under way (Cooper and Spencer 1978:151). Collaboration is so extensive that in South Australia a special project has been deemed necessary just to identify and document the 'myriad activities' of the Central Northern Adelaide Health Service's Women's Health and Safety Unit, which includes Dale Street Women's Primary Health Service, Northern Women's Primary Health Care Service and the Northern Violence Intervention Program (MacKenzie 2009:6).

---

1   Much of the pioneering community health centre infrastructure established in the 1970s has now been disbanded. After the Fraser Government handed back responsibility, most State and Territory governments have presided over a dismantling process, as part of an exercise to shift costs to the Commonwealth. Without community health centres, citizens will primarily get their services from general practitioners in private practice, subsidised by the Commonwealth through Medicare. Queensland never established a comprehensive community health centre network, due mainly to the vehement opposition of organised medicine in cooperation with the conservative government that held power there until 1989. Victoria has retained the most extensive community health centre infrastructure, although centres have lost at least some of their independence. The Aboriginal community-controlled health sector, however, has been maintained and has managed to expand in some jurisdictions.

At the most fundamental and perhaps most important level, according to one of the principles of women's health, health workers collaborate with clients and families in arrangements where power is shared. The 'health worker as expert' model is supplanted with one that aims to empower and enhance the self-esteem of those seeking advice and care. Both the expertise of professionals and the expertise of individuals and family members are recognised. As Radoslovich (1994:51) argues, 'women's health centres believe in empowering women to take control of their health…To achieve this, the services have adopted particular styles which differ from traditional service models'.

Women in centres and services support each other and work with agencies in the wider community. In the early days, they provided strong support for groups trying to establish new services. They share information and experiences, work together to address service problems and act politically to influence public policy. In collaborative partnerships, they produce a broad range of community health, outreach and education services designed to meet multifaceted needs, especially the multiple needs of disadvantaged groups. By working together at the local level with other service providers and agencies, the resources of the community are mobilised and appropriate community-development projects are generated. The teams of health professionals employed by most women's health centres, including nurses, dieticians, counsellors and psychologists, for example, are generally well equipped through their training and their approach to health, to facilitate community participation and community development (Baum and Keleher 2002:36). Ongoing collaboration has, however, always been hampered by scarce resources and the pressure to respond to women's immediate needs (Broom 1990:121). For many centres and services, demand is so heavy that the capacity to operate beyond day-to-day provision is limited. Nevertheless, an amazing array of informal interactions and collaborations characterises the work of the sector.

The move towards multi-agency cooperation and collaboration in health mirrors changes that are taking place in the way Organisation for Economic Cooperation and Development (OECD) countries are governed. Since World War II, the complexity of policymaking processes and the interdependence of the agencies have increased in Western countries in response to globalisation. A large literature has emerged on what is called 'collaborative' or multilevel governance (see, for example, Leo and Enns 2009; Sorensen 2004; Stein and Turkewitsch 2008). Growing international interaction has increased the number of intergovernmental actors and agencies involved in policy, as well as expanding their roles. At the same time, there has been a proliferation of NGOs, both national and international, so that governments now collaborate in decision making with a variety of agencies, public and private, including corporations, unions, NGOs, members of social movements and individuals (Gray

2010).[2] Collaborative governance has been defined as a 'governing arrangement where one or more public agencies directly engage non-state stakeholders in a collective decision-making process that is formal, consensus oriented, and deliberative and that aims to make or implement public policy or manage public programs and assets' (Ansell and Gash 2007:2).

Health sector partnerships, often complex and multilateral, can be seen as a form of collaborative governance. Acknowledging the importance and ubiquity of partnerships and the varied forms they take, VicHealth has attempted to develop a typology, producing a fact sheet and the Partnerships Analysis Tool to assist practitioners in their work. Partnerships, VicHealth argues, usually move along a continuum depending on the level of commitment and degree of joint action. At one end is networking, which involves exchange of information for mutual benefit but is not time consuming and does not necessarily involve further cooperation. Coordination is the next stage on the continuum. Here, information is exchanged and activities are altered for a common purpose, involving more time and requiring greater levels of trust than networking. Cooperation, the next point on the scale, involves a sharing of resources for common purposes as well as information exchange and a shift in activities. More time and higher levels of trust are needed, and perhaps detailed agreements. Collaboration is identified as the most complex and committed type of partnership. As well as having the features of the other three types, collaboration involves a willingness to increase the capacity of another organisation and to share turf. High levels of trust are needed because risks are involved but, offsetting this, there is a possibility of highly beneficial outcomes (VicHealth n.d.[a], n.d.[b]).

While the VicHealth categorisation is helpful in terms of conceptualising different partnership forms, in practice, many women's health activities cannot be neatly classified. Political action, for instance, can be rather one-sided at least initially but might develop into a cooperative endeavour. For example, Victorian women's health centres engaged in a local-government capacity-building project in 2008. First, efforts were made to ensure that candidates standing for election had information about women's health. Next, candidates were asked to commit to an action plan, called Safe, Well and Connected: Victorian Local Government Action Plan for Women's Health 2008–2012. Endorsement of the plan entailed commitment to the development of local women's health strategies, addressing issues such as mental illness, disability, intellectual disability, violence, family friendly workplace practices and the concerns of women carers, lesbians and culturally diverse women (Hudson 2010; Women's Health in the North web site). As well as not fitting into any one type of partnership, joint endeavours often change over time. An interaction might begin as networking, for example,

---

2   A recent book explores the impact of changing governmental architecture and processes on the efforts of women's movements to influence public policy in different countries. See Haussman et al. (2010).

but develop into committed collaborative activity as linkages are established and trust deepens. Nevertheless, the VicHealth framework is a useful organising tool for a discussion of the way women work together and with other agencies for health.

Networking

Information sharing—the purpose of networking according to the VicHealth typology—is a basic aspect of women's health work. Aboriginal women find that value and empowerment flow from networking together to share health information. Gatherings also enable them to address difficult issues, such as violence, meet health providers, extend their networks and affirm their cultural and spiritual values (Adams et al 2002; Pearse 2002). Centres and services develop networks, partly to fulfil the needs of their own clients but sometimes to assist with service provision for clients from other organisations, often in a two-way information exchange. For example, Women in Industry Contraception and Health (WICH), Victoria (now the Multicultural Centre for Women's Health), shared information with Adelaide Women's Community Health Centre in the late 1980s, when Adelaide was interested in introducing programs based on WICH models. It also checked translations for the Victorian Domestic Violence Education Task Force and for the Prostitutes Collective. It has been consulted about curriculum development by the Broadmeadows TAFE and about migrant women's information needs by the National Women and AIDS Campaign. In addition, organisations visit the centre to learn about its work and from its experience. In 1989, WICH was a member of the Victorian Women's Health Services Providers Group, Non-English Speaking Background (NESB) Women's Health Services Funding Group, the Women's Health Forum, the Coalition against Depo-Provera and the Occupational Health and Safety Commission's NESB Workers Advisory Committee (WICH Annual Report 1989).

Sometimes what is nominally called a network operates more as a system of coordination or cooperation in VicHealth's terms. For example, Western Australian alcohol and drug agencies formed Wanada, a network that spreads across that State. Member agencies provide education, advocacy, community development, prevention, treatment and support services. Members include women's health centres and Aboriginal health services and corporations. Wanada is a member of Community Sector Services and provides services for its member organisations, including child care for clients and interpreter services—a much larger role than suggested for a network in the typology (Wanada web site). In another example, the Government of Victoria took the lead in developing integrated family violence networks in 1989. Community groups, including women's health centres and sexual assault and domestic violence services, formed regional networks under the program. Other network members include representatives from criminal justice, housing and community health. The main aim is to provide a more coordinated system, geared towards the protection of victims. In 2006, there were 20 partnerships, funded to provide integrated services, involving 70 organisations. Clearly, such activity involves more than an exchange of information. Similarly, the Alice Springs Women's Shelter convenes the Central Australian Family Violence and Sexual Assault Network, which comprises 26 government and non-governmental agencies. As well as sharing information, the network is involved in planning and advocacy (Commonwealth of Australia 2008b).

Cooperation

According to the VicHealth typology, cooperative activity includes information sharing, alteration of activities for common purposes and resource sharing. A great deal of women's health action fits into this category. From the early days, activists shared information and worked together for common benefit. The collective that later set up the Leichhardt Women's Community Health Centre (LWCHC) gave assistance to similar groups in Adelaide and Canberra, as well as others in Sydney, and produced the controversial booklet *What Every Woman Should Know* (Broom 1991:2). As mentioned, women in other States travelled to Leichhardt, the flagship centre, to learn from experiences there and, for their part, Leichhardt women travelled locally and interstate, as requested, to assist new centres. In the process of planning for a refuge and a women's health centre, Western Australian women had regular contact with, and support from, Leichhardt. Adelaide women had similar support (Radoslovich 1994:14). Leichhardt became a model for the health centre movement and cooperation was a hallmark of its operations.

Similarly, when the Hobart Women's Health Centre opened with precarious, short-term funding in 1987, women from Liverpool Women's Health Centre visited to provide training. HealthSharing Women in Victoria and Women's Health Statewide, Adelaide, supported the new centre by providing health information leaflets. There were also links with women in WICH, through which advice on appropriate services for immigrant and refugee women was channelled. A similar set of cooperative interactions took place between women establishing new refuges, who were able to learn from services already in place. The pattern of supporting new initiatives sometimes attracted the support of outside groups. In establishing Ngalawa Wingara in Liverpool, many different groups worked together in what became a full-scale collaboration. Ngalawa Wingara means 'to sit and think' and is an Aboriginal women's healing space, a beautifully landscaped area beside the health centre, with stones, plants, mosaic decorations and a rock pool. Clients and community women use the space for quiet time or to meet and talk. A steering committee of local women worked with health workers and the South Western Sydney Area Health Service, using the talents of a local artist, to set up the space. Assistance was supplied by local businesses, including nurseries. The artist worked closely with the steering group and received support from a group of Hoxton Park elders.

Women's health centres and services continue to cooperate in the establishment of new groups and services, as in the early days. Women's Health Victoria (WHV), the Breast Cancer Action Group and other Victorian women's health services established BreaCan in 2003. Originally funded as a pilot by the Victorian Department of Human Services, the service provides holistic support, information sessions, library resources, exercise programs, complementary therapies and opportunities for women to interact with trained peer-support volunteers, all of whom have themselves experienced cancer or cared for someone with cancer. The service is State-wide, confidential and provided without charge. In 2007, BreaCan expanded its activities to include women with gynaecological cancers. It subscribes to the philosophy that the best services are delivered in collaboration with partners and has formed a research partnership with the Key Centre for Women's Health in Society at Melbourne University (now the Centre for Women's Health, Gender and Society). BreaCan is community managed and receives operational funding from the Victorian Department of Health (BreaCan 2009).

Cooperation in the sense of sharing or creating resources for mutual benefit takes place when State-wide services provide a range of resources for the sector. For example, Women's Health NSW has produced a non-governmental women's health service training program that can serve as an orientation tool for new workers and aims to increase knowledge and skills about outcomes-based planning. Women's Health Queenslandwide provides comprehensive web-based health information, a library service and a range of education courses for professionals. Education courses have also been developed for schools, corporate-sector women and community members. Like its sister organisations, WHV produces extensive resources. All these agencies undertake advocacy for the whole sector. In South Australia, the Family Medicine Program at the Royal Adelaide Hospital established a women's health training module, in cooperation with femocrat women's advisers and community-level women's health groups.

A recent cooperative venture in Melbourne took the form of an Indigenous Women's Health Day, organised by Women's Health West and a number of mainstream health services, including the Western Melbourne Division of General Practice and North West BreastScreen. Held at the Western Suburbs Indigenous Gathering Place, a two-way exchange of information took place, during which Aboriginal women discussed their health concerns. Community women were able to meet healthcare providers, helping to build a sense of trust. Women's Health West continues to collaborate with the Gathering Place. The service also works with African women, Bosnian women, young women and women with disabilities, and has programs addressing emotional wellbeing, violence prevention and mental health, to name a few. All of these endeavours involve cooperation with a range of local agencies (Women's Health West web site).

Cooperation also takes place between Aboriginal community health services and other agencies. For example, in Victoria, the Gunditjmara Aboriginal Cooperative and the South Western Centre against Sexual Assault (CASA) worked together on a successful project to raise awareness about family violence and sexual assault. An evaluation of the project found it had produced 'increased and more relevant community education' and that the mutual learning from informal liaison among the workers in both organisations had been 'most fruitful'. Moreover, cooperation continued after funding ran out (South Western Centre against Sexual Assault 2003–04:49–50).

Cooperation is also strong among domestic violence agencies. The North Queensland Domestic Violence Resource Service (NQDVRS), itself a product of joint endeavour, and the Coalition on Criminal Assault in the Home North Queensland applied to the Queensland Government for funding to establish the Domestic Violence Resource Service for Townsville and Mount Isa in 1993. The service works closely with the Women's Centre and Sera's Women's Shelter and provides student places for James Cook University, TAFE and students from overseas. It has also established a partnership with the Queensland Police Service, which aims to provide better responses to domestic violence (NQDVRS 2009:1). The NQDVRS, the Sunshine Coast Domestic Violence Service and the Gold Coast Domestic Violence Service recently ran a one-year pilot to trial a support program for women and children staying in their homes after perpetrators had been required to vacate.

Sometimes women's health centres join forces with other agencies to help meet the health needs of rural women. For example, Women's Health Statewide in South Australia identified rural women's health as a priority and attended major country events, such as field days, to raise awareness of issues and provide information. It worked with groups such as the Women's Information Service, Women's Legal Services and the Working Women's Centre in these ventures. Country visits were coordinated with the work of local health workers. Ways of enhancing rural health work were explored, which often involved maintaining extensive relationships with country personnel over a period of years. The Women's Shed Project in Oodnadatta, near the Simpson Desert, is a partnership between the Northern and Far Western Regional Health Service, Dunjiba Council and Oodnadatta Health Service. A preventive health program, it uses the arts as a medium of communication.

Women's health groups regularly take up one another's issues, especially when a threat to existing rights or infrastructure is perceived. As an example, women concerned with violence took up the abortion issue towards the end of the Howard Government period (1996–2007), when the preservation of existing services came under threat, as represented in statements by the Health Minister, Tony Abbott, and the Prime Minister. In response, Issue 19 (2007) of the journal *Women against Violence* focused almost entirely on issues of pregnancy counselling and abortion, naming government pronouncements as 'the violence of misinformation'.

Collaboration

Collaboration sits at the complex end of the partnership continuum in the VicHealth framework. As well as information and resource sharing, collaborators must be willing to increase the capacity of one or more outside organisations to achieve common purposes. Again, much of the activity of the women's health movement falls into this category. Groups have worked together extensively to enhance mutual capacity building, often with outside agencies, including trade unions, family planning associations and political parties.

The Immigrant Women's Speakout Association in New South Wales provides a good example. It has established connections with other agencies, including the NSW Domestic Violence Network. Staff serve on a number of outside advisory and steering committees, including the Violence against Women Regional Reference Group, Family Planning Australia, Women's Health in Industry Program Steering Committee and the Australian Domestic and Family Violence Clearinghouse Advisory Committee. Similarly, Women's Health NSW, formerly Women's Health and Information Resource and Crisis Centres Association (WHIRRCA), has long experience working in collaboration with other NGOs to enhance capacity. In 2008–09, the Female Genital Mutilation Advisory Committee, the NSW Council of Social Services and the Primary and Community Health Working Group of NSW Health were among the committees on which it served. Other groups with which it is linked include the Multicultural Disability Advocacy Association of New South Wales, the NSW Police Domestic and Family Violence Stakeholder Forum, Reproductive Choice Australia (RCA) and the Royal Australian College of Physicians Health Consumers and Community Partnerships Forum (Women's Health NSW web site).

A recent example of a multi-partner project intended to produce information for mutual benefit is the Gender, Workplace Injury and Return to Work Research Project conducted in South Australia in 2003–04. The steering committee was drawn from a range of stakeholders and researchers. The aim was to explore people's experiences following workplace injury and return to work, to shed light on obstacles and to find out whether men's and women's experiences are the same or different. Project initiators included the Working Women's Centre, the Office for Women, the Australian Manufacturing Workers Union, the Equal Opportunity Commission, Dale Street Women's Health Service, the Migrant Women's Lobby Group and a community representative. During the research process, views were canvassed among employers, managers, OHS/rehabilitation coordinators, unions, health and safety representatives and trainers, claims agents and case managers (WorkCover Corporation and the Working Women's Centre 2005).

The promotion of cultural sensitivity has been furthered through collaboration. In 1981, LWCHC joined with refuges, Family Planning NSW and government agencies to organise a conference to promote the employment of immigrant women in established services and to encourage ongoing interaction between groups providing services in immigrant communities. In addition, it worked with Annandale Neighbourhood Centre and the Leichhardt Council to produce a 10-week health project for immigrant girls at the local high school (Stevens 1995:49). A Queensland example of intercultural collaboration is the formation in 1993 of the non-English cultural background (NECB) Women's Health Reference Group, to provide information and to advance the health of immigrant women in the Logan and North Albert areas. Members of the reference group were the Logan Migrant Neighbourhood Centre, Logan Women's Health Centre, Logan Hospital and the South Regional Health Forum. The reference group lobbied successfully for a NECB health worker for the Logan Women's Health Centre and held cultural awareness workshops and seminars.

Major collaborations have also been undertaken in the sexual assault field. Recently, the Australian Research Council funded a joint project between the NSW Rape Crisis Centre and the University of Western Sydney, which investigated the possibility of promoting ethical, non-violent relationships between young men and young women (Carmody and Willis 2006). From this research, a six-week education program for young people was piloted and developed, with the aim of creating opportunities for learning new ways of negotiating sexual intimacy and promoting ethical, non-violent skills. In 2009, funding provided by the Commonwealth's Respectful Relationships Program was used to train educators and run groups with young people in New South Wales and Queensland. Collaborators include the AIDS Council of New South

Wales (ACON) and the National Rugby League in Queensland. Influence has crossed the Tasman: the New Zealand Ministry of Justice provided funding in 2010–11 for the program to be run in New Zealand.

Collaboration with Communities

Community-development projects are a standard part of the work of women's health centres. Meeting complex needs involves day-to-day collaboration with other service providers and agencies to try to ensure that a full range of services is available. Women's health workers recognise that no one agency can effectively meet more than a fraction of a community's health needs. For example, domestic violence services must interact with local doctors, local hospitals, mental health services and so on, when clients need medical assistance. Similarly, cooperation with housing authorities, local councils, social service agencies and possibly local charities might be necessary. The Immigrant Women's Health Service (IWHS) in the western suburbs of Sydney works with multiple agencies to help meet the needs of its clients. It has facilitated the establishment of support groups for women from 19 cultural groups, which meet regularly at the centre. Other community-development projects include the Ethnic Communities Sustainable Living Project and a support group for Vietnamese working women. Among the agencies with which it collaborates are Women's Health NSW, the Smith Family, the Serbian Orthodox Welfare Association, Playgroup Australia, Miller TAFE Outreach, Granville TAFE, the Multicultural Respite Network, Fairfield City Council, Liverpool City Council, Fairfield Division of General Practice, the Benevolent Society, Australian Quarantine Inspection Service, Fairfield Hospital, Liverpool Hospital, Fairfield Migrant Resource and the Wetherill Park Police, to name only some (Immigrant Women's Health Service web site).

Women's health centres also participate in community efforts to rectify environmental degradation. From the early 1980s onwards, for example, in the Dale Street area, concerned residents mobilised in response to problems such as dust, noise, factory emissions and spills of copper chromium arsenate and chlorine gas. Centre workers had noticed increases in the incidence of bronchial disease and ear, nose and throat problems. Dale Street thereupon employed local women to document the health problems being experienced and develop strategies to deal with them. The report was presented to a large public meeting, which included representatives of government and industry. Subsequently, a favourable public policy response emerged.

Dale Street Women's Health Centre has been involved in a number of other community-development projects (Radoslovich 1994:68–70). For example, it was noticed that many local women worked at home as piece workers. The centre responded with a support project called 'Outwork: Reaching an Invisible

Workforce' in the second half of the 1990s. Information was assembled and distributed about OHS issues, rights and entitlements under safety legislation and workers' compensation arrangements (Tassie 1997:185). As part of the project, the centre worked extensively with individuals and organisations, including employers, doctors, community workers and community groups representing women from different cultural backgrounds.

OHS Meets a Social View of Health

Extended collaboration took place between feminists in different agencies with the ultimate aim of overhauling OHS regimes that had been in a state of neglect for decades (Irving 1979; Pearse and Refshauge 1987:646). Until the 1970s, OHS was not seen as a health issue. Rather, it consisted of a narrow, prescriptive regulatory regime, focusing largely on particular industries, such as mining, manufacturing and construction. Just as medical research had focused on male bodies, investigations into safety and conditions of employment concentrated on the safety of men. At the time, women were seen as a low-risk, part-time or temporary workforce. The occupations considered appropriate for women were supposed to be safe and were therefore seen as outside the ambit of OHS. One of the views of the day was that there was no need to include women in OHS discussions because they could always avoid health problems by staying at home or working in another industry. For example, the report of the Williams Inquiry into OHS in New South Wales in the early 1980s failed to discuss the problems of either migrants or women, dismissing each with a one-line mention (Dimech 1982:18). It was not until 1985 that women's occupations were included in the industrial death registration system (Skues and Kirby 1996; Shoebridge and Shoebridge 2002:7). Immigrant women were in a particularly vulnerable position. Their representation in union structures was virtually non-existent yet as a group they were severely affected by work-related injuries and they constituted the majority of those suffering from RSI, for example.

Workers' health action groups were formed in most jurisdictions from 1977 onwards. Many women unionists saw health from a social perspective and worked to broaden the meaning of OHS, arguing that it should be much more than a set of minimum safety standards. Rather, employers should have a 'duty of care' to provide a safe, healthy place of work, one that would not only prevent the high incidence of industrial injuries but would also contribute to physical, mental and emotional wellbeing. The notion of a healthy workplace was influenced by ideas from industrial democracy and included the establishment and resourcing of participatory structures where workers would exercise responsibility and discretion.

Women unionists also worked to increase their representation in union structures, trying to ensure their election as union officials—a process assisted by funding grants from the Whitlam Government. A critical mass of female officials meant being able to raise and pursue issues not previously raised inside a union and being able to establish collaborative links with women's organisations, community organisations, political parties and other relevant agencies outside (Shoebridge and Shoebridge 2002:10). Working women's centres and women's health centres were collaborators in the many coalitions that were formed in the 1980s and 1990s around OHS issues.

After the main health issues were identified, women pressed for OHS provisions to be incorporated in industrial awards. A preventive focus required that hazards are eliminated 'at the source' rather than compensation being provided after the event. Seeing OHS as an industrial democracy issue, an argument was made that union-elected health and safety representatives should have powers to inspect workplaces, draw attention to conditions needing improvement and stop work if conditions were considered dangerous (Pearse and Refshauge 1987:636–42).

Women unionists argue that working life affects the rest of life and is therefore crucial to health. They raised problem issues, such as the availability of flexible working arrangements to fit with family responsibilities and union provision of child care, arguing that child care is an industrial issue. Other specific problems are working with chemicals, stress, sexual harassment, RSI and compensation in the case of injury. Violence in the workplace is identified as a problem, especially in nursing homes and hostels, where staff care for people with dementia and intellectual disabilities. Stress became a more urgent issue in the 1990s, when job insecurity increased and many women and men did not know whether they would have a job the following week.

The women's health movement in most States and Territories had good working links with women in the union movement. In many cases they knew each other through overlapping memberships of political parties and unions and a few sat on policy committees. So while women in trade unions played a crucial role in advancing women's OHS, in turn, the broader women's health movement supported workers' health and was a force in shaping a context conducive to workplace reform.

Liverpool Women's Health Centre was a pioneer in recognising OHS as a women's health issue. In 1975, the Industrial Health Group was formed on the discovery of a high incidence of musculoskeletal workplace injuries particularly among immigrant women. About the same time, the trade union arm of the women's movement lobbied for federal funding for the Melbourne Working Women's Centre, which was set up in 1976. Through the centre, OHS issues were advanced, along with issues around equal pay and conditions of work (Pearse and Refshauge 1987:639). The musculoskeletal and RSI conditions that disproportionately affected immigrant women workers had previously been put into the 'too hard basket', participants remember. Through collaboration between members of advocacy networks, however, information about injuries was publicised and changes in conditions of work were slowly achieved.

In Western Australia, women unionists championed the principle that employers are responsible for providing safe working environments. They had close ties with women's health centres, academics, health policy professionals, workers' health centres in other jurisdictions, including the Lidcombe Workers' Health Centre, and with international organisations. They felt that they had good access to policymakers under Labor governments and succeeded in getting improved OHS arrangements written into policy. Union representatives sat on the health policy committees of the ALP, which was an opportunity not available under Liberal governments. A women's OHS committee was established in the Trades and Labour Council in the early 1980s and the first paid female officer was appointed in 1983. The incumbent Labor Government met the costs of the position. The committee was wound up in 1988 but the principles it promoted found their way into Australian Council of Trade Unions (ACTU) policy and then into the policies of Work Safe Australia. One Western Australian union instituted an immigrant workers' health project in the 1980s, which consisted of a team of five to six women who visited workplaces over a period of six months to talk about health and health rights to women in their own languages. A shortage of resources, however, limited the extent to which such work could be undertaken.

OHS was a major issue for Queensland women in the 1980s. The Brisbane Women's Health Centre shared premises with the Union of Australian Women which contributed to a cross-fertilisation of ideas. The Women in Trade Unions Network was formed in 1985 and it became the centre of a large, diverse, feminist network, which included the Queensland Workers' Health Centre. Membership was restricted to unionists but there was close collaboration with domestic violence and rape crisis networks and other relevant agencies. Helen Abrahams, a medical practitioner with specialist qualifications in occupational health and long experience in women's health in Adelaide and later in rural New South Wales, was Director of the Workers' Health Centre from 1982 to 1991.

The network, more resembling a full-scale collaboration in VicHealth terms, saw its major task as persuading the trade union movement to take more interest in women's issues. The Queensland Nurses Union used OHS issues as a vehicle to further this aim. The network met monthly, inviting expert speakers to talk on issues such as rape and domestic violence. Both the Workers' Health Centre, which had outreach services in workplaces, and the Brisbane Women's Health

Centre worked together extensively in relation to immigrant women's health. A drive was undertaken to increase union membership of the Workers' Health Centre.

Another agency that collaborated to pursue women's health issues was the Trade Union Training Authority (TUTA). TUTA provided training in representation and negotiation skills for unionists at all levels. It also ran education courses about industrial relations systems and sessions on working women's issues, including sexual harassment, which was a notoriously difficult issue to pursue either in the workplace or in the courts (Thornton 1984; Working Women's Centre 1980). Workers from the Brisbane Women's Health Centre participated in teaching and women from community organisations availed themselves of TUTA courses in order to learn negotiation and meeting skills.

Bernadette Callaghan, Queensland Secretary of the Federated Clerks Union in 1983, was the first woman elected to the Queensland Trades and Labour Council after which women's health became one of the areas of the council's work. For example, it lobbied the Queensland Government to fund the Brisbane Women's Health Centre in the mid-1980s. The Federated Clerks Union participated strongly in the Women in Trade Unions Network but officially it never differentiated between men's and women's health; however, because women constituted a majority of members, OHS issues were able to be raised.

The Queensland Workers' Health Centre was heavily involved with other agencies in OHS campaigns in the 1980s, including campaigns against RSI. An aggressive educational campaign was undertaken and brochures developed. An unsuccessful RSI test case was mounted but, eventually, the campaign to bring about safer processes of work was successful. Noise was identified as a safety issue and the centre backed a union campaign against it. Action was also taken concerning the problems facing women outworkers.

A major campaign identified sexual harassment as a serious workplace issue. Women unionists had posters and brochures produced, forums were held, meetings organised and resolutions passed. Despite opposition from the national body of the clerks union, which banned the posters, the campaigns were successful in articulating and gaining a level of acceptance of the problem as a women's health issue. At the time, there was no anti-discrimination legislation in Queensland.

Because the Queensland union movement was generally conservative, opportunities for women to generate debate about access to abortion were limited; however, after the Bjelke-Petersen Government authorised a police raid on the Greenslopes Fertility Control Clinic in 1985, union members were persuaded to participate in a protest rally at City Hall.

In South Australia, there were cooperation and collaboration between the women's health movement, the community health movement, trade unions and the Working Women's Centre, which was established in 1979. In a relatively small community where people knew each other, the union movement enjoyed a particularly good relationship with the women's movement. There were both formal links, through organisations such as the SA Coalition for Workers Health Action, and informal links—for example, overlapping memberships of political parties and other organisations.

The SA Coalition for Workers Health Action, established in 1984 to promote a preventive approach to OSH, had a membership drawn from trade unions, the women's health movement, the Working Women's Centre, the community health and welfare sectors, allied health workers and others. It was a member of the Australian Coalition for Workers Health Action, which lobbied for legislative change, changes to workers' compensation arrangements and for a workers' health centre. It did not get the centre but it did get the legislative reform. As in other States, in South Australia, RSI became a major issue. Word-processing pools had been introduced into the public sector without consultation with unions. There were no guidelines for use; there was no ergonomic furniture and no awareness of the health implications of overuse. Women providing word-processing services were required to have a keystroke rate of 18 000 words per hour, which was monitored by a machine. At the end of the week, those who had under-performed were counselled. The result was what was described as an 'epidemic of RSI', which especially affected immigrant women. The unions, in close cooperation with women's health centres and the Working Women's Centre, demanded 10-minute rest breaks, a reduction of the key stroke rate to 12 000 words per hour and ergonomic equipment. Sympathetic practitioners were needed for referral but were difficult to find, so women were referred to Adelaide Women's Community Health Centre where staff became expert in the intricacies of RSI. Similarly, in other States and Territories, women in unions worked with the women's health movement and other groups to promote a more expansive view of OHS.

Meanwhile, women unionists were working to increase their voice at the national level. In 1975, they demonstrated outside the ACTU Congress, demanding that working women's issues be put on the agenda, which was part of a major campaign to press the council to adopt a Working Women's Charter. A charter was adopted two years later, followed by the council-sponsored Working Women's Charter Conference in 1978. The Women's Committee of the ACTU was established in 1977. It focused on issues such as child care, RSI, flexible working hours and parental leave. After an intense struggle, the 1981 ACTU Congress made a historic decision to support women's right to free, safe, legal abortion (Hague and Milson 1982:15). The first woman was elected to the executive in 1983 and, shortly afterwards, the Working Women's Policy was produced and endorsed.

The ACTU now campaigns regularly on issues of importance to women workers, including pay equity, paid parental leave and sexual harassment, and supports strategies to promote compliance with the *Equal Opportunity for Women in the Workplace Act 1999* (ACTU 2009; Burrow 2008).

In summary, a long collaboration, played out differently in different settings, took place between groups concerned with women's health at work. Problems were articulated, the meaning of OHS was expanded and it was given a place on Australian political agendas. Legislative reform has been achieved in all jurisdictions. In South Australia, both major political parties made OHS election promises before the 1983 election. Reform legislation was introduced in that State in 1986 and the Occupational Health and Safety Commission was established, with the Women's Advisory Committee and provision for women's representation on all other committees. The Labor Government in Western Australia took reform action from 1983 onwards, in response to women's advocacy, producing a discussion document that suggested that the focus of OHS be changed from safety to health. Legislative change was subsequently developed through a tripartite process and became law in 1987. When Labor lost office in 1993, however, much of the reform was overturned.

Australian OHS legislation now provides for worker-elected health and safety representatives—one of the demands of women in the 1970s and 1980s. Representatives have been given broad powers in most jurisdictions, including the right to order that work be stopped if conditions are considered unsafe. All State and Territory legislation provides for the establishment of health and safety committees, on which both employees and employers are represented, and everywhere inspectors have wide powers. Arrangements, however, still vary from jurisdiction to jurisdiction (National Research Centre for OHS Regulation web site) due to differences in political culture and the incumbency of governments (Pearse and Refshauge 1987:640).

Occupational health and safety was officially recognised as a priority women's health issue in the first NWHP—a tribute to women unionists and their collaborators who worked hard to bring hidden problems to public attention and to have appropriate responses embedded in legislation and public policy.

A Note on Working Women's Centres

Several Working Women's Centres were established in the 1970s and 1980s to provide work-related support for women, including those from diverse cultural backgrounds and those disadvantaged in regard to workplace bargaining. All 'formed strong partnerships with other community organisations, government agencies, universities and unions and are experts on women and industrial relations issues' (Queensland Working Women's Service 2007–08:9). In 1975, the first two Working Women's Centres were established, one in Melbourne and the other in an industrial suburb of Newcastle, NSW: the Hunter Region Working Women's Centre. The former was the first trade union women's research and advisory centre in Australia, set up under the auspices of the Australian Council of Salaried Professional Associations. It campaigned for women to take a more active part in trade union and political life and for women's issues in employment, including family friendly policies. It also advocated for reproductive health rights, including abortion and general women's health issues (The Australian Women's Register, Working Women's Centre at Melbourne 1975–84). The Hunter region centre was a multipurpose centre but health has always been the major focus of its work. From the beginning, it was funded from disparate sources, including the Commonwealth Health and Hospitals Services Commission (HHSC) (Broom 1990:15–16).

The Working Women's Centre was established in South Australia in 1979 by bureaucratic process. It has always received State funding but is managed by a community board. It collaborated closely with women's health activists. Working Women's Centres were established in 1994 and 1995 in Queensland, Tasmania and the Northern Territory, with combined Commonwealth/State funding. All collaborated extensively with the women's health movement, as discussed, and all were primarily concerned with the interests of women who were not represented by a union. They provided advice, information and support. Among the range of OHS issues dealt with are RSI, outwork, family friendly practices, workplace bullying and sexual harassment.

The Workers' Health Centre was established in Lidcombe, Sydney, in 1977 with the support of progressive trade unions and Leichhardt Women's Community Health Centre but with no government funding. While not exclusively a women's centre, it campaigned regularly on key women's health issues as part of its core work to raise the profile of workers' health issues. It was able to organise migrant women to take action on RSI and made a detailed submission to the Williams Inquiry into OHS in New South Wales in the early 1980s (Dimech 1982:16). Working Women's Centres and Workers' Health Centres have regularly worked with the women's health movement on an 'as needed' basis.

Working Women's Centres came under funding threat and were forced to curtail the services they provided when they opposed the Howard Government's industrial relations policies, especially the WorkChoices legislation of 2005. The New South Wales centre closed towards the end of that year, after a long and unsuccessful struggle to retain Commonwealth funding without curtailing its services. The Tasmanian centre closed in August 2006, when the funding contract it was offered by the Commonwealth stipulated that the money was for 'the provision of information on WorkChoices only'. Women in the Australian

Services Union were unable to persuade the Tasmanian Government to meet the Commonwealth funding shortfall. Three centres, however—those in the Northern Territory, Queensland and South Australia—survived the Howard years, only to be told in 2008, under a Labor government, that Commonwealth funding might be terminated. Months of time-consuming campaigning, letter writing and meetings with departmental officials took place before short-term funding was again secured.

Partnerships

Partnerships are located at the complex collaboration end of the VicHealth continuum. They are often a blend of hierarchy, and market and network forms of participation and are generally thought of as voluntary. The concept of partnerships, suggesting that participants are in relatively equal positions, appears regularly in recent government reports, reflecting its acknowledgment as an intrinsic element of preventive health care (Baum and Keleher 2002:36). The National Preventive Health Taskforce discussion paper *Australia: The healthiest country by 2020* envisages partnerships as a key element of almost every type of preventive healthcare strategy (Commonwealth of Australia 2008a).

Because one of the principles of women's health is empowerment, building and promoting strong, collaborative partnerships is a favoured way of working (Women's Health in the North web site). Since 2000, health partnerships have been established in Victoria where there are now 31 Primary Care Partnerships (PCPs). More than 800 agencies, including women's health centres, are involved. A central aim is to 'facilitate coordination of the provision of a broad range of services between GPs, community nurses and therapists, youth workers, home carers and people in numerous agencies' (Government of Victoria 2002). Victoria has instituted the Aboriginal Health Promotion and Chronic Care Partnership, in which government agencies and Aboriginal community health centres work together on multiple projects.

As part of the Victorian Primary Care Partnership strategy, all women's health and community health centres have health-promotion plans for 2009–12. Victoria has also established partnerships in violence prevention. Lauded as the first whole-of-government approach in Australia, Partners in Prevention is a network of Victorian professionals who work with young people. Established in 2007, the network is funded by VicHealth and managed by the Domestic Violence Resource Centre Victoria (DVRCV). Members meet four times a year to share resources and information and are involved in a variety of programs, including Relationships Education and Awareness for Life, a schools program aimed at supporting young people to experience positive, rewarding relationships. Feeling Safe Being Strong is a primary-school prevention project run by Bethany Community Support, and Respect Protect Connect is a secondary-school peer-education program run by Women's Health in the South-East in partnership with the South Eastern Centre against Sexual Assault. Other projects include performance pieces and online information and resources (Partners in Prevention web site).

Part of the Victorian Government's aim in pursuing partnerships appears to be to save money through better management of the rising incidence of chronic disease in an ageing population and less use of expensive hospital, medical and residential care. Such an overriding objective is likely to undermine the autonomy of partners. And so a study has found: one evaluation of the Primary Care Partnerships detected a reasonable level of collaboration but there was limited capacity for agencies to follow their own priorities at the local level (Lewis 2009). At the same time, early evaluation has suggested that better health outcomes will follow (Hahn 2002).

Partnerships in violence prevention have also been established in South Australia. The Western Collaborative Approach (WCA) is a partnership developed in 2005 among 21 key agencies in the area of the Central Northern Adelaide Health Service. Among the groups involved is Dale Street Women's Primary Health Service. The project, which includes Aboriginal people and organisations, makes use of 'Change Champions'—men who are prepared to actively oppose violence against women and disrespectful ways of speaking. It has a reference group, a leadership group and key area focus groups (Johns 2009:7).

The Hobart Women's Health Centre has been involved in a recent partnership with government and other agencies, which examined the health needs of women from diverse cultural backgrounds. The aim was to improve access to quality services through the establishment of permanent regional migrant and refugee women's health worker positions. Existing State-wide networks were used to facilitate consultation and to provide support and feedback on completion. Project steering committee members were drawn from relevant branches of government, women's health and rural health services, multicultural organisations, the Royal Hobart Hospital, TAFE Tasmania, the University of Tasmania and Devonport City Council (Valencia 2007).

In New South Wales, the Aboriginal Health and Medical Research Council (AH&MRC), while mindful of the principles of Aboriginal self-determination, supports partnerships with government, along with collaboration between relevant governmental departments with responsibility for Aboriginal health. Formal partnerships with the NSW Government, under which the parties were to enjoy equal status, were struck in 1995, 1997 and 2001. The aim was to ensure that the health expertise of Aboriginal communities was channelled into health policymaking processes. As part of the strategy, partnerships were put in place at regional and local levels where health plans were developed. AH&MRC also participates in formal and informal partnerships with peak organisations involved in the delivery of health care for Aboriginal people.

Conclusion

So many and varied are the forms of collaboration that it is impossible to differentiate between types with precision, although VicHealth makes a valiant attempt. In community-based health care, cooperation and collaboration are central parts of everyday operations, and women's health groups have found strength in working together, supporting each other wherever possible. They have formed networks, associations, coalitions and service-provider groups and have worked at all levels of political systems to try to change policies and so improve women's health. Women unionists worked collaboratively to revolutionise the meaning of occupational health and safety and to put the new version on political agendas. Expectations about what constituted decent working conditions were raised and women's rights to control their bodies eventually became ACTU policy.

One of the distinguishing features of the joint ventures, partnerships and collaborations being developed in the different health systems is that they have a population-health focus rather than a focus on individual treatment. Evidence shows that interventions at the level of community care improve population health; however, only a very small proportion of Australia's total health budget is spent on population-focused programs. In 2008–09, 3.2 per cent of total Australian health spending was devoted to community health (some of which is not population focused since individual services are also provided). Another 2.1 per cent was spent on public health, defined by the Australian Institute of Health and Welfare (AIHW) as activities that 'focus on prevention, promotion and protection rather than on treatment, on population rather than on individuals, and on the factors and behaviours that cause illness and injury rather than the illness and injury itself' (AIHW 2011:2). Total spending on community health and public health combined therefore was 7.3 per cent of the total health budget and has been stable over the past decade (AIHW 2010c:119). Although health promotion and prevention have been on the Commonwealth policy agenda since 2007, no major investment in health has so far been made.

The next chapter presents case studies of two issue-specific sections of the movement: the maternity-care reform movement and the abortion rights movement. In the first, there has been less collaboration with other parts of the movement than we might expect. In the second, collaboration bubbles forth almost spontaneously when a threat is perceived or an opportunity presents itself, such is the centrality of reproductive health rights in the women's health movement.

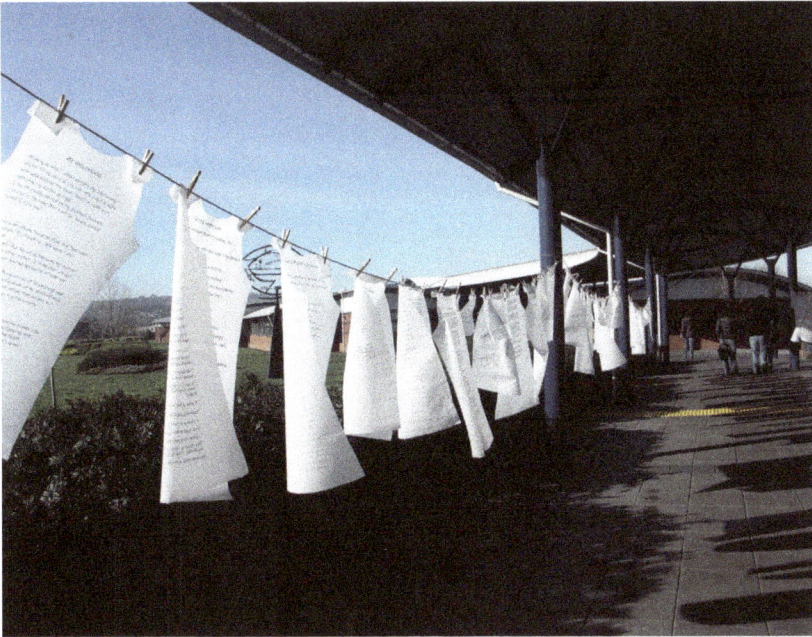

Women hang their health concerns out to dry at the Women on Top Health Forum, Launceston, June 2008.

Photo: Tracey Wing

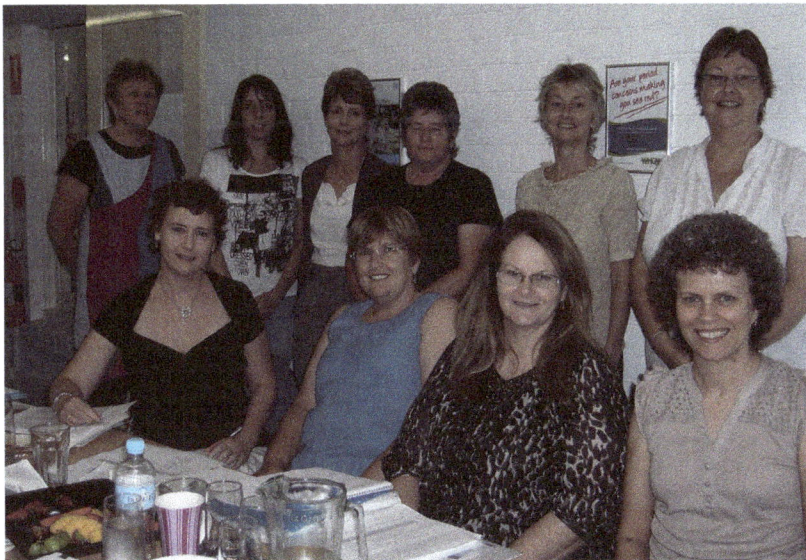

Members of the Queensland Women's Health Services Alliance meeting in Brisbane, February 2011. Front row from left: Kris Saunders, Selina Utting, Robyn Liddell, Maree Hawken. Back row from left: Cathy Crawford, Belinda Hassan, Cathy North, Greta Brennan, Ruth Tidswell, Kathy Faulkner.

175

Photo: Queensland Women's Health Network

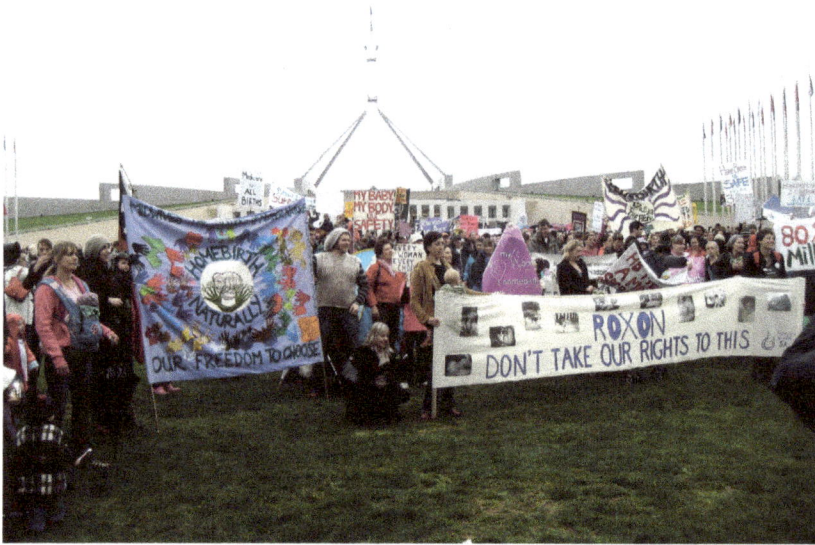

The 'Mother of All Rallies', organised by Maternity Coalition. Approximately 3000 women demonstrate in support of expanded maternity-care choices outside Parliament House, Canberra, 7 September 2009.

Photo: Maternity Coalition

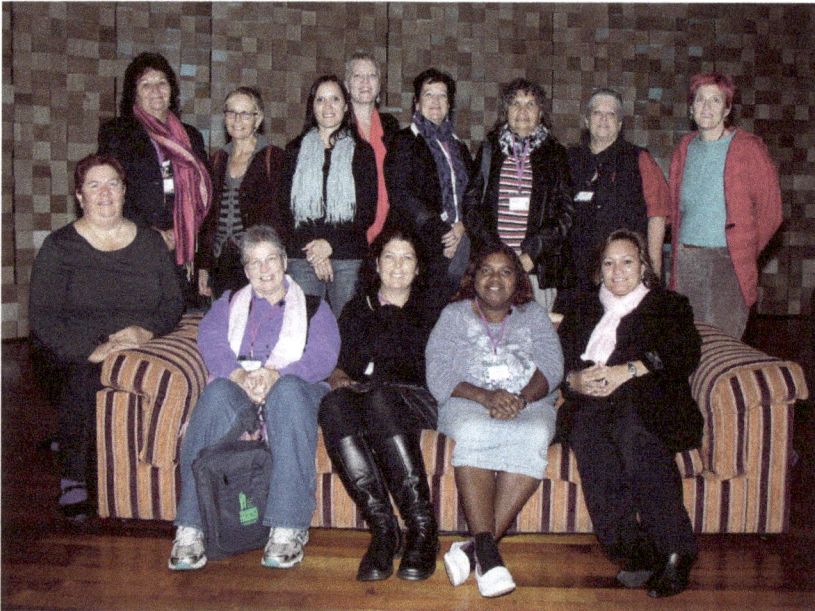

An NT contingent at the Sixth AWHN National Women's Health Conference, Hobart, 2010.

Photo: Tracey Wing

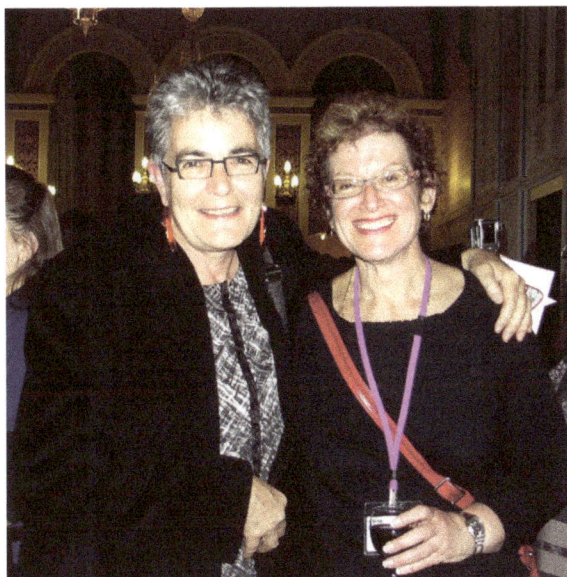

Marilyn Beaumont, formerly Executive Director, Women's Health Victoria, with Professor Karen Grant, University of Manitoba, at the pre-conference reception, Government House, Hobart, 2010.

Photo: Tracey Wing

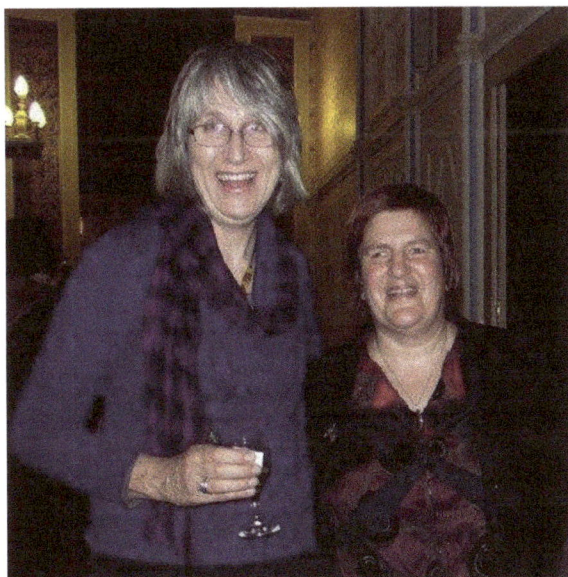

Former AWHN convenors Helen Keleher (1999–2005) and Celia Karpfen (2006–07) at the pre-conference reception, Government House, Hobart, 2010.

Photo: Tracey Wing

6. Women's Reproductive Rights: Confronting power

No book about the modern women's health movement and its impact on public policy in Australia would be complete without including the work of the maternity-care reform movement and the abortion rights or pro-choice movement. These two groupings have laboured long and hard to establish women's reproductive health rights and to ensure women's access to a full range of options. Both have campaigned for women's rights to control their own bodies and for rights to the information necessary to participate in decisions about their own care. Both have worked to undermine patronising attitudes, to change public opinion and to counter unnecessary medicalisation. And both struggle in the face of staunch resistance from some of the most powerful forces to be found in politics. In the first case, the movement is confronted by sections of the medical establishment, whose power and position it challenges. In the second case, anti-choice forces, including but not restricted to powerful religious organisations, mobilise to resist any proposal to liberalise existing laws. Considering the strength of the interests mobilised against them, women have made important gains in both areas but there are still major reforms to be achieved.

I use the term groupings to describe the two movements because in both cases organisational linkages, internal and external, are loose and fluid. The early maternity reform groups were not closely associated with either the women's movement or the women's health movement. Many members did not support feminist goals, while conversely mothers' rights were not a pressing issue for most feminists. As more women came to identify as feminists in the maternity-care reform movement from the 1970s onwards, differences in priorities and strategies became divisive. Internal dissension and the absence of strong working links with the women's health movement have undermined effectiveness. Abortion law reform, on the other hand, has been a galvanising force in the women's and women's health movements. Because pro-choice activists are to be found in numbers in all feminist organisations, there is less need for dedicated abortion law reform groups than there was in the 1960s and early 1970s. If a threat to existing rights or a window of policy opportunity for goal advancement is perceived, women's groups quickly and easily form activist coalitions. The strong consensus among feminists about the importance of a woman's right to control her own body helps to explain why gains have been possible notwithstanding powerful, well-resourced opposition.

The Maternity-Care Reform Movement

Members of the maternity-care reform movement, like those of the broader women's health movement, saw themselves as agents of social change. They demanded that women's agency and women's bodies be respected and they worked for an extension of women's rights. They challenged the unquestioning acceptance of medical dominance and scientific knowledge that had become entrenched in the post–World War II period. Information about pregnancy, childbirth and breastfeeding, they argued, was abysmally hard to come by when it should be freely available. Moreover, maternity care should be more holistic, should show greater respect for birthing women and their right to make informed decisions and should be delivered in continuous, trusting, collaborative partnerships.

Childbirth, most members of the movement argue, is a normal life event, the province of women for millennia. From the late nineteenth century onwards, it was gradually taken over by a predominantly male medical profession and progressively and unduly medicalised. By the 1960s, dissatisfaction began to be voiced in Australia and most Western countries about aspects of the birthing process, including women's lack of control and authority. Like the women's health groups that mobilised a little later, mothers' groups had dual objectives: they wanted to improve information and services for women and influence public opinion to promote structural changes in the organisation of care. They called for fundamental reform of the rushed, impersonal, hierarchical and medicalised environments that characterised the labour wards of the day (Gosden and Noble 2000:71–2; Reiger 2001:1–84). In most jurisdictions, with the possible exception of some Aboriginal women, there was little choice but to have one's baby in a hospital, with its attendant 'preparations', the most unpopular of which were enemas and pubic shaves. Support persons, including husbands, were generally banished, women were given drugs they did not want and often left alone during labour. Mothers and babies were separated, supplementary bottle feeding, which has a depressing effect on lactation, was common, and family members, including fathers, viewed newborns through nursery windows.

Prenatal services in the 1960s mostly took the form of medical checks; care of the medical kind was provided by general practitioners and private obstetricians. Information about lactation was scarce and rates of breastfeeding were falling dramatically (Reiger 2001:15–36). In line with international thinking, calls were made for a change of direction towards more natural childbirth. Women should be at the centre of the birthing process, there should be less reliance on analgesics, more freedom of movement permitted during labour and persons able to provide emotional support should be allowed to be involved. Employing a rights approach, maternity-care reform groups argued that women were entitled to have their voices heard, their needs recognised, their bodies respected and their childbearing capacities valued (Reiger 2001:37).

Partly in response to these claims and partly due to broader changes, a series of accommodations was won. Gradually, hospital practices were modified and labour wards made more woman and family friendly. Traditional labour wards were refurbished and efforts made to make them look less like hospitals. Breastfeeding gained acceptance, even in public (at least until the 'baby' becomes a toddler). By the early 1980s, birth centres, with more women-friendly practices and more homely atmospheres, were being established in major metropolitan hospitals, despite initial opposition from some obstetricians and midwives (Andrews 2000:23; Reiger 2001:187–262). The medical dominance of childbirth, however, remained almost entirely intact despite the recognition of midwives as autonomous professionals in several countries and by bodies such as the World Health Organisation (WHO) (Reiger 2000:56).

Maternity-Care Reform Groups

In Australia, the movement was led by the Childbirth Education Association (CEA), which had been formed in 1961 as the Association for the Advancement of Painless Childbirth, and by Parents Centres Australia. The Nursing Mothers Association (NMA),[1] now the Australian Breastfeeding Association, began in 1964 as a support group but also lobbied to change rigid hospital practices that militated against successful breastfeeding. A plethora of new groups supporting homebirth and maternity reform was established from the 1970s onwards, including Homebirth Access Sydney, Homebirth Australia, Maternity Coalition, the Homebirth Network of SA, Mothers and Midwives' Action Victoria, Natural Parenting Melbourne, Blue Mountains Homebirth Group, Hunter Home and Natural Birth Support, Birth Choices South West WA Inc., Nimbin Birth and Beyond and Joyous Birth, to name just a few. Homebirth Australia is the peak body for homebirth awareness and promotion.

Other birthing-related groups include the Caesarean Awareness Network of Australia, Caesarean Awareness Recovery Education Support SA and friends of birth centres in different States.

The Maternity Coalition (MC) was formed as an advocacy and information-sharing organisation in Victoria and New South Wales in the late 1980s to influence the State government inquiries into maternity care that had been set

---

1 Reiger (2001) provides a detailed account of the activities of the NMA, later the Nursing Mothers Association of Australia, and the CEA.

up. In the mid-1990s, it clarified its goals and philosophy, working to support both consumers and midwives as participants in all aspects of policy and health decision making and in service delivery. It is committed to the promotion of normal physiological birth and breastfeeding. In 1997, it established its own journal, *Birth Matters*, and began to expand beyond the original two States. In 2011, it is a national, non-profit, umbrella organisation, with some 500 individual and organisational members. It argues for women's rights to access to the maternity care of their choice, including community-based midwifery care, and it strongly promotes continuity of care throughout pregnancy, birth and for six weeks postnatally (MC 2008; Newman et al. 2011).

At the same time and in line with international developments, Australian midwives began to organise in what has been called the 'rebirth' of midwifery. Midwives sought to regain their traditional role as autonomous professionals, caring for women in childbirth, independent of both medicine and nursing. They developed their own competency standards, codes of ethics and their own models of care. As Reiger (2000:53) describes it:

> [T]his involves a shift away from a medical/scientific framework and hospital-centric practice towards one emphasising holistic care, the value of intuitive as well as technical knowledge, a collaborative partnership with women and new forms of work organisation. The re-emergence of midwifery away from medical dominance reflects the influence of the feminist critique of medicalised reproduction.

The National Midwives Association was formed in the late 1970s and became the Australian College of Midwives Incorporated (ACMI) in 1987. It has branches in all States and Territories. Other professional groups include the Midwives Action Group, the Australian Society of Independent Midwives, Midwives Australia, the Australian Private Midwives Association, Midwives in Private Practice and the Home Midwifery Association of Queensland. Part of the project to reclaim midwifery was to gain independence from nursing through a separation of education programs. Since the incorporation of midwifery into nursing in earlier decades, a general nursing qualification had been the prerequisite for postgraduate midwifery training. Associations of midwives in the States and Territories, supported by groups such as the MC, set about the task of changing policy to permit the introduction of direct-entry Bachelor of Midwifery degrees. Prospective midwife practitioners would then have a choice of education pathways. Rather than a fragmented medical model, a holistic, continuous model of care is generally promoted. Maternity reform activists want to change present arrangements under which a woman might encounter upwards of 20 midwives and doctors, with none of whom she has a close relationship, during the course of pregnancy and birth (Vernon 2011:3).

A Divided Movement

The maternity-care reform movement in Australia has experienced significant divisions and persistent cleavages alongside commitment to and enthusiasm for change. Breastfeeding and childbirth reform groups faced internal divisions from their inception. They split regularly on personal and philosophical grounds, which sapped energy and limited the materialisation of a national voice. The homebirth movement has been particularly prone to serious divisions on a range of philosophical issues, including disagreements arising from the coexistence within the movement of several strands of feminism (Gosden 1998; Reiger 2001:84–108). Moreover, for the most part, the Australian maternity-care reform movement and the feminist women's movement have largely worked separately (Reiger 2001:264). Unlike the US situation, for example, in Australia, the maternity reform advocates of the 1960s and 1970s did not see themselves primarily as feminists. Although they worked hard to promote women's rights, many were socially conservative (Reiger 2001:176). And while not anti-feminist, some members were primarily committed to childrearing as professional mothers and were not particularly interested in feminist goals, which they saw as stressing achievement in the public sphere. Some, especially in the NMA, feared that promoting women's workforce rights could downgrade their work as mothers in the home.

On the feminist side, childbirth, lactation and mothering have not been major issues, partly due to concerns that such a focus would lead back to essentialism (Reiger 1999b). Economic independence has always been a high priority, however, as well as disruption of the public–private split so that women can participate in both spheres. Work-related issues were therefore emphasised, including accessible child care, education and training opportunities and equal pay. Despite differences, however, there were, and still are, many issues of shared concern, including women's rights to control their own bodies, unnecessary medicalisation, the male medical takeover of reproductive and other health services, patronising attitudes, the inappropriateness of many treatments and the paucity of information.

Given so much commonality, it is perhaps surprising that collaboration has not been closer. In the United Kingdom, the United States and New Zealand, in contrast, links have been close and productive (Garcia et al 1998; Kitzinger 2005). One stumbling block in the Australian context is divergent views about what constitutes access and equity. The issue of private, fee-for-service midwifery practice remains contentious both inside and outside the maternity reform movement. Services provided on a fee-for-service basis are generally not accessible to those on low incomes even when they are publicly subsidised. The introduction of private, fee-for-service maternity care would create the same access and equity problems that currently plague the medical-care system, unless midwifery fees were set by government. Access to services is a critical issue in the general women's health movement and important to those in the homebirth movement who are committed to the availability of public-sector birth care for all Australian women 'across barriers of class and culture' (Gosden 1998:47).

In the fullness of time, however, some of the differences between the early maternity-care reform groups and feminist groups narrowed. According to Reiger, many maternity-care activists became radicalised through their campaign work, including encounters with hospital systems and medical professionals. Many others were influenced by the increasingly feminist stance taken by the homebirth groups that were being formed, sometimes from among their own ranks (Reiger 2001:159–83). On the other side, as they became established, women's health groups began to take a keener interest in maternity care and related issues, such as postnatal care. At the level of service provision, women's health centres responded to the maternity-care needs of their clients. For example, the Leichhardt Women's Community Health Centre (LWCHC) provides a range of reproductive health services, which includes postnatal services and information and care in relation to postnatal depression (LWCHC web site), and Women's Health West in Victoria works with diverse groups of African women and girls through the Family and Reproductive Rights Education Program (Women's Health West web site). The outcome of this convergence was that by the 1980s, maternity-care and birthing issues were on the agendas of both the women's health and the maternity-care reform movements and had found their way into the first NWHP (Andrews 2000:16). For the most part, however, the two movements continued to move forward along parallel pathways—a direction at least partly shaped by limited resources. Unfunded advocacy organisations run by volunteers, whether they be young mothers or women in paid work, find it difficult to manage the workload within their own groups. Time constraints often mean that the establishment of collaborative links is beyond their capacity.

Maternity-Care Reform Becomes a National Issue

As discussed, the political context of the 1980s was favourable for the advancement of women's issues. Concerns found their way onto party political platforms—a process assisted by increasing numbers of female politicians and bureaucrats. The development of the NWHP and the National Agenda for Women in the second half of the decade involved extensive consultation with women, stimulating debate and raising expectations that governments would take effective action to raise the status of women. In this context, the combined impact of advocacy by so many maternity reform and women's health groups created a set of pressures that governments were unable to ignore. In the two decades following the mid-1980s, upwards of 30 major inquiries into Australian maternity care, some specifically focusing on services for Aboriginal women, were undertaken in the States and Territories. Maternity reform groups were able to influence the inquiries, gaining representation on steering committees and working parties in some cases and providing consumer representatives in others.

Maternity care also attracted the attention of two high-level national health agencies in the 1980s: the Medicare Benefits Review Committee and Australia's premier medical research institution, the National Health and Medical Research Council (NHMRC). The latter body took the unprecedented step of establishing the Working Party on Homebirths and Alternative Birth Centres in 1986. A report released the following year endorsed the right of women to choose where to give birth and urged hospitals to modernise their premises and practices. A subsequent publication, the *Statement on Homebirths* (1989), again supported birthing choices. As an advocate of birth centres and home births while simultaneously endorsing the importance of the role played by specialist obstetricians, the NHMRC placed itself in a contradictory position. In 2000, on the advice of its Health Advisory Committee, both the 1987 and the 1989 documents were rescinded (Andrews 2000:28–9).

The Medicare Benefits Review Committee was established in 1984 to assess aspects of the operation of the newly reintroduced national health insurance scheme, Medicare, and to consider whether benefits should be extended to cover the services of selected allied health professionals. In general, the committee did not support the extension of fee-for-service private practice. It suggested instead that the Commonwealth should fund States and Territories to allow allied health services—such as dietetics, occupational therapy, physiotherapy, podiatry and speech pathology—to be provided as part of their community health programs. Allied health professionals would be remunerated by salaries or on a sessional basis (Commonwealth of Australia 1986a:343–90). In this context, the committee recommended against an extension of Medicare benefits to the services of private practice midwives; however, it supported the expansion of birth centres in hospitals, the provision of public funding for midwifery services outside hospitals and it recommended a pilot homebirth program to assess feasibility, safety and costs (Andrews 2000:28).

The State and Territory inquiries of the late 1980s and early 1990s placed a broader range of birthing issues on the various policy agendas (Reiger 2001:281, 2006); however, no State or Territory embarked upon major structural reform. The implacable opposition of the Australian Medical Association (AMA), the

Royal Australian College of Obstetricians and Gynaecologists (RACOG) and the College of General Practitioners presented an almost insurmountable obstacle. In 1989, the two colleges issued a joint statement disregarding NHMRC evidence and emphasising their concerns about the safety of homebirth (Reiger 2001:278). At stake, of course, are the economic interests of the profession, which has recognised the profitability of the maternity 'industry' since the 1920s (Norling and Woodhouse 1998:19).

Another obstacle to action is concern about cost, which is always at the forefront of State and Territory health policymaking because health is the major expenditure item, consuming approximately one-third of sub-national budgets. And while savings are possible from moving service provision out of acute-care hospitals into community settings, federal financial arrangements are a strong disincentive to such experimentation. In the case of maternity care, the Commonwealth funds most of the cost of services provided by obstetricians and general practitioners through Medicare. In the absence of additional Commonwealth money, the States and Territories are reluctant to introduce new midwifery services for which they would not otherwise have to pay, although the additional expense would be partly offset because there would be fewer hospital midwives. The general approach for Australian governments is to try to shift costs onto the other level wherever possible. It is not customary to freely assume expenses that are the responsibility of another government. Moreover, the prevailing managerialist thinking of the day resulted in the frequent restructuring of government departments, which often dislodged key policymakers, including femocrats. Under the circumstances, action was taken on only a few of the recommendations of the various reviews.

Movement at the Local Level

Some scattered innovations, however, began to be undertaken at the local level. By the mid-2000s, team-based midwifery was being trialled in several major hospitals in capital cities in an attempt to increase continuity of care. There are small publicly funded midwifery programs in Perth, in the northern suburbs of Adelaide and in rural Victoria. The Perth program mainly provides homebirth services, the Adelaide program targets low-income mothers, including Aboriginal mothers, and the rural Victoria program is designed to care for young mothers who do not access antenatal services, including young women with mental health issues, drug and alcohol dependence and the like. A successful midwifery-led birthing facility operates from the Mareeba Hospital in far north Queensland. According to Boxall and Flitcroft (2007), system-wide reform is more likely to be introduced when policymakers are able to refer to sufficient examples of successful and popular, midwife-led, locally based programs. At this stage, however, most of the hospital-based initiatives, which are hybrid models, do not achieve high levels of continuity of care because deeply ingrained practices such as working in shifts are retained.

One Step Forward

Forward movement, albeit on a small scale, came from the Commonwealth in the form of the Alternative Birthing Services Program (ABSP), initially called the Birthing Options Program, which was introduced in 1989. The ABSP was heavily influenced by the views that Australian women expressed when they were consulted for the NWHP and several State-level inquiries. Insufficient information, especially for immigrant, Aboriginal and rural women, lack of control of the birthing process, lack of control over place of birth and difficulties with continuity of care were all major concerns. Stress, depression and family disruption were reported by Aboriginal women who are often required to leave their communities up to six weeks before the birth of their babies. Rising levels of birth interventions, including caesarean sections, inductions and forceps deliveries were raised as concerns and women reported that interventions often proceeded without consultation or discussion. 'Most birthing women are healthy and wish to experience normal deliveries in an environment of their choice', the NWHP argued (Commonwealth of Australia 1989:22). The NHMRC's 1987 finding that homebirths were not less safe than hospital births was noted (Commonwealth of Australia 1989:20–7).

In developing the ABSP, the Commonwealth was not thinking only about women's health needs; the program also had a number of perceived advantages. Structural changes in maternity care would reduce the cost to Medicare because midwifery-led services would be cheaper than specialist-dominated, hospital-based services and would provide genuine competition for obstetricians, which should keep downward pressure on their fees. It might also encourage specialists to concentrate on high-risk births, where their skills are needed. Shorter hospital stays would not only save money but would free up beds that could be used to reduce waiting lists. At the same time, midwifery-led programs would offer women more choices (Commonwealth Department of Community Services and Health quoted in Andrews 2000:26–7).

The ABSP was an eight-year program announced concurrently with the first NWHP. The stated objectives were to encourage the sub-national jurisdictions to promote greater choice and to promote cost effectiveness in birthing services through expanded birthing centres and the provision of homebirth services. The policy supported midwifery-led models of care and included an option through which the States and Territories might address Aboriginal women's birthing issues. In providing a public subsidy for homebirth, the Commonwealth was attempting to make services available to low-income women who had not previously been able to afford private fees. Midwives were to be independent but were not to be private fee-for-service practitioners. Rather, they would be employed by sub-national health services on a salaried or contract basis, as had been recommended by the Medicare Benefits Review Committee (Andrews 2000:31–6).

The ABSP met with vehement opposition from the medical profession. The AMA President of the day, Bruce Shepherd, claimed that the guidelines discriminated against doctors and RACOG announced that it did not support homebirth as a safe option. Moreover, it opposed midwives operating independently of doctors and hospitals. In the event and in order to accommodate the position of organised medicine, the program was modified in its second four-year phase. The emphasis remained on midwifery-led services but homebirth was removed altogether from the objectives, even though trials had begun in South Australia and Tasmania as part of the first phase. The second phase placed more emphasis on community-based midwifery and left the States and Territories to choose whether to pursue homebirth options. Sub-national jurisdictions were specifically encouraged to develop appropriate services for Aboriginal and Torres Strait Islander women, especially in relation to ante and postnatal care (Andrews 2000:37–42).[2]

Despite the many perceived policy advantages, the ABSP was never a major program. Indeed, it has been described as 'largely symbolic' given that only $15.3 million was allocated to cover reforms in all States and Territories over eight years (Andrews 2000:27). Nevertheless, a national program, however small, can be seen as a positive outcome following two decades of women's advocacy. Non-medical approaches to childbirth were put on the national policy agenda for the first time and birth centres that had been considered radical 15 years earlier gained legitimacy and were expanded. The status of midwives and midwifery-led practice was enhanced, especially in birth centres, where midwives gained responsibility and greater autonomy. The ABSP played an important role in supporting innovative services, including those at Alukura for Aboriginal women and a publicly funded midwifery service, the Community Midwifery Program in Western Australia, which includes homebirth. It was the first Australian public policy to seriously challenge the entrenched medical domination of maternity care. As Andrews (2000:38) argues, the program

> Explicitly challenged the hegemonic medical model of childbirth that constructed pregnancy as pathological and always a risky business...

---

2   This 'encouragement' was something of an abnegation of responsibility because the Commonwealth has full constitutional power to make laws in relation to Aboriginal people. Space limitations preclude a discussion of the initiatives taken under the ABSP, which are reviewed in Andrews (2000).

The medical hegemonic discourse advocated medical surveillance for all women so that the few who might really need intervention were not overlooked. The ABSP approach argued that all women could choose to have a natural, normal birth free of intervention and that measures should be in place for those few women who may need medical intervention or assistance in the case of an emergency.

The ABSP experience also shows that policy change in fields where strong vested interests hold sway is most likely to take place in very small, incremental steps.

Two Steps Back

The dozen years following the conclusion of the ABSP were not conducive to the promotion of midwifery-led maternity care at the national level. On the contrary, the Howard Government strengthened medical dominance in the health system generally in a number of ways. First, the proportion of Australians holding private insurance who were therefore able to afford private hospital services was increased at considerable expense to the public purse, beginning with a $2 million publicity campaign to promote private insurance in 1996. Then, in 1998, after lesser measures had failed to increase coverage, a 30 per cent public subsidy for private premiums was introduced. When this measure also failed, the Commonwealth changed longstanding policy, permitting private insurers to charge higher premiums to new subscribers as they grow older. Lifetime Health Cover, as this scheme is called, was accompanied by what amounted to scare tactics in the 12 months leading up to its introduction. An $8.7 million, taxpayer-funded publicity campaign urged people to 'Run for Cover', with the result that the numbers of Australians covered by private insurance increased by 50 per cent (Gray 2004:34–8). Higher private insurance coverage, among other things, means more financially rewarding fee-for-service private hospital work for specialists, including obstetricians.

The second windfall for certain groups of specialists, particularly obstetricians and those providing in-vitro fertilisation (IVF) services, came in the form of the Extended Medicare Safety Net (EMSN). Introduced in 2004, the EMSN was supposed to reduce out-of-pocket expenses for citizens; however, an independent review in 2009 found that, overall, the additional Commonwealth expenditure had not lowered costs for patients but had rather increased provider incomes. Moreover, funding was of most benefit to high-income citizens. The 20 per cent of Australians living in the most affluent areas had received 55 per cent of benefits whereas the 20 per cent living in the least affluent areas had received only 3.5 per cent (Commonwealth of Australia 2009f:vi). In 2007, 31 per cent of total benefits under the scheme were paid for obstetrical services and 22 per cent for IVF procedures. The EMSN was found to have had an inflationary impact, forming the basis for steep rises in medical fees, with the most profound effect in the areas of obstetrics and IVF. Between 2003 and 2008, obstetricians reduced their in-hospital fees by 6 per cent while they increased their out-of-hospital fees by 267 per cent.[3] During the same period, in-hospital fees for IVF services were reduced by 9 per cent but out-of-hospital fees were increased by 62 per cent. The review team came to the conclusion that doctors were able to calculate that their patients would qualify for the EMSN and therefore felt 'fewer competitive market pressures to contain their fees' (Commonwealth of Australia 2009f:63, 73).

Thus, the introduction of structural changes that increased private insurance coverage and underpinned fee increases far in excess of inflation served to further embed private obstetrical practice. Under such circumstances, it was unlikely that collaborative or shared care arrangements with midwives would flourish. Other actions by the Howard Government that demonstrate its lack of interest in promoting alternative models of maternity care were its return of the ABSP, along with the NWH Program, to the States and Territories in 1998 and its failure to invite midwives to the National Forum on Medical Indemnity Insurance, chaired by the Minister for Health and Ageing, Senator Kay Patterson, in 2002.

Despite the unpromising national political climate, maternity-care reform groups continued to work for change. MC consciously looked to expand and invited members Barbara Vernon and Justine Cairns to join its executive—a move that heralded a period of major advance for the organisation (Newman et al. 2011:85–6). Realising the need for unity, efforts were made in 2002 to form a cohesive front. The National Maternity Action Plan (NMAP), a detailed document supported by research evidence, was written by the leaders of MC and endorsed by a broad coalition of consumer and provider groups. It was launched in all jurisdictions and it called on governments at both levels to support publicly funded, community-based midwifery care in urban, regional and rural areas. The plan pointed out that the right to choose a midwife as a leading carer is available to women in a number of OECD countries[4] and that scientific evidence shows good outcomes for both mothers and babies.[5] Midwives are in the best position to provide continuity of care from early pregnancy until babies are four to six weeks of age, the NMAP argued, and continuity of care

---

3   This number is not a typographical error.
4   Publicly funded, midwife-led care is readily available in New Zealand, the Netherlands, Britain and Canada.
5   In the Netherlands, childbirth has never been as medicalised as in other OECD countries. In 2007, 41.5 per cent of women remained in primary care throughout pregnancy, labour, birth and during the postpartum period, receiving care from a midwife or a general practitioner; 31.3 per cent gave birth at home. Women are very positive about the quality of the care they receive and intervention and pain relief use is very low compared with that in similar countries (Weigers 2009). A recent study of more than half a million Dutch

has been shown to result in fewer obstetrical interventions, such as caesarean sections. Therefore, as well as providing choice and appropriate care for women, midwifery-led services would save health dollars (MC web site). The launch of the NMAP marked the beginning of a period of strong unity within MC. When in 2003 obstetricians threatened to close their practices in response to high indemnity insurance premiums, the then President of MC, Dr Barbara Vernon, welcomed the announcement, issuing a media release claiming that pregnant women would be better off with fewer obstetricians in private practice.

The National Maternity Services Review

Maternity activists attracted the attention of the ALP in opposition, which announced that it would develop a national maternity services plan should it win office in 2007. Another development that put maternity care on the national agenda was the inquiry of the Productivity Commission into the health workforce which reported in 2005. It recommended 'a shake-up' of the health industry to break down inefficient professional boundaries and promote flexibility (Lane In press). Momentum also came from the Maternity Services Inter-Jurisdictional Committee, set up by the Australian Health Ministers Advisory Council (AHMAC), which increased dialogue across jurisdictions. Picking up consumer lobbying around the NMAP, it put forward a framework to advance primary maternity service provision (AHMAC 2008).

In government, Health Minister, Nicola Roxon, established a National Maternity Services Review led by the Commonwealth's newly appointed Chief Nurse and Midwifery Officer, Rosemary Bryant. The review, which began in 2008, was asked to examine the full range of possible maternity services and to seek information on a number of key issues, such as successful models of care for rural and remote communities and the aspects of the Australian system that fuelled high intervention rates. Submission writing was facilitated by the intensive work of MC and other groups and the review received a record number of more than 900 submissions[6]—more than twice as many as the National Health and Hospitals Reform Commission, which sat at much the same time. Submissions pointed to familiar problems, such as the extremely limited birthing options for women living in rural and remote areas, exacerbated by the closure of more and more rural birthing units because of lack of medical staff. The NSW Midwives Association, the Menzies School of Public Health and the Australian Indigenous

women by British researchers found that there is no difference in the perinatal mortality rate during the first week of life between homebirths and hospital births. The number of babies who die or need neonatal intensive care is the same in both groups at seven per 1000 births (de Jonge et al. 2009).

6   Submissions to the review can be found at <http://www.health.gov.au/internet/main/publishing.nsf/Content/maternityservicesreview-submissions>

Doctors Association stressed the problems facing Aboriginal and Torres Strait Islander women whose babies have poorer perinatal outcomes. These submissions argued what experienced practitioners had known for years: that giving birth far from home disrupts the link between birthplace and land, separates families, causes additional and unnecessary stress and is culturally inappropriate and unsafe.[7] Also frequently mentioned were difficulties experienced in obtaining continuity of care and the inappropriate utilisation of acute-care hospitals for healthy birthing women, resulting in the overuse of technologies that should be reserved for women with complications.

The Australian College of Midwives' submission presented 13 reasons for Australia's high intervention rate, including the absence of consistent, professionally endorsed, evidence-based guidelines for appropriate practice. David Ellwood, Professor of Obstetrics and Gynaecology at the School of Clinical Medicine, the Canberra Hospital, made a personal submission, focusing on intervention rates, the adverse impact of the private health insurance subsidy on public hospital services and the need for a national approach to maternal and perinatal morbidity and mortality reporting. 'The inexorable rise in the caesarean section rate is something which needs to be addressed as a matter of some urgency', Elwood argued. He noted that the rate is significantly higher in the private sector and commented that it is 'an odd situation' when women can choose elective caesarean sections and be financially supported for doing so but Aboriginal women are unable to choose to birth naturally on their own country. He argued that an appropriate response would be to increase the availability of midwifery-led care. Ellwood also drew attention to the adverse impact of the EMSN on the capacity of public hospitals to attract medical staff. Incomes are so good in the private sector, he argued, that it is possible to work part-time and still ensure a reasonable income. Policies need to be changed 'so that full-time employment in the public sector is more competitive with the kinds of incomes which are now possible in the private sector' (Ellwood 2008).

On the positive side, submissions drew attention to a number of successful local innovations. These include the midwifery-led Belmont Birthing Service in New South Wales, which provides education and preparation for birth, parenting sessions, breastfeeding information and continuity of care. The service is for all women in the Hunter region and is linked closely with John Hunter Hospital's obstetric services where medical support is available when needed. The Malabar Community Midwifery Link Service, run by the Sydney Royal Hospital for Women, is located in an area with a large Aboriginal population. It is considered to be culturally appropriate, is available to people living in surrounding suburbs and to Aboriginal women from outside the area. Its high standard of service has

7   See, for example, Australian Indigenous Doctors Association (2008); Baldwin-Jones (1989); Cox (2009); Fitzpatrick (1995); Menzies School of Health Research (2008).

been recognised (Homebirth Access Sydney submission). Another successful model of care has been developed by the Orange Aboriginal Medical Service, which has links with local professionals, including allied health professionals, and the Orange Base Hospital.

Submissions to the review by medical unions supported the status quo. It was argued that Australia had a high standard of safety for mothers and babies that would be jeopardised if medical control were undermined. Intervention rates had increased but this was a phenomenon in all OECD countries largely because mothers are older and there is a higher incidence of obesity and related illnesses. The AMA supported expanded funding arrangements for midwives but only if midwives were medically supervised. The idea of independent midwives as autonomous professionals is anathema:

> Highly interventionist government agendas to advance an ideological cause are likely to create problems in the delivery of maternity services and exacerbate tensions in interprofessional relationships…The government should not introduce any publicly funded arrangement which is based on independent midwife care for mothers and babies in Australia or use public funds to establish separate streams of midwife led maternal care on the one hand and medical led maternal care on the other. (AMA 2008)

The Royal Australian and New Zealand College of Obstetricians and Gynaecologists (RANZCOG)[8] argued for a collaborative model in which obstetricians, general practitioners, midwives, anaesthetists, paediatricians, pathologists and allied health professionals would work together. It opposed independent midwifery practice 'where one particular professional group or individual works in isolation'. Instead, it proposed a 'Private Collaborative Model', under which private midwives and private obstetricians or private general practitioners would work together within a framework of agreed protocols and guidelines.

The review released its report, *Improving maternity services in Australia*, in February 2009 (Commonwealth of Australia 2009g). It made 18 recommendations that it suggested the Commonwealth, States and Territories might consider during the development of the proposed National Maternity Services Plan. A key recommendation was that the importance of the midwifery role should be recognised and choice should be enhanced by expanding the range of maternity-care models on offer. Consideration should be given to changing Commonwealth funding arrangements, and professional indemnity insurance for midwives should be supported. Other recommendations included the development of national multidisciplinary guidelines for collaborative models

---

8   RACOG amalgamated with the Royal New Zealand College of Obstetricians and Gynaecologists in 1998.

of care, the expansion of birth centres and the provision of more comprehensive information for pregnant and breastfeeding women. Four recommendations related to improving services for Aboriginal women and increasing cultural awareness (Commonwealth of Australia 2009g:57–9). Homebirth, however, was dismissed on the grounds that it is the preferred choice of relatively few women (Commonwealth of Australia 2009g:15–21). In welcoming the report, Minister Roxon said that it brought better services for mothers and babies 'one step closer'. She noted the widespread concern expressed about high rates of medical intervention, high rates of postnatal depression and the relatively low rates of breastfeeding (Gordon 2009).

Responses to the report followed predictable lines, with midwifery and nursing groups welcoming the endorsement of an expanded role for midwives but expressing reservations about the failure to consider the homebirth option in more depth. The Commonwealth responded with a very modest $120.5 million maternity reform package as part of the 2009–10 Budget. Under the package, the patients of eligible midwives and nurse practitioners[9] would have access to specified Medicare and pharmaceutical benefits. The Commonwealth would underwrite a new professional indemnity insurance scheme for midwives and nurse practitioners, deliver more services to rural and remote locations through the Medical Specialist Outreach Assistance Program, increase scholarships for general practitioners and midwives and introduce a 24-hour, seven-day-a-week telephone help and information service (Jolly et al. 2009:8–10).

Legislation to facilitate the new arrangements was introduced into Parliament in June 2009 and had a turbulent passage. The Senate referred it to the Community Affairs Legislation Committee for inquiry—an outcome that had been partly shaped by MC, which had lobbied parliamentarians extensively in order to gain more scrutiny of the proposals. MC had organised the 'Mother of All Rallies' in September at which approximately 3000 homebirth supporters had converged on Parliament House. It was also at least partly responsible for the unexpected support for expanded options shown by a number of speakers in the Senate. Another round of public hearings was held and more submissions received. After considering the most controversial issues, particularly homebirth, the committee satisfied itself that the legislation was sound, that it did not remove existing rights and would not make homebirth unlawful. It recommended that the Bills be passed; however, Commonwealth amendments attempting to clarify the meaning of 'collaborative arrangements' resulted in referral to the Community Affairs Legislation Committee yet again, provoking more controversy and generating more submissions. The committee concluded that the proposed collaborative arrangements would allow a flexible approach to

---

9   The Australian Nursing Federation has argued for access to Medicare benefits and prescribing rights for nurse practitioners since the 1990s but the proposition has been vigourously opposed by medical unions.

practice across the country and recommended that the Bills be passed. Senator Rachel Siewert, of the Australian Greens, produced a dissenting report arguing that it is unnecessary to legislate for collaborative arrangements since they are already encoded within regulatory frameworks (Senate Community Affairs Legislation Committee 2010). In the event, the Commonwealth did not proceed with its amendments and instead negotiations were held with stakeholders to work out details. The Senate finally passed the legislation in March 2010.

As promised, the National Maternity Services Plan has been developed and endorsed by the Australian Health Ministers Conference to cover the five-year period from November 2010. The plan's vision is stated as follows:

> Maternity care will be woman-centred, reflecting the needs of each woman in a safe and sustainable quality system. All Australian women will have access to high-quality, evidence-based, culturally competent maternity care in a range of settings close to where they live. Provision of such maternity care will contribute to closing the gap between health outcomes of Aboriginal and Torres Strait Islander people and non-Indigenous Australians. Appropriately trained and qualified maternity health professionals will be able to provide continuous maternity care to all women. (Commonwealth of Australia 2011c:3)

The plan confirms that Australia is a safe place to give birth, except for Aboriginal and Torres Strait Islander women. It also confirms the comparatively high rate of interventions in Australia, which in 2007 was 5.2 per cent above the OECD average. It notes that interventions in the private sector are 'substantially higher' than the average (Commonwealth of Australia 2011c:9). Actions agreed for the first year include the facilitation of increased access to midwifery-managed models of care, investigation by the States and Territories of options for the provision of publicly funded homebirths and identification of the characteristics of culturally competent maternity care for Aboriginal and Torres Strait Islander women (Commonwealth of Australia 2011c:61–9). It is too early to assess the effectiveness of the plan but its success will at least partly depend on the provision of sufficient Commonwealth funds to induce the States and Territories to themselves shoulder the costs of services that would otherwise be paid for mostly by the Commonwealth through Medicare.

The new maternity-care arrangements became fully operational on 1 November 2010. Medicare rebatable services can now be provided by eligible midwives for care during pregnancy, labour and birth in a hospital—as long as the midwife has admitting rights—and for home-based postnatal care for six weeks after birth. Routine tests can be ordered and specified drugs prescribed. The Commonwealth is underwriting professional indemnity insurance for all eligible midwives, which has not been available since 2001 when a crisis in the insurance industry resulted in the withdrawal of existing policies for midwives. A small window is therefore open for the development of new care models. Private obstetricians may enter into arrangements with midwives that allow them to provide continuity and team-based care, before, during and after birth, although the price might be prohibitive for many women. Choices for Aboriginal and Torres Strait Islander women might be expanded, allowing them to birth 'on country' or closer to country but only if midwives and doctors willing to collaborate are available. Midwifery Group Practices (MGPs), where hospitals employ midwives to look after women through all the stages of pregnancy and birth, might be expanded. Currently, MGPs, located largely in metropolitan areas, are in their infancy and are unable to meet demand. The new legislation will allow the establishment of private MGPs, provided collaborative arrangements can be negotiated, but accessibility will be an issue (Vernon 2011:36).

There are, however, a number of hurdles to be overcome before significant change emerges. In the first place, few midwives currently have the qualifications and experience to become Medicare eligible. Second, the States and Territories have the capacity to place barriers in the way of successful implementation because they, rather than the Commonwealth, have the power to grant the legal right to prescribe under the Pharmaceutical Benefits Scheme. They also have the power to grant or withhold hospital visiting rights for midwives. In the past, some jurisdictions have granted visiting rights; others have not (Vernon 2011:36). Moreover, State and Territory governments do not have full power in this area because decisions are made at the level of the individual hospital board where doctors have considerable influence. Further, it is not known what stance private hospitals will take in relation to visiting rights. Without visiting rights, a midwife cannot care for a woman in hospital during labour and birth, thereby severely disrupting continuity of care.

The Commonwealth initiatives have met with a mixed response from the maternity-care reform movement. The Australian College of Midwives and the Australian Nursing Federation (ANF), for example, endorse those aspects of the reforms that support private midwifery practice (ANF 2009; Australian College of Midwives 2009). Most groups, however, are disappointed that the Commonwealth is not underwriting indemnity insurance for homebirth midwives, thus virtually excluding homebirth from the reforms.

The new measures do not make homebirth unlawful but indemnity insurance is a condition of registration for midwives, as for other professionals. Transitional arrangements providing exemption from this requirement are due to expire towards the end of 2011, when homebirth will become illegal. One concern is that homebirth will then be driven underground (Commonwealth Department of Health and Ageing n.d.; Jolly et al. 2009:10–13).

The groups within the movement that have worked to achieve an independent midwifery profession are extremely disappointed with the requirement that to become 'eligible', midwives must enter into collaborative arrangements with one or more doctors. Under the new arrangements, doctors must approve of a woman's care and may revoke that approval at any time. This gives medical practitioners control over the way midwives work and control over women's choices, at least indirectly. It certainly negates midwifery's claim to independent professional status. As Lane (In press) argues, 'genuine collaboration fails to flourish under vertical structures'. In her view, we now have a 'militarised form of collaboration where midwives are now more firmly relegated to subsidiary status than ever before by legislative decree'. Critics question the need for contracts and agreements between private medical practitioners and midwives, arguing that the existing regulatory framework ensures collaboration between team members. A study of existing team-care projects in three States shows that midwives collaborated routinely but that many visiting doctors 'resisted authentic collaborative practices' (Lane In press). It has been pointed out that independent midwives who might wish to practice in rural and remote areas will be unable to do so if there is no doctor close by (Barclay 2010:1).

In summary, the path towards maternity-care reform is littered with conflict. Consumers mobilised to assert the rights of birthing women, midwives struggled to become independent professionals, while groups within the medical profession worked to preserve their sphere of practice. Despite intense opposition, however, public policy has been modified and opportunities for incremental expansion of midwifery practice have been created. The movement has achieved a modification of practices associated with childbirth and breastfeeding and has contributed to attitudinal change over many years. Maternity care is, however, as medicalised as ever. The structure of health financing, along with entrenched cultural norms, provides inducements for women to seek medicalised childbirth. Further, the reforms do not provide women with choice of carer, choice of birth location or the right to make their own decisions about care—rights that New Zealand women gained in the 1990s. As a recent analysis argues:

> [O]bstetrics, despite increased [numbers of] women entering the profession, continues to act as an institutional bastion of male domination of women, overriding women's agency in childbirth and maintaining masculine 'medicine'…while alternative 'birth models that work', emphasising interaction, holistic care and the integrity of organisms, struggle for legitimacy and support. (Newman et al. 2011:91)

A Woman's Right to Choose

Some of the strongest collaborations between Australian feminist groups have taken place around reproductive rights, particularly the right to safe, affordable abortion. Building on the work and achievements of existing abortion law reform associations, the advent of the second-wave women's movement saw the formation of multiple groups ready to campaign for a woman's right to access abortion and a full range of contraceptives and abortifacients. Some groups formed to campaign specifically for sexual and reproductive rights. Others were established with a broader agenda but welcomed the chance to work with like-minded groups. Pro-choice groups have worked with each other, with women's health centres and services, with most groups in the women's movement, with family planning associations and with groups with a wider focus, such as the YWCA. Along with campaigns against violence, the struggle for reproductive choice has been a unifying force in the women's movement (Goldrick-Jones 2002:123), although as mentioned, many Aboriginal women do not share the majority view.

Throughout history, women have looked to termination as a response to unwanted pregnancies despite restrictive legislation and unconscionable practices; however, prior to the 1960s, abortion was not politicised in Australia. In contrast with the English situation where the Abortion Law Reform Association was founded in 1936, in Australia, groups had not yet mobilised to call for the liberalisation of old laws (Siedlecky and Wyndham 1990:66). In the United Kingdom, after years of intense debate, the *Abortion Act* was passed in 1967 legalising abortion up to 28 weeks' gestation. At the same time, pro-choice groups had mobilised in the United States and some jurisdictions had begun to liberalise their laws. These debates spread to Australia where interest in reform began to be articulated. At the time, governments presided over criminal codes that retained abortion and regimes that taxed contraceptives and excluded sex education from schools.

After the passage of the UK legislation, the Australian Humanist Society promoted the establishment of abortion law reform associations, which by 1971 were set up in all States and the Australian Capital Territory. In the meantime, changes had taken place in two jurisdictions as a result of cases where doctors were charged with procuring abortions. In 1969 in Victoria, the Menhennit ruling set out the conditions under which abortion could be lawfully performed, which included the necessity 'to protect a woman from serious danger to her life or her physical or mental health'. Three years later in New South Wales, a similar judgment was made by Mr Justice Levine. The definition of mental health was extended to include the effects of economic and social stress. Neither the Menhennit nor the Levine rulings changed the law, as such. The first State to reform its abortion law was South Australia, where legislation was passed in 1969 making abortion lawful when a medical practitioner considers that continuing the pregnancy involves a risk to the life, physical or mental health of the mother or when there is a substantial risk that the child will be seriously handicapped. The Northern Territory passed similar legislation in 1974, while there were two unsuccessful attempts to introduce legislative reform in Western Australia in the late 1960s and early 1970s (Siedlecky and Wyndham 1990:78–86).[10]

Feminists Step up to the Plate

From the early 1970s onwards, feminists formed groups dedicated to the twin tasks of abortion law reform and the provision of support for women who needed it. Early groups included the Women's Abortion Action Coalition, set up in 1972 in Melbourne, and the Abortion Information Service, opened in Perth in 1974, which was subject to a police raid early in its existence. A raft of groups was formed in Adelaide in the early 1970s, including The Body Politic, concerned with contraception, abortion and health, and the Adelaide Abortion Referral Service, which later became the Counsellors' Collective. A Women's Right to Choose, which held public meetings every few weeks, was another Adelaide group.

In Sydney, Control set up an abortion information, referral and counselling service at Women's House, in 1973. Pregnancy testing and contraceptive advice were added later. It lobbied doctors to reduce their fees for abortion and encouraged them to introduce their own counselling services and to provide contraceptive advice. All workers were voluntary and rostered themselves to provide services in the evenings and on Saturday afternoons (Stevens 1995:27). An associated group was the Women's Abortion Action Campaign (WAAC), formed in Sydney in 1972, and in Adelaide and Brisbane in 1973. WAAC's purpose was to campaign for the repeal of abortion laws and it organised a National Conference on Contraception and Abortion attended by more than 400 women in 1975 (Siedlecky and Wyndham 1990:86). Control, Queensland, also known as the Women's Pregnancy Advisory and Abortion Referral Service, was set up in 1977 and operated with the support of Women's House.

No account of the early campaigns for reproductive rights would be complete without mention of the work of Jo and Bertram Wainer in Melbourne. Jo Wainer was the inaugural Secretary of the local Abortion Law Reform Association. As she remembers it, the group had no language with which to discuss reproductive rights and had to invent it. The Wainers gathered information about backyard

---

10   Siedlecky and Wyndham (1990) provide a detailed historical account of Australian struggles for women's reproductive rights until the 1980s.

abortion networks, police corruption and professional abortionists, which they publicised through every available avenue. In 1969, Bertram Wainer, a general practitioner, devised a scheme through which police corruption could be exposed, and afterwards, agitated for a public inquiry. Test cases were organised to explore the extent of the Menhennit ruling. Because lucrative business dealings were being exposed, threats were made against the Wainers' lives. Bertram Wainer was evicted from his surgery and censored by the AMA. In 1972, he established Australia's first open abortion clinic, in St Kilda, and in subsequent years both Wainers continued to campaign (Wainer 2006:1–18).

Coalitions and Collaborations

One of the first major collaborative projects between women's groups took place in 1982 when the Right to Choose Coalition was formed by WEL, the Union of Australian Women, the Women's Abortion Action Committee, the Australian Union of Students Women's Department, the Working Women's Centre, Melbourne, the Melbourne Unitarian Church, the ALP Status of Women Committee and the Women's Right to Abortion Committee. The coalition produced a monthly newsletter called *Freedom to Choose*. The Women's Abortion Action Coalition also formed in Melbourne and collaborated with interstate groups.

Since the 1970s, activism far too extensive to document here has continued in all Australian jurisdictions, generally involving coalitions of women's groups. An account of women's experiences seeking abortion in Queensland, Tasmania and South Australia between 1985 and 1992 has been written by Lyndall Ryan, Margie Ripper and Barbara Buttfield (1994). The work of one of the major actors, Children by Choice, Queensland, was described briefly in Chapter 2. The remainder of this chapter provides an overview of recent collaborative action, including unsuccessful attempts to secure access to medical abortion, and brief accounts of the three successful campaigns to remove abortion from sub-national criminal codes.

The Mifepristone Debacle

Access to medical abortion is available in most OECD countries including the United States but in Australia its use remains illegal in several jurisdictions. Medical abortion can improve access for the hundreds of thousands of women who live far from a surgical facility and it is considerably cheaper than surgical abortion. Availability would increase choice for women, some of whom might be attracted by greater privacy. The retention of abortion in criminal codes restricts availability and can have disastrous consequences for individuals: in 2010, a young Queensland couple was tried for procuring an abortion, using medicines imported from the Ukraine.[11]

Some of the problems that the women's movement has faced when trying to achieve reform can be attributed to the structure of the Australian political system, where a single senator can achieve a strong bargaining position if her/his vote is critical for the government of the day. Brian Harradine, Independent Senator for Tasmania from 1975 until 2005, was one such and he used the opportunities that presented to the full. Over the years, he made several attempts to have access to contraception and abortifacients reduced, to have Australia's overseas aid regulated so that abortion and contraceptive provision would be restricted[12] and to abolish the Medicare rebate for abortion. In this last crusade, he was unsuccessful.

In the early 1990s, RU-486, also known as mifepristone, was available in Australia, as part of international trials; however, the anti-choice movement staged an intense campaign against it and in 1996 Senator Harradine proposed legislation that required the Commonwealth Health Minister to approve the importation, evaluation, registration and listing of certain abortifacient drugs and, furthermore, to table approval in both Houses of Parliament within five sitting days. Despite women's movement protests and the work of many parliamentary women, the legislation was passed. Labor Party Senator Rosemary Crowley wrote to AWHN expressing disappointment that she had been 'unable to persuade a majority' of her colleagues to oppose the amendment. With the new requirements in place, pharmaceutical companies did not seek approval to market the drug from the Therapeutic Goods Administration (TGA)—a process that is expensive, would provoke political controversy and might result in approval being overturned in Parliament.

This was still the situation in 2006 when, following initial moves by Australian Democrats Senator Lyn Allison and some fancy footwork and face-saving manoeuvres by the Howard Government, a Private Member's Bill to override the Harradine amendment was introduced from the Government's own ranks by Nationals Senator Fiona Nash. The Bill was opposed by Health Minister, Tony Abbott, and the Prime Minister. Senator Nash enlisted the support of Senators Judith Troeth (Liberal), Claire Moore (Labor) and Senator Allison in drafting and sponsoring the legislation (Dowse 2009). A massive support campaign was organised by pro-choice groups. Twenty NGOs, including AWHN, Sexual Health and Family Planning Australia, the Australian Reproductive Health Alliance,

---

11   After waiting for almost two years for a trial in an overstretched court system, the couple was acquitted.
12   The restrictions on overseas aid remained in place until March 2009, when, in response to heavy lobbying by the women's movement, the women's health movement, the Greens and others, the restrictions were overturned.

Women's Health NSW, the Public Health Association of Australia and WEL, formed a new coalition: Reproductive Choice Australia (RCA). RCA worked to inform the debate in the media, on the Web and in public forums. It produced fact sheets, wrote letters and held health information sessions. It monitored the media, responding to all significant arguments. There were more than 1000 media articles in the 12 months preceding the passage of the legislation. Pro-choice members of the Senate supported an inquiry into the proposals, which extended the period of controversy. After the Prime Minister announced that a conscience vote would be permitted, RCA systematically lobbied Members of the national Parliament. The Bill passed through both Houses in February 2006. Ninety per cent of women senators, regardless of party, voted for the Bill, but only 46 per cent of men. It was passed in the House on a show of hands because the Government anticipated the outcome and did not want a division to be called (Dowse 2009).

The 2006 amendment removed the power of the Commonwealth Health Minister over the importation of abortifacients, returning authority to the TGA; however, medical abortion is still not freely available because pharmaceutical companies have not applied to import and distribute the relevant drugs. Individual doctors or groups of doctors may apply to the TGA for approval to import and distribute but this type of strategy is hampered because abortion remains in the criminal codes of four States and one Territory.

Working to Liberalise Laws

After more than 40 years of activism, the liberalisation of abortion law has been achieved in fewer than half the Australian jurisdictions. When criminal charges were laid against the Queensland couple in 2009, women's groups moved swiftly into action. Intense controversy erupted, especially in Queensland, where Labor was in government and a woman, Anna Bligh, was Premier. A new coalition, Pro Choice Qld, was established. Large rallies were held, support flowed in from groups around the country and the Government was urged to remove abortion from the State's criminal code, once and for all. Those Queensland doctors who were facilitating medical abortions suspended operations as fears about illegality re-emerged. State cabinet approved legislative changes in November but only to make mifepristone lawful under the same circumstances as surgical abortion—that is, where there is a serious health risk to the mother. Agitation for decriminalisation continued but at the end of 2009 Premier Bligh made it clear that her government had no plans to act. Any reform legislation would have to be introduced as a Private Member's Bill and she would not bind her colleagues to any particular position (Elks 2009). That situation prevails in 2011.

In three jurisdictions—Western Australia, the Australian Capital Territory and Victoria—however, women have succeeded in having abortion removed from the criminal code. In each case, women's groups mobilised and worked closely together. In the Western Australian case, controversy broke out in 1998 when two medical practitioners were arrested for performing an abortion, after a child had repeated family discussion in a classroom 'news' slot. The view of the authorities involved was that the correct interpretation of Western Australian law was that abortion was legal only in life-threatening situations. Upon the arrests, hospitals and clinics cancelled abortion lists and the ANF advised members not to participate in procedures. Amid rallies and speeches, two Bills were introduced into Parliament. A member of the Opposition Labor Party, Cheryl Davenport, introduced an abortion repeal bill into the Upper House, while Attorney-General, Peter Foss, introduced a less radical Bill into the Lower House. Unrestrained debate took place over a period of weeks, during which one member made a three-hour speech! Both Bills eventually passed both Houses; however, the Upper House responded by ruling the Foss Bill out of order, leaving only the Davenport Bill before the Parliament. There followed a period in which a host of amendments, some seriously restrictive, was proposed. On 6 May 1998, however, the Lower House passed the Davenport Bill, which made abortion legal in cases where a woman has given informed consent. On 21 May, the legislation was passed in the Upper House. The relevant sections of the Western Australian Criminal Code were repealed and replaced with a new section that makes it unlawful for anyone other than a medical practitioner to perform an abortion. While the campaign for complete repeal failed, termination is now lawful where a woman has given informed consent.[13]

The first jurisdiction to achieve complete decriminalisation was the Australian Capital Territory, after feminist campaigns spread over more than 30 years. The legislation in force when self-government was handed down required that all abortions be carried out in a public hospital. Women went on a waiting list, and afterwards, appeared before a committee, which included a psychiatrist, to establish eligibility or otherwise. Most women who could afford it chose to travel interstate rather than be part of the waiting list/committee process. A coalition of local feminist groups, Options for Women, was active on an as-needed basis in the Territory from the 1980s onwards, agitating for reform. Members included Sexual Health and Family Planning ACT (SHFPACT), the ACT Women's Health Network (ACTWHN), WEL, the YWCA and representatives from a range of services, such as the Rape Crisis Centre, the Domestic Violence Crisis Service and various refuges. After the election of a Labor government led by Rosemary Follett, in 1991, the Minister for Health, Wayne Berry, introduced legislation that allowed a freestanding clinic to be established. The legislation had a

---

13   For a discussion of legal complications that could emerge from the legislation see Stephen (n.d.).

difficult and protracted passage because not all members of the Government supported it but it was eventually passed. Subsequently, SHFPACT borrowed a large sum of money to set up Reproductive Health Services Proprietary Limited (RHS), adding a fraught responsibility to its list of duties.[14] Establishment was supported by the Health Minister, who made secure premises available at peppercorn rent, giving ACT women access to a feminist-run service that met with the ethical code of the Abortion Providers' Federation of Australia.

In 1994, Minister Berry had a Crimes Amendment Bill prepared, which sought to repeal the three relevant sections of the Criminal Code. Intense campaigns by pro and anti-choice forces followed. The proposal was set aside in preparation for the 1995 election, which the Labor Party lost. In 1998, under a Liberal minority government, which provided another institutional window of opportunity, a counterattack was launched by Independent Member of the Legislative Assembly, Paul Osborne. He introduced a Bill with the stated intention of reducing the number of abortions. Termination was to be permitted only in cases of 'grave medical risk' or 'grave psychiatric risk', with teams of doctors to be on hand to make assessments. Again, groups of ACT women took to the streets, holding rallies, speaking to the media and lobbying. At the same time, pro-choice members of the Government worked to have the more restrictive provisions of the legislation amended. The modified *Health Regulations* (*Maternal Health Information*) *Act* was passed into law in 1994, causing enormous problems for the board of RHS. The legislation required that women undergo a 72-hour 'cooling off' period between their first contact with a doctor and a termination. This requirement was both demeaning and particularly difficult for women living in surrounding rural areas. Another requirement was that information, including pictures of unborn foetuses, be provided to all women seeking an abortion. In the event, legal opinion was obtained that advised that 'provision' did not mean requiring women to open and read mandated material provided in large brown, sealed envelopes. Had staff been required to show foetal pictures to clients, the RHS Board would almost certainly have decided to cease operations. The legislation remained in place while the Liberal Party held government.

Prior to the 2001 election, Wayne Berry, in opposition, released draft legislation for the repeal of both the abortion provisions of the *Crimes Act* and the Osborne legislation. Candidates were questioned by WEL and other women's groups about their attitudes to the proposed legislation at pre-election gatherings. Labor was returned to government at the October election and, in early December, the two Bills were introduced into the Assembly. Options for Women was brought

---

14   RHS caused continual difficulties for its parent association throughout its 12 years of existence. Apart from ACT Government legislation, which at one time threatened to close the service, there were successive legal cases to be handled, as challenges came thick and fast, requiring that a lawyer be appointed on retainer. That the legal situation played havoc with the organisation's capacity to obtain affordable insurance was only one of many problems.

out of abeyance to conduct a support campaign. All the customary strategies were used, with perhaps one addition: for several weeks, information stalls were set up in major shopping centres on Saturday mornings. A roster was developed and women from a variety of organisations went together in pairs, hauling fold-up tables and boxes of papers, posters and pamphlets. The most common response from members of the public was 'You're joshing me! Are you for real? Abortion is illegal?'

As in the Western Australian Parliament, the ACT Assembly was the site of various manoeuvres, including the introduction of alternative legislation by an anti-choice member. When the time came to vote, no-one could predict what the result would be but indications were that it would be extremely close. And so it transpired: the Assembly was deadlocked at eight votes to eight, until Helen Cross of the LPA, who had not divulged her position, voted with the six Labor members, one Green and one Democrat to pass the two Bills on 21 August 2002. Cross took the view that retention of abortion in the Criminal Code was archaic. Although members were free to exercise a conscience vote, Cross was ostracised and later expelled from her party. The Osborne legislation was repealed and all mention of abortion was removed from the *Crimes Act 1900*. The Australian Capital Territory became the first Australian jurisdiction where abortion is regulated under health legislation like any other medical procedure. The dogged determination of Berry and his assistant, Sue Robinson, made a huge contribution to the outcome, as did Helen Cross, of course, the only member of the LPA who supported the reform.

The most recent success took place in Victoria, where abortion was also removed completely from the Criminal Code, in 2008. The Victorian campaign was a long, carefully planned collaboration between many pro-choice groups, demonstrating the relative ease with which momentum can be mobilised on this issue. The process began in response to the increasingly hostile pronouncements about women's reproductive rights made by members of the Howard Government, including the Prime Minister and the Health Minister, Tony Abbott. In 2005, representatives from women's health and reproductive and sexual health groups met and agreed to work proactively to protect women's rights, forming the Association for the Legal Right to Abortion (ALRA), which was later incorporated. The association had a broad-based membership and its major objective was to have abortion removed from the Criminal Code through a campaign that would last as long as necessary. The approach chosen was to educate politicians, members of the media and the community about the problems that arose from the criminal status of a medical service that many women use. Health professionals and their organisations were encouraged to make their views public.

ALRA strategies included meeting all Victorian Members of Parliament, questioning them about their attitudes to reform legislation and inviting them to join the ALRA. In the first year, seven ALRA briefing papers were written and made available on the web site, which had links to the extensive resources on the WHV web site. A comprehensive range of information papers, including 'What MPs need to know about termination of pregnancy', was produced and disseminated. Resources were developed to facilitate community participation in the lead-up to the 2006 election. A table of Victorian parliamentarians was drawn up that included their concerns and voting intentions. All parliamentarians were provided with information and key women in all parties were approached for support. Health movement members met regularly with their local Members of Parliament.

Through the four-year campaign, all briefing papers were reviewed annually and new papers were written in response to issues that emerged from MP interviews. In 2006, ALRA and WHV staged a forum, capitalising on an SBS documentary on the life of Dr Bertram Wainer. Media and communication expertise was obtained and spokespeople were given media training. Activists were careful not to make decriminalisation an issue for the 2006 election as part of a deal with the Premier but they strongly supported pro-choice candidates. Immediately after the November election, campaigning recommenced. The Royal Women's Hospital, the Centre for Women's Health, Gender and Society, Melbourne University and WHV cooperated to stage a conference at the end of November that produced an advocacy tool, *Abortion in Victoria, Melbourne Declaration*. ALRA calculated that there were sufficient supporters in Parliament to pass decriminalisation legislation. The following month, WHAV formed a new group, the Abortion Law Reform Women's Health Services Campaign Organising Group. Its activities included letter writing, media releases, creating copy for newsletters, meeting with parliamentarians, keeping a list of supporters and facilitating local electorate activity. Its work was coordinated by WHV and it made an important contribution to the campaign.

In July 2007, Labor parliamentarian Candy Broad announced her intention to introduce a Private Member's Bill seeking decriminalisation, amid a storm of protest. By this time, however, a number of key professional bodies, including RANZCOG and the AMA supported decriminalisation. The private Bill was withdrawn in August after Premier, John Brumby, made a commitment to pursue reform and asked the Victorian Law Reform Commission (VLRC) to provide advice on legislative options by March 2008. The Premier argued that it was essential that the law reflect contemporary community standards. The commission held multiple meetings with different groups and received more than 500 submissions. Its report was released in March but remained cabinet-in-confidence until June.

As in other places, campaigning was intense. WHV continued to produce evidence-based resources for general campaign use. Yet another broad coalition, ProChoice Victoria, was formed, which included the Multicultural Centre for Women's Health, RCA, the Doctors Reform Society of Australia and Marie Stopes International. It helped to organise rallies and forums, it lobbied, wrote letters to *The Age* newspaper and participated in radio and television interviews. An active web-based advocacy tool was established. Anti-choice campaigners targeted pro-choice MPs with messages and letters in an effort to change minds and picketed the entrances to termination facilities. At one point, a 2000-person anti-choice rally was held and the city was draped with posters depicting foetuses at different stages of development. At another point, the Roman Catholic Archbishop threatened to shut down the maternity and emergency departments of Catholic hospitals if the Bill were passed. In the meantime, ALRA and WHV continued a strategy of quiet approaches to parliamentarians and encouragement of active community participation. Community watching networks were formed in different electorates which fed information back to WHV about anti-choice activity.

When the VLRC report was tabled in Parliament, activism intensified. The report recommended three options, two that would leave the situation unclear and conditional and a third, model C, which would provide for lawful abortion on the basis of a woman's informed consent. Parliamentarians who supported option C were encouraged to make their position known and WHV kept a list.

In August, the Minister for Women's Affairs, Maxine Morand, introduced the Abortion Law Reform Bill 2008 into the Parliament. Based on model C, the legislation proposed to fully decriminalise abortion during the first 24 weeks of pregnancy, after which women would need the permission of two doctors, who may approve the procedure if they considered it medically appropriate, taking into account a woman's current and future physical, psychological and social circumstances.

Within Parliament, more than 40 amendments were moved in the Lower House, most of which sought to impose a variety of restrictions, such as making counselling compulsory. Similarly, in the Upper House, more than 70 amendments were put forward. In the event, a conscience vote took place on 11 September and the Victorian Abortion Law Reform Bill passed, unamended, in the Lower House by a vote of 49 to thirty-two. The Bill passed unamended into law in the Upper House late on the night of 10 October 2008 by a vote of 23 in support and 17 opposed (Bullimore 2008; Oliver and Hawkins 2008). Marilyn Beaumont, Executive Director of WHV, described the ensuing scene at Parliament House as follows:

Those present to witness this history in the making were dignified and respectful of the Parliamentary protocols but only until we had made our way from the Council Chambers. Tears, hugs, clapping and speeches were some of the range of responses and emotions visible in response to the stunning outcome for women's health in Victoria. Our joining together with so many organisations and individuals in advocacy for abortion to be removed from the *Victorian Crimes Act* and for abortion to be regulated as a health service has been a monumental achievement. (Personal communication, 13 October 2008)

Conclusion

Activists in the maternity-care and abortion law reform movements have worked tirelessly for more than 40 years to advance women's reproductive health rights. The task has been made gargantuan in both cases because powerful opposing interests have countered feminist campaigns at every turn. With only their own skills and the support of female colleagues and sister groups, women have had to try to match the arguments and campaigns of the resource-rich groups pitched against them. The maternity-care reform movement turned the personal into the political when members challenged the medical model of pregnancy and childbirth care that became entrenched after organised medicine achieved the subordination of midwives in the first half of the twentieth century. Like the early abortion law reformers, the issues of respect for women's bodies and women's rights to information and self-determination had to be articulated and drawn to public attention. Language had to be invented to express concepts and concerns not previously discussed in public. In both cases, like activists in the rest of the women's health movement, women thought of themselves as social change agents, part of a movement that would raise the status of women and improve the conditions of their lives.

In both domains, there are major achievements to celebrate but the reforms are incomplete. Health financing arrangements and cultural norms provide incentives for women to seek medically dominated care and the prospects of independent midwifery practice and access to homebirth in the short term look bleak. Abortion remains in the criminal code in five jurisdictions and medical abortion, which has been available in comparable countries for more than a decade, is available to only a tiny number of women in a few special cases. In a policy area where powerful groups have a lot to lose from change, incremental reform rather than radical restructuring is, however, the order of the day. The women of both movements can therefore be justly proud of the reforms they have achieved. In the next chapter, the main policy responses to the women's health movement at the State and Territory level are examined.

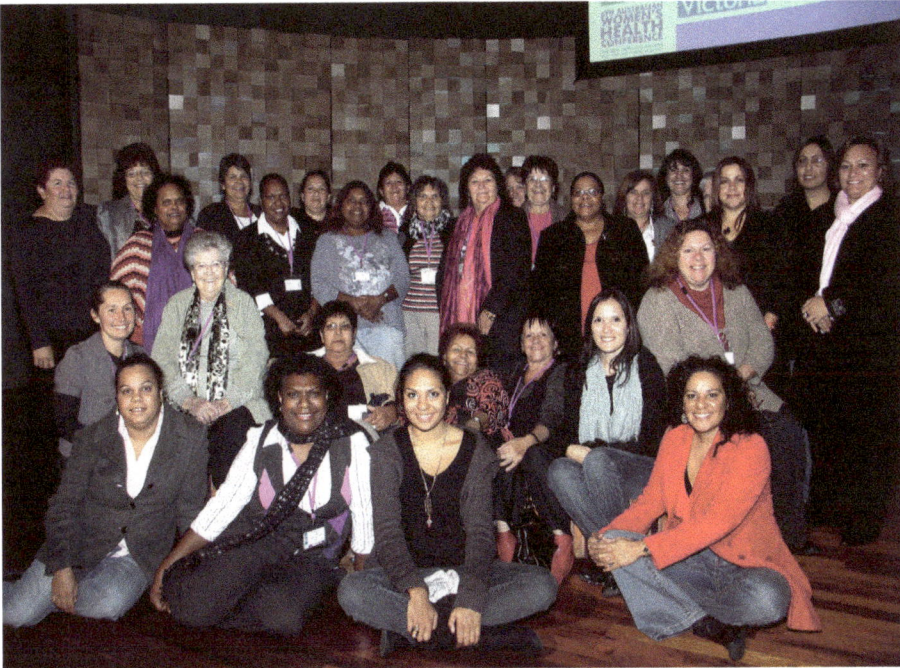

Members of the AWHN Aboriginal Women's Talking Circle at the Sixth AWHN National Women's Health Conference, Hobart, 2010.

Photo: Tracey Wing

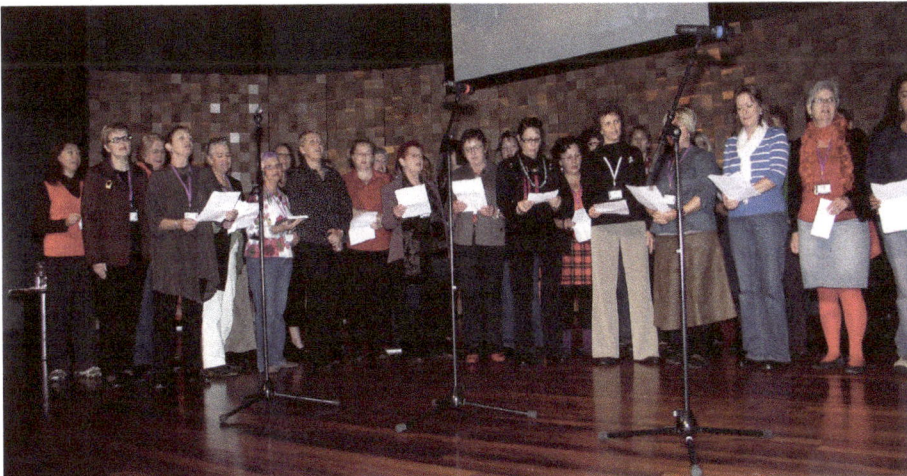

The Sixth AWHN National Women's Health Conference Choir, on stage, Hobart, 2010.

Photo: Tracey Wing

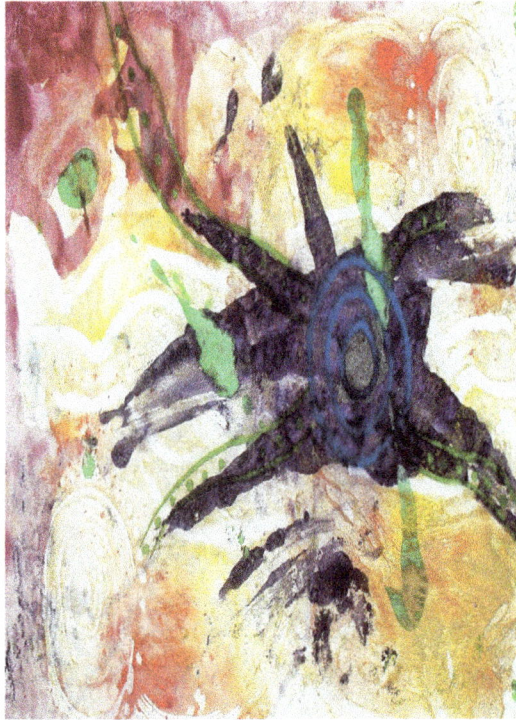

National Aboriginal and Torres Strait Islander Women's Health Strategy

"This image is of my woman's site on Country where I live. It is where I travel to for maintaining my mental, emotional, spiritual and physical well-being. Within this place I can speak with my inner self and to my ancestors. It is where I seek clarity, guidance and reassurance, and affirm my Aboriginal identity." Pamela Croft Warcon

The National Aboriginal and Torres Strait Islander Women's Health Strategy launched at the Sixth AWHN National Women's Health Conference, Hobart, 2010.

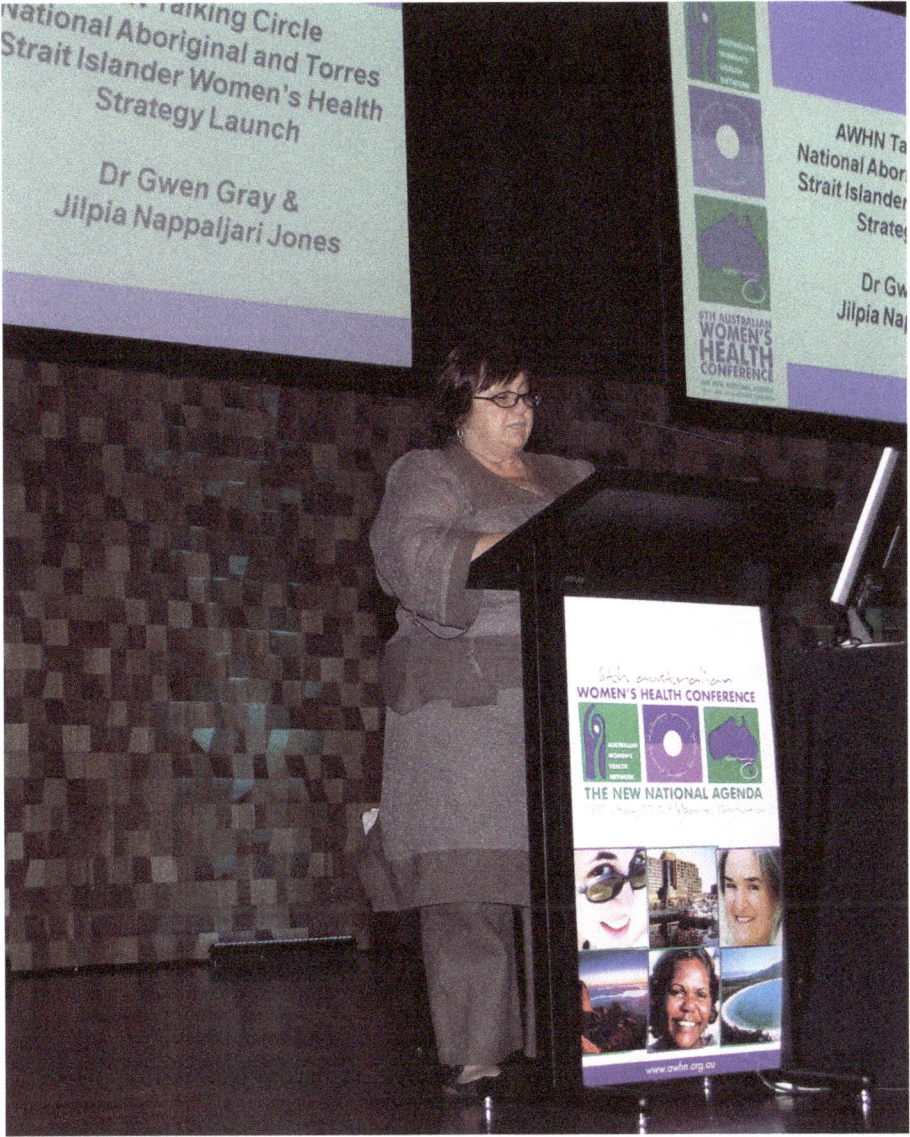

Sandy Angus, co-author, speaking at the launch of the National Aboriginal and Torres Strait Islander Women's Health Strategy, Hobart, 2010.

Photo: Tracey Wing

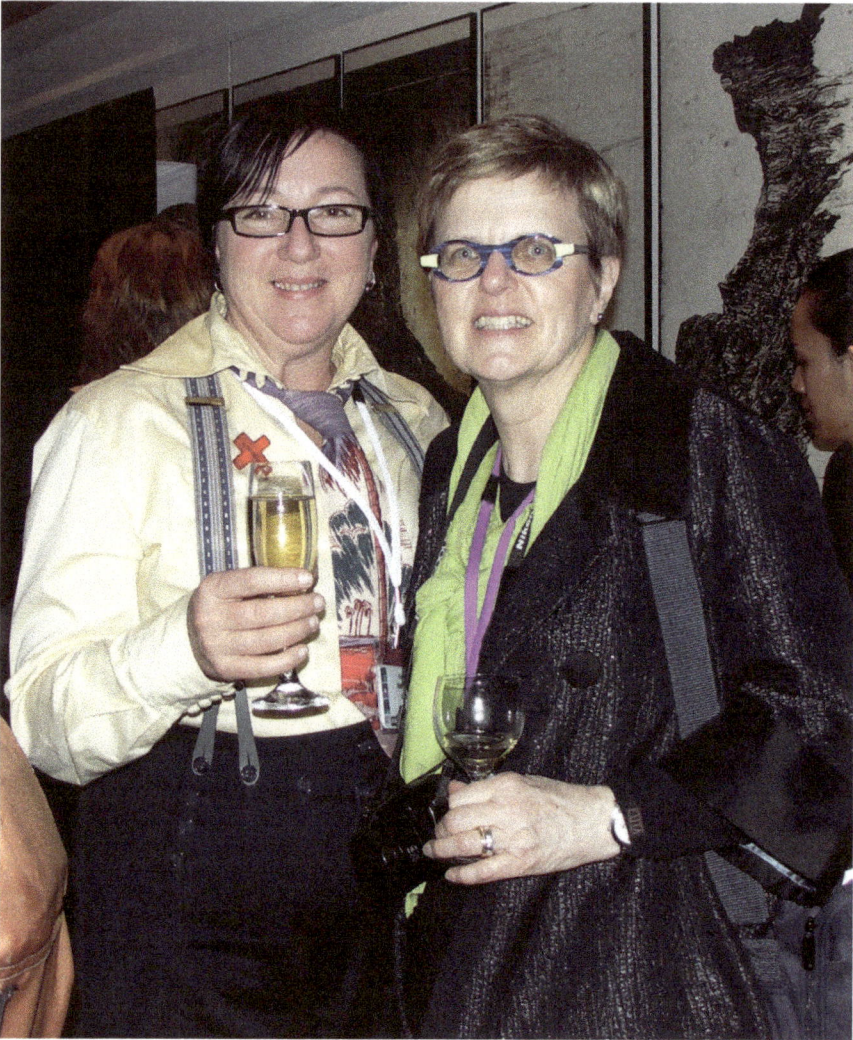

**Kelly Bannister, Conference Convener, with keynote speaker,
Professor Lorraine Greaves, British Columbia Centre of Excellence for
Women's Health, at the pre-conference reception, Government House,
Hobart, 2010.**

Photo: Tracey Wing

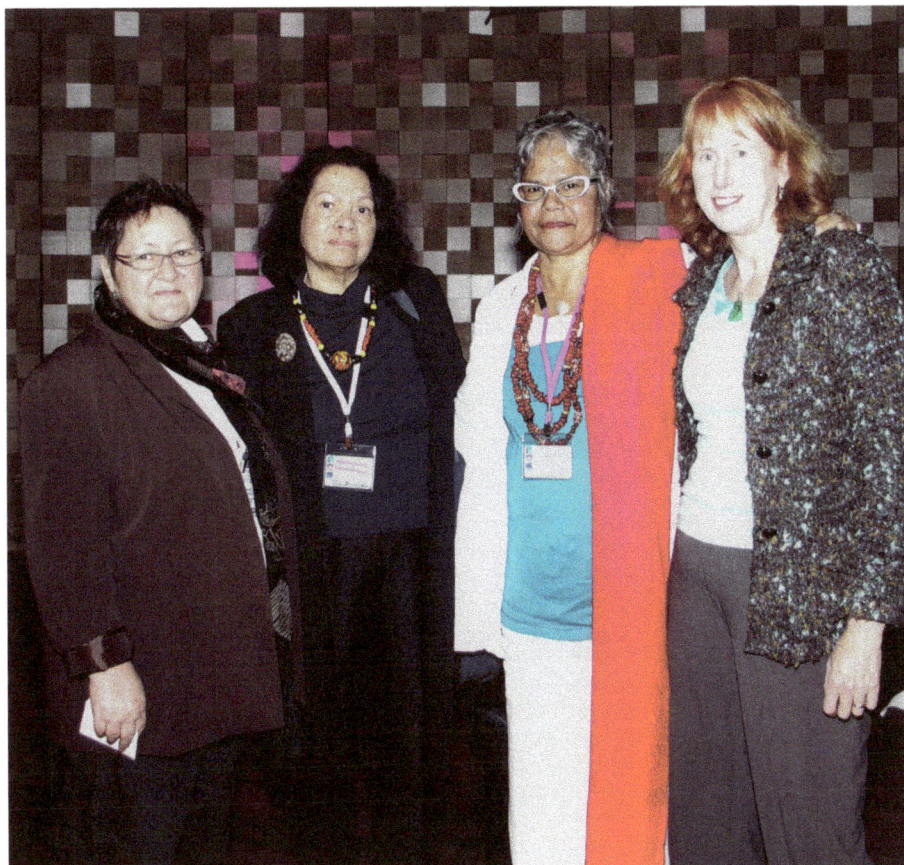

At the Sixth AWHN National Women's Health Conference, Hobart, 2010. From left: Denele Crozier and Jilpia Nappaljari Jones, AWHN committee members, with Jo Willmot and Fran Baum, keynote speakers.

Photo: Tracey Wing

7. Policy Responses: States and Territories

> The 1980s saw 'unprecedented feminist activism around public policy development in health'. (Schofield 1998:128)

If setting up separate services for women was difficult, the objective of influencing public policy was probably even harder. Consider the circumstances: groups of feminists, easily dismissed as part of a lunatic fringe, spoke about taboo subjects in public and circulated a radical critique of an esteemed institution—namely, the medical-care system. Persuading people of the validity of their claims was not easy. First, issues and concerns had to be identified and articulated. Sometimes a new language had to be developed with which to discuss issues previously hidden from view. Explanations had to be developed about why things were as they were. Meetings had to be held, agreements forged, position papers written and arguments disseminated in public places. Coalitions of support had to be created and maintained. Bureaucratic hostility was common and often a majority of political party members opposed, did not understand or were not interested in women's health perspectives. In some jurisdictions, women's health was seen as synonymous with abortion, which could be counted on to raise intense opposition. The social health perspective was new and often not well understood so that many health bureaucrats tried to incorporate women's health initiatives into the conventional medical paradigm. This came about partly because of familiarity with past practice and partly because bureaucracies do not like to establish organisations over which they have little control. Incorporating women's health into the medical model would also maintain trouble-free relations with organised medicine and avoid political fallout. Influencing public policy was not achieved easily.

The advocacy of the women's health movement, however, built up such momentum by the 1980s that political parties felt they could not afford to ignore it, especially as opinion polls were showing that the 'women's vote' was a force to be reckoned with. The decade can be seen as a golden age in the development of women's health policies, centres and services. As well as general women's health policies, strategies to confront domestic violence were formulated and reforms implemented. Prior to and feeding into the development of the NWHP in the second half of the 1980s, most States and Territories had initiated inquiries into women's health and/or developed their own policies. At the same time, women's health policy machinery was introduced in all jurisdictions and at the Commonwealth level. These new institutional arrangements assisted policy and program advancement; women's health advisers and the units they ran were crucial in the many-pronged struggles for policy influence that followed. Sexual assault was the hardest issue to bring out of the wings and position on the policy stage.

New South Wales

The establishment of health policy machinery and the development of policy progressed steadily in New South Wales under the Wran Labor Government (1976–86), even if persuading it to make up the funding being withdrawn by the Commonwealth was a struggle. A Women's Coordination Unit was established in the Premier's Department in 1977, followed by the establishment of women's units in key departments to work with the Coordination Unit—a hub-and-spoke model as advocated by WEL. The Women's Advisory Council, the main channel through which community views were fed into government, was established in the same year. The council consulted with women, paying special attention to rural areas. As in all consultations with Australian women, here, health emerged as a major concern and became an element of the reform agenda. The council recommended that more women's health centres be established, more birthing choices be developed, better contraceptive information be made available and that participation in health decision making be facilitated.

New initiatives, however, took several years to develop, despite persistent lobbying by movement members. In June 1984, the Women's Health Policy Review Committee was established. The Women's Health Unit, with a staff of three to four, headed by the Women's Health Advisor, Carla Cranny, was set up in 1985. Most staff members were experts in particular fields and had links with grassroots women's groups. By the mid-1980s, the Wran Government had made a clear commitment to women's health action.

The Policy Review Committee was charged with identifying the main women's health issues, assessing the adequacy and accessibility of existing services and determining appropriate funding mechanisms. Its final report was presented in November 1985 and formed the basis of an approach termed 'a policy in action' in the absence of a formal policy. Extra funds were provided for rural and public hospital sexual assaults centres, and, as discussed, some unfunded health centres received funding for the first time. By 1986, 19 women's health centres, including Jilimi (later renamed Waminda), were being funded by the State Government. Women's health coordinators were installed in each of the health regions, along with women's health educators and approximately 60 women's health nurses, who were trained to provide sexual, reproductive and breast health services. With increased capacity, women's health centres were seeing more than 80 000 women each year (NSW Women's Advisory Council to the Premier 1987:187–9).

Bureaucratic resistance to separate women's health services remained, nevertheless, even in New South Wales, which has the longest experience and the most centres. One of the arguments against centres was that NGOs needed to deliver better services than the mainstream in order to justify a funded existence.The mix of services provided in the two sectors is too different to compare quality in any straightforward sense. During this time, NGOs were evaluated and measures put in place to ensure financial accountability. Some centres found the requirements of intricate record keeping and statistical collection onerous, particularly given the straitened financial circumstances in which they found themselves. Differences in the power of stakeholder groups were clear: women's services were required to account in detail for the trivial funding they received whereas multimillion-dollar hospitals were able to report in broad-brush terms.

In 1988, the Labor Government was replaced with the neo-liberal-leaning Greiner Liberal Party Government, which quickly set in place a review of all NGOs funded by the Health Department. Although the women's health sector feared it might lose support, it had established its legitimacy to the extent that the Premier endorsed the principles of the NWHP in a women's policy statement in 1990. In 1995, the government changed hands again and the Carr Labor Government was elected. A women's health discussion paper was produced in 1998, and a policy document, *A Strategic Framework to Advance Women's Health*, indicating directions until 2003, was released in 2000. The document confirmed a commitment to a social view of health and other principles of the NWHP, including intersectorality. The four key strategic directions identified were adoption of a gendered approach to health, collaboration to address social determinants, advancement of women's health research and the application of a health-outcomes approach, based on measurable indicators. In April of the same year, the Gender Equity in Health statement was released, which recognised gender as an important determinant of health. It presented an overarching framework for promoting women's and men's health (NSW Health Department 2000:1).

The Women's Health Outcomes Framework was subsequently developed and released in 2002. It provided a guide to measuring and monitoring conventional health outcomes and prioritised mental health and the prevention of violence against women, as well as preventive health measures, such as smoking cessation. Influenced by the principles of the NWHP, it acknowledged the social health perspective and the importance of health promotion, disease prevention, equity of access to appropriate and affordable services and a strengthened primary healthcare system (Women's Health Unit 2003).

In January 2010, the interim Women's Health Plan, 2009–2011, was released. Priority action areas include violence, the Aboriginal Family Health Strategy, the improvement of the health of pregnant women, and the health of immigrant and refugee women and women living in regional, rural and remote areas. Each Area Health Service is required to implement and monitor the plan. The plan suggested that 2010 was a time of transition because the Commonwealth would soon release a new NWHP. A full review of New South Wales policies for women is to be held in 2012 (NSW Department of Health 2010).

Queensland

The Bjelke-Petersen Government, including the Health Minister in the early 1980s, Brian Austin, was not interested in women's health. Leisha Harvey, only the second woman in Queensland to hold a cabinet position, took the health portfolio in 1987 and, after intense lobbying, agreed to set up the Women's Health Advisory Council. The Women's Health Forum was held, attended by 400 women, as part of Queensland consultations for the NWHP; however, there had been no further policy progress when the Government lost office in 1989. By then, community consensus about the importance of women's health had emerged. Nevertheless, the new Labor Government took time to act, partly because supporting women's health apparently meant supporting access to abortion in the minds of some parliamentarians. Jude Abbs, first Interim Convenor of AWHN, was an ALP member and introduced women's health as an issue. Because policy development on women's issues lagged behind other jurisdictions, there was a sense that time had to be made up. Former Women's Health Adviser Janet Ramsay describes her experience at Queensland Health as trying to do 20 years' of policy development in two years.

The Queensland Labor Party had formed a women's policy committee, which saw women's health as a priority issue, with special emphasis on the needs of women in rural and remote areas. By this time, diverse groups of community women were well organised in Brisbane and in regional towns and were ready to assume responsibility for managing women's health projects. Networks had been formed, meetings and forums were held and expectations were high.

The Women's Health Unit was established in 1991, with between five and eight permanent, designated women's health policy positions (Gray 1999:210). Between 1989 and 1995, Anne Warner, Minister for Family Services and Aboriginal and Islander Affairs, was the only woman in the Queensland cabinet,She was only the second ALP woman to be elected to the Parliament and the first to hold a ministerial portfolio. so her office tended to operate as a centre of women's issues.

A discussion paper, *Towards a Queensland women's health policy*, was developed in 1992 followed by a consultation process across the State and in the Torres Strait Islands. The Royal College of General Practitioners, strongly opposed to the discussion paper, did its own survey to try to show that women did not really care about the sex of general practitioners or about women's health issues. The Queensland Medical Women's Society also voiced opposition. Members were upset, for example, about a proposal to train women's health nurses. Within government, it was felt that the support of organised medical groups was necessary, so extensive negotiations were held.

Queensland Health received 138 written responses to the discussion paper, which was followed by a green paper with the same name. The Goss Government was committed to hearing from Queensland women about health priorities but some members counselled caution at this point, as it was realised that consultation creates expectations. The green paper provoked considerable controversy and the abortion issue was again raised. To get cabinet approval, which was extremely difficult in any case, the 'A' word had to be avoided at all costs.Even Family Planning Queensland felt it had to hold itself aloof from the abortion issue for self-protection. After a politically fraught passage during which the need for separate women's health services was questioned extensively, the Queensland Women's Health Policy was launched in November 1993.

The 1993 policy was never reviewed or updated, nor was it properly monitored. Despite the existence of a relatively well-staffed women's health unit, little research or statistical collection was carried out. These omissions were put down to lack of central direction and coordination. Within government, there was talk about partnerships with the community sector but no real action was taken to develop connections or concrete programs. In 1996, the Women's Health Unit was formally abolished.

In 2001, Queensland still had no access and equity policies and no bilingual health workers, except in women's health centres and services. Women advocating for the employment of interpreters in health agencies were told that there were not enough migrant and refugee women to justify the effort. Although women's health never had a high profile within government, members of the movement feel that it was gradually accepted as a legitimate area of public policy. Moreover, the principles of women's health are thought to have influenced the direction of Queensland primary healthcare policy due to compatible principles and philosophies.

South Australia

> The State health bureaucracy appears to have had an unfavourable view
> of the women's health centre from the start. (Auer 2003)

In the late 1970s, women's groups in South Australia had mobilised and were campaigning for separate women's health services. The Liberal Party won government at the 1979 election and Jennifer Adamson (later Cashmore), a supporter of a feminist health perspective, became Minister for Health for the next three years. Gaining support within government and the bureaucracy, however, was not easy. It took until the middle of 1982 for the minister to be given authority to request the South Australian Health Commission to develop a women's health policy. A working party was set up and consultations undertaken but the policy had not been written when the Government lost office.

Labor women had responded to grassroots agitation by establishing a women's policy committee within the party in 1978. On gaining office in 1982, a major task was to finalise the women's health policy. A philosophical framework supportive of women's health was accepted within the party and the importance of opening channels of communication with women so that they could contribute to policy was emphasised.

The Adviser on Women's Health, Liz Furler, who reported directly to the minister, was appointed in January 1984. Health Minister, John Cornwall, who supported separate women's health services, proposed that she become a member of the Health Commission Executive, but 'at least a dozen reasons were advanced over so many weeks by the existing members of the executive as to why such an appointment would not be "appropriate". Most of them relied on the fact that her position did not carry Executive Director status' (Cornwall 1989:45). At the time, there were no women in senior executive positions at the commission. When the minister insisted, the Adviser on Women's Health was 'grudgingly admitted' but she was 'never accepted into the inner sanctum. Nor was her "pushiness" ever forgiven' (Cornwall 1989:44–5).

In August 1984, the *Report of the Working Party on Women's Health Policy* was released, which was the first women's health policy in Australia. Women's health, however, had no natural home in the bureaucracy and it took time to decide where responsibility should be located. Indeed, it took four years to identify which area should take responsibility for immigrant women's health. According to one femocrat involved in the processes, the South Australian Health Commission resisted all changes recommended in the policy because bureaucrats did not want to deal with an assortment of small agencies. Under the circumstances, it was not hard to get the policy endorsed but it was very difficult to get a commitment to implementation, maintenance and proper funding.

In spite of the obstacles, a number of valuable projects were undertaken after the release of the report, including the establishment of new women's health centres, as discussed in Chapter 3. The representative Women's Health Consultative Committee to the Health Commission was appointed to advise on issues raised in the policy. Aboriginal, immigrant and older women, women with disabilities and single mothers were represented, together with women from general practice, nursing and the voluntary sector. A program of seminars on women and health was initiated in regional and rural areas. Abortion services were improved, along with responses to child sexual abuse. Equal opportunity for women within the health system became a central issue.

The new Social Health Unit was established in 1986, which was seen as integral to the Government's social justice strategy. The Adviser on Women's Health became the Director and her office was transferred. The new unit had a staff of eight, including an Aboriginal project officer. It was not directly responsible for women's health and its creation gave rise to considerable controversy. Some members of the movement wanted a more direct focus on women's health and discussion was rekindled about whether it had been a good idea to work with 'the state' after all. In the event, the major supporters of the Social Health Unit, Minister Cornwall and the Director, Liz Furler, both moved away before the unit had time to make an impact. After their departure, the staff and resources of the unit were slashed.

In 1988, the metropolitan women's health centres worked together to produce a five-year strategic plan, developing strategies around key issues (Radoslovich 1994:62). Under the Brown Liberal Government, however, elected in 1993, the independence of women's health centres was lost. Inspired by the neo-liberal objectives of increased efficiency and expenditure reductions, the regional centres were amalgamated with community health centres to form regional community health centres, while Adelaide Women's was amalgamated with the Women's and Children's Hospital, as discussed above. Severe budgetary cuts were used to 'encourage' cooperation (Radoslovich 1994:104–5). The changes accorded with the longstanding Health Department position of strong opposition to separate women's health centres.

The Olsen Liberal Government released a consultation paper in 2000, as the first part of a project to develop the Department of Human Services Policy and Planning Framework for Women's Health and Well-Being. A key initiatives paper, *Women's health and well-being*, setting out a snapshot of existing projects, was released in 2001. The Government changed hands in 2002. The

Women's Health Ministerial Advisory Council was established by incoming Health Minister, Lea Stevens, in 2003 and a new Women's Health Policy was launched in 2005. It describes itself as 'a policy like no other' because 'it is about all of us—the whole health system and the South Australian community. It is about changing health for women, changing health for everyone—but it starts with women.' The policy takes a social determinants perspective and suggests structural reform to achieve a focus on prevention and primary health care, aiming to achieve 'health for all' (Government of South Australia 2005). Based on the policy, the Women's Health Action Plan was written and, in 2009, Women's Health Statewide produced an evaluation, 'Women's Health Action Plan Report Card'. While a number of programs and strategies were introduced in key women's health areas, the major reforms envisaged in the 2005 policy did not proceed.

Tasmania

In Tasmania, where hospitals have been the central health institution for decades, awareness of the importance of primary health care was slow to develop. Many people saw community health as an extension of hospital care into the home situation, with hospital staff providing the service (Shaw and Tilden 1990:29). The women's health movement was therefore without an important band of community health allies and, while the movement was strong, those with authority in health policymaking took a long time to respond to the new ideas. As one femocrat has argued, the road to women's health in Tasmania has been 'a twisted and convoluted one: a step or two forwards, some backsliding and a few quantum leaps' (Personal communication).

The election of a Labor government and the launch of the first NWHP in 1989 heralded a positive period for women's health and brought renewed energy from community groups. Money was made available for a Women's Health Forum, as a means of generating input to the NWHP, under which funding was provided for a women's health senior policy officer position. Research on women's health needs in regional areas was also funded, along with the Hobart Women's Health Centre. In subsequent years, various small projects were supported and funding was directed towards the development of a Tasmanian women's health policy, which was launched in 1994. In the mid to late-1990s, a discrete women's health program was developed within the Department of Health and Human Services. Regional coordinators were appointed and an information service was established. A manager was appointed in 1999 to oversee the program and all positions were made permanent in the same year.

During the early 2000s, the Women's Health Program became part of the Population and Health Priorities Unit within Population Health, alongside other priority areas, such as Aboriginal health, immigrant health, youth health and men's health. Since that time, there has been a focus on health equity, diversity and gender mainstreaming. Although it works to improve mainstream services, the Women's Health Program aims to achieve change at the level of population health and is structured around a regional outreach model.

According to the evaluation of the NWHP, the Tasmanian Women's Health Program developed within a context where there had been a philosophical shift from traditional illness orientation towards a social view of health with a focus on primary health care (Commonwealth of Australia 1993:45). The program was maintained until 2011 when State finances became stressed. The budget announced funding cuts across portfolios, including a $100 million reduction in health funding. The implications for women's health are not clear at the time of writing but it is anticipated that a leaner program will result.

Victoria

In Victoria, the Cain Labor Government was elected to office in 1982. Although the new Premier regarded the women's policy machinery set up under the previous Liberal Government with suspicion (Sawer 1990:162), Mary Draper was appointed Women's Adviser in 1983. One of the issues she discussed with the Premier was a women's health policy. A group of women parliamentarians and femocrats, in response to grassroots activism, identified women's health as a key issue and agreed that the development of a policy should be a priority.

A number of crosscutting forces operated. Within the Labor Party, support for separate women's health services was weak and, even among female members, opinion was divided. The party's Health and Welfare Policy Committee did not favour separate women's services, arguing that community-based services were important but they did not have to be separate. Many officers within the Department of Health were hostile; the view that women's health was a waste of time and money was strong. As in other States, in Victoria, health bureaucrats tended to oppose government funding for community groups on grounds of increased complexity and accountability problems. On the other hand, there was a commitment to community consultation and an awareness of lagging behind other jurisdictions on women's issues. Victoria was certainly lagging behind New South Wales, perhaps rekindling ancient rivalries. Female politicians and femocrats were able to use these forces to advantage, assisted by opinion polling that showed the electoral importance of attracting the women's vote. Kay Setches and her colleagues, who included Joan Kirner and Carolyn Hogg, are said to have been known as the feminist mafia.

The Labor Party's health platform for the 1985 election was headed by policy for hospitals and made no mention of women's health. Under these circumstances, many avenues had to be used to promote the development of a formal women's health policy. An intense struggle ensued, which included women parliamentarians persistently lobbying the Premier. Senior bureaucrats, no matter how resistant, are likely to be responsive to the wishes of the minister and, in 1985, David White, who supported women's health, became Health Minister. Jenny Macklin, later to become a Commonwealth minister and Deputy Leader of the Labor Party, was a member of the minister's staff and her work is regarded as pivotal in the struggle for a positive outcome.

The strongest resistance to separate services was gradually eroded and an in-principle agreement was reached that the Health Department should develop a policy. Minister White announced the establishment of the Ministerial Women's Health Working Party, under the leadership of Kay Setches, who later joined the cabinet. Before entering Parliament, she had been coordinator of the Maroondah Women's Refuge. A discussion paper was distributed and consultation was undertaken with thousands of Victorian women.

Many senior parliamentarians, however, were not convinced that funding community-based women's health services was a wise move, nor that electoral advantage would follow. A number of others were simply not interested. The Cain Government perceived itself as having inherited a poor financial situation and wanted to prove itself as a sound financial manager.This cannot, however, be considered a serious justification for inaction, since the amounts of money so far allocated to women's health are too small to have a serious budgetary impact, irrespective of jurisdiction. After another intense struggle, it was agreed to set up the Victorian Women's Health Program, as outlined in Chapter 3. In the event, funding was approved in 1987 prior to the release of the working party's final report, *Why women's health, Victorian women respond*.

The Women's Health Policy and Program Unit was established in the Health Department to implement the changes. The two major policy directions were long-term structuring of general health services to reflect women's health issues and the provision of separate services (Women's Policy Coordination Unit 1987:68–9). A women's health centre was established in each region, and specialist community-based women's addiction services and services for young women were set up under the new program.

By 1990, the Cain Government was in crisis, the budget deficit was high and some financial institutions were deeply unstable. Divisions emerged within the ALP about an appropriate response. There were attempts to regenerate momentum and to identify important issues for the 1990s but energy was low and the party's policy committees were in decline. Although a dynamic leader, Joan Kirner, took over in 1990, the Government was unable to regain its electoral strength and it lost office to the Liberal Party under Jeff Kennett in 1992.

Social policies and programs were not Kennett Government priorities but reigning in expenditure was. Shortly after the election, the health budget was cut by 12 per cent. The traditional bureaucratic distaste for separate women's health services once again emerged in proposals to 'integrate' women's health centres into primary care services. The number of people working on women's health in the bureaucracy was reduced. In 1997, however, Health Minister, Rob Knowles, asked the Ministerial Advisory Committee on Women's Health to begin the development of a women's health plan for Victoria. A round of consultations followed and, in 1998, the Department of Human Services and the Ministerial Advisory Committee on Women's Health jointly sponsored a women's health conference as part of the policy development process. The conference met with an overwhelming response (Beaumont 1998:6–7.) A women's health plan was written before the Government (unexpectedly) lost office, after which the plan was abandoned. Overall, the Kennett Government era has been described as a 'policy vacuum' for women's health (Johnstone and Bachowski 2000:4).

The incoming Bracks Labor Government was elected on a platform of commitment to women's issues. The Ministerial Advisory Committee on Women's Health and Wellbeing was established, chaired by Caroline Hogg. After a discussion paper and further consultations, the four-year Women's Health and Wellbeing Strategy was launched in 2002. The strategy focused on the needs of women with the most disadvantages, particularly in the areas of safety and security, mental and emotional health and participation. Upon the expiry of the strategy, a group of women's health providers collaborated to write a new policy proposal, *Women's Health Matters: From policy to practice, 10 point plan for Victorian women's health, 2006–2010*. The plan was endorsed by 30 women's health and community groups. The aim was to attract the attention of political parties in the lead-up to the 2006 election. The document successfully influenced priority setting.

In 2009, WHV released a second 10-point plan for the period 2010–14, which builds upon the 2006 document and suggests policy directions, including increased funding for women's services (WHV web site). In Victoria, the women's health movement has had considerable success in building a positive partnership with the State Government in recent years.

Western Australia

The Burke Labor Government came to power in Western Australia in 1983 with a clear agenda to promote the status of women. Deborah McCulloch, former women's adviser to the Premier of South Australia, was employed as a consultant to help develop women's policy machinery. The Women's Advisory Council, which had a strong women's health focus, was set up in the first year. It is said that the Government initially listened carefully to the council's advice. Liza Newby, who later led the national consultation for the NWHP, was appointed Director of Women's Interests in the Division of the Department of Premier and Cabinet. In 1986, the small Women's Health Unit was established within the Health Commission, headed by Thea Mendelsohn.

The Working Party on Women's Health was set up, which produced a report in 1986. At the time, Ian Taylor, an ally of women's health, was Health Minister. A women's health conference was held to which Liz Furler was brought from Adelaide as a keynote speaker. Hundreds of women from all over the State attended, demonstrating the high priority women placed on health. Regional forums and workshops were held, which were also well attended. Minister Taylor attended all the forums and took time to talk with women about their health needs, sometimes for a whole morning. In the meantime, the Women's Advisory Council pressed hard to get the recommendations of the working party accepted; however, the 1986 draft policy was never endorsed.

Infrastructure gains were made in 1988–89, when funding was approved for rural sexual assault centres in Bunbury and Geraldton, and the embryonic women's health centres in Fremantle and Kalgoorlie were provided with small amounts of funding; however, progress was slow. The Women's Health Unit had only one permanent position, supported by a continuous flow of temporary staff. The situation was exacerbated because the unit could not get information about the availability of finance. Over time, the influence of the Women's Advisory Council waned.

Keith Wilson, no friend of women's health, took over as Health Minister in 1988 when grassroots women were highly mobilised and were campaigning for a network of women's health centres. The minister strongly opposed separate services and did not support reproductive choice. His early actions included cuts to the core funding for the WA Family Planning Association. About this time, Women's Health Care House was given three months' notice to quit its premises, which were earmarked to be bulldozed. Requests that the minister provide a building were ignored until centre staff wrote an article for the Western Australian *Sunday Times*. Premises were offered the following day.

Within the Labor Party, Minister Wilson is said to have been a 'majority of one', who regularly threatened to resign if the health portfolio were taken from him. Carmen Lawrence, as Premier, supported her Health Minister publicly in what is reported to have been an extremely difficult time within the party. Under the circumstances, Labor women could do little to influence the Government's approach.

Within the Department of Health, women's health became known as 'the poisoned chalice' because association might end a public servant's career. The result was that few women in the bureaucracy were willing to be advocates. By 1990, it appeared that Western Australia alone might not join the NWH Program. The Women's Health Adviser was told to develop a new set of reference groups and to focus on introducing changes to the mainstream health system, rather than plan separate services.

A number of alternatives to separate women's health services were considered, including well women's clinics that would be run from general practitioners' offices—doubtless a suggestion from medical unions. Another proposal was to use the NWH Program money to employ women's health coordinators. In 1990, the matched funding requirement was used to oppose acceptance of the program, transforming it into a 'States' rights' issue in an effort to gain political traction.

The Women's Advisory Council continued to press the Government to join the NWH Program, supported by community groups. A well-attended meeting, addressed by Premier Lawrence, was called by WEL to increase the pressure. Staff in the Commonwealth Women's Health Unit exercised discretion, keeping open the opportunity for Western Australia to join after it could have been closed. Eventually, in March 1991, more than a year late, Western Australia joined the program, after which most of the State's women's health infrastructure was established. Observers are of the view that if it were not for Commonwealth money, Western Australia would have a very small women's health infrastructure.

Any attitudinal changes within government or the bureaucracy at the time of joining were ephemeral. Participants reported a quick reversion to a policy of 'what the Government thought women's health should be'. In summary, after an initial burst of positive action under the newly elected Burke Government and Health Minister Taylor, women's health initiatives were resisted in government circles, despite strong pressure from parliamentary women, women in the bureaucracy and women in the community. Moreover, absurdities appeared regularly. For example, male doctors were given responsibility for managing the Alternative Birthing Services Program, funded under the NWH Program. King Edward Hospital for Women henceforth became known informally as King Edward Men's Hospital for Women. Under the circumstances, struggling to infuse the primary care system with women's health principles was thought to be much too hard, given the massive groundswell of support that is needed to support structural change, and movement members selected their goals strategically. In the middle of the 1990s, the Women's Health Policy Unit was reduced to two bookcases.While the claim is colourful, it is only a slight exaggeration. In 1995–96, a senior manager had responsibility for women's health, in addition to five other portfolio areas. She was able to spend on average only one-sixth of her time on women's health (Gray 1999:210).

The Australian Capital Territory

The process of developing a women's health policy in the Australian Capital Territory was stimulated by the announcement of the forthcoming NWHP but interrupted by the introduction of self-government in 1989. Some of the regular opponents, who feared a policy would legitimate an abortion service, were active. At the time, the Australian Capital Territory had a relatively extensive network of community health centres—a legacy of the Whitlam Government's constitutional authority in the jurisdiction. Some people held the view that community health centres could adequately meet the needs of womenThis is not an entirely unreasonable view, given appropriate women-focused arrangements. (Broom 1991:80–1). A women's health adviser position was established in the mid-1980s by the then ACT Health Authority. Marilyn Hatton was appointed and work began on a women's health directory and a formal policy. At the same time, a small women's health service was set up by the Health Department. The distribution of the draft policy was delayed, pending expected initiatives to be outlined in the NWHP. *Women's Health Development in the ACT* was released in November 1990 in draft form but the document was never finalised or formalised.

The first ACT Government was headed by the first Australian female head of government, Rosemary Follett, who set up the Women's Health Advisory Committee (WHAC) in 1989. The ACT Women's Health Network (ACTWHN) was represented on the committee through its six-year existence. WHAC regularly consulted with ACT women about their health needs and monitored policy developments and changes, including the controversial alternative birthing services program. Under the Follett Government, legislation was changed to allow abortions to occur in facilities other than a public hospital, as discussed in the previous chapter. Under the Carnell Liberal Government (1995–2000), the importance of women's health was downgraded. Meetings of the WHAC ceased and, more seriously, Canberra's relatively extensive network of community health centres was progressively dismantled.

Labor was re-elected in 2001, under the leadership of Jon Stanhope, who remained in power until 2011. A five-year women's plan was produced, with an excellent health section setting out key principles. Substantial investment has been made in transitional housing for families in crisis, for example, including designated properties for women and children escaping domestic violence. But, as elsewhere, a serious shortage of low-cost housing remains. In 2008, the Government embarked on a consultative review of the Women's Health Services Plan—a process assisted by a widely representative steering group. A paper, *Health status of women in the ACT*, was released in 2008 as a guide to the review. The 2008–09 Budget announced that $1 billion would be spent on an overhaul of the ACT public health system, including $200 million to be spent specifically on women's services. The $90 million Women's and Children's Hospital is under construction in 2011, along with a new community health centre in a newly settled, densely populated suburb. Existing community health centres are being expanded and refurbished.

The Northern Territory

Despite the small population of the Northern Territory, a strong women's movement emerged from the 1970s onwards that tended to be involved in all women's issues. The Family Planning Association was set up in 1973 by Jo Parish, Lyn Reid and members of WEL. At the time, key people in the Northern Territory Government supported women's health and money was made available to support interstate training for family planning staff. In 1974, legislation, which passed by one vote, made abortion in a public hospital lawful up to 14 weeks' gestation if there was a danger to the health of the mother or if there was a danger of serious deformity. Early government support for women's health faded, however, and, as we have seen, funding was withdrawn in 1980 from the centres that women had established in Darwin and Alice Springs.

After pressure from WEL, the Office of Women's Affairs and Women's Adviser position were introduced in 1983. The office was a policy coordination unit, located in the Chief Minister's Department, and it works across government. The Women's Advisory Council was later established. There was only one woman in the Legislative Assembly at the time and no women in cabinet, so that these institutions, which were relatively well resourced, played important roles.

As word about the possibility of the NWHP circulated, Northern Territory community women began to mobilise more strongly. A submission was written to the National Agenda for Women requesting funding for a women's health conference, as a mechanism to begin formulating a Territory position. The application was successful and small working groups were formed. The conference was held in 1989 and attracted a large contingent of Aboriginal women. The proceedings were published and distributed to key players, including the Chief Minister and senior bureaucrats. Widespread ignorance about women's health was revealed when, after the proceedings were circulated, the Women's Adviser received numerous calls asking what women's health was all about.

When the Territory began to implement the NWH Program, there was no infrastructure in place, apart from Congress Alukura and family planning clinics in Darwin and Alice Springs (Commonwealth of Australia 1993:46). A struggle ensued between the Government and the women's health movement about how the program money would be spent. The Government wanted to spend most of the money on consultations, whereas the movement wanted a Northern Territory women's health policy and the establishment of a women's health adviser position. Staff at the Office of Women's Affairs felt pressured by colleagues, who did not understand the notion of a separate focus on women's health or did not see value in such a perspective. Nevertheless, members of AWHN Top End Branch felt they had been able to influence decision making. At the time, Carmel O'Loughlin, Director of the South Australian Office for Women, was employed as a consultant. She raised issues at senior levels of the Health Department and managed to have these concerns accepted—testimony to the centrality of the femocrat role in the right circumstances.

An advisory committee, consisting of one Commonwealth officer, one Northern Territory officer and two NGO members, including an Aboriginal woman, was set up in September 1991 to oversee the implementation of the program. The women's health movement proposal for a women's health adviser position was rejected outright at first but a change of chief minister and a turnover of senior bureaucratic staff brought a change of direction. The Women's Health Adviser was appointed in 1992 and the Women's Health Strategy Unit (WHSU), with one funded position, was created. The Women's Health Policy was released later the same year. The policy has eight objectives, which include the reorientation of mainstream health and welfare services to enable them to be more responsive to the needs of women. One of the aims is to provide 'direction for the development of specialised women's health services' but there is no mention of community-based women's health centres (Government of the Northern Territory 1992).

The mobilisation of community women and the influence of the NWHP are reported to have been the springboards for action that resulted in a Territory policy. In turn, the policy provided a framework within which women employed in the Government could work. Community women also found it a useful tool for keeping pressure on political representatives, allowing them to argue for action on the issues that the policy enunciated. In the event, most of the NWH Program money in the Northern Territory was used to provide sexual and reproductive health information.

The WHSU, with its single women's health advisor, now manager, position, has been retained. In 2001, in response to the increasing incidence of heterosexually acquired HIV infections by young women, the unit conducted a pilot project, in partnership with the AIDS/STD Program of the Centre for Disease Control. The aim was to increase awareness of the dangers of HIV among young heterosexual women. Evaluation of the project was positive, except that the target group thought the campaign could have been more effective had it been targeted at young men as well (WHSU 2003). In 2004, the Health Department embarked on a large project to assemble in one place all available information on the health and wellbeing of Northern Territory women, with the aim of providing a resource for policymakers, researchers and health professionals. The result was a report, *The Health and Well-Being of Northern Territory Women: From the desert to the sea*, released in 2005. The report is set within a social determinants framework. The WHSU envisaged that the report would form the basis for a revised Northern Territory women's health policy (Department of Health and Community Services 2005:2). In 2008, *Building on Our Strengths, A Framework for Action for Women in the Northern Territory*, was released. Overall, however, Northern Territory support for women's health centres and programs has been comparatively weak.

Violence against Women Becomes a Policy Issue

Significant changes have been achieved in public policy and the law in relation to violence against women since the 1970s, when domestic violence was a private matter, apprehended violence orders (AVOs) were almost unheard of and 'good wives' suffered in silence. Even among professionals, including marriage guidance counsellors, the existence of violence in marriage was not acknowledged and scarcely appeared in the professional literature (Mugford 1989). Under the circumstances, feminists had to identify the most pressing issues and draw attention to basic but unrecognised anomalies, such as the plight of women and children trying to escape violence who were ineligible for public housing because the 'family' already had a public tenancy.

All States and Territories, where primary responsibility for criminal justice is located, have taken policy action, as activism made violence against women 'one of the rediscovered crimes of the 20th century' (McFerran 2007:1). The survey below is indicative only, capturing a few of the main policies, papers, programs, projects and statements of intent that have been produced over the past 30 years. A review of the main policies and programs currently in operation across Australia can be found in the background paper *Time for action*, produced by the National Council to Reduce Violence against Women and their Children (Commonwealth of Australia 2009a).

The Wran/Unsworth Labor Government in New South Wales (1976–88) supported refuges by filling the funding gap left by the Commonwealth and funding new refuges from its own resources (McFerran 1990:1). New South Wales was the first State to introduce legal reform intended to improve the remedies available to women experiencing violence. The Task Force on Domestic Violence was set up, which reported to the Premier in 1981, and was followed by the *Crimes (Domestic Violence) Amendment Act 1982*, which implemented many of the task force's recommendations. All States and Territories In Queensland and the Northern Territory action was slower. subsequently enacted similar legislation, the main thrust of which was to define the range of offences that constitutes domestic violence and to make AVOs available in cases of violence or where violence is feared. The onus of proof was changed to the civil standard of the 'balance of probabilities', breach of a protection order became a civil offence, rules were made to provide for the compelling of witnesses, police were encouraged to lay charges and their powers of entry to a dwelling were extended. This round of legislation was influenced by US, Canadian and British reforms (Mugford 1989).

Further legislative reform took place in New South Wales in 1987, extending the definition of domestic violence. In 1991, the NSW Domestic Violence Strategic Plan was developed, as an attempt to coordinate government services. Reports in the first half of the 1990s drew attention to the uncoordinated nature of the response and, in 1996, another report, *New Directions in Reducing Violence Against Women*, was released by the Department for Women and the Premier's Council for Women. This was followed in the same year by the NSW Strategy to Reduce Violence Against Women (VAW Strategy), the objective of which again was to try to provide a coordinated, whole-of-government response, focusing on prevention. A new set of central and regional State structures was put in place. Actions under the VAW Strategy include the Staying Home Leaving Violence pilot project in Bega and eastern Sydney, which was extended in 2009 to six other locations. In 2008, the Government produced a discussion paper, *NSW domestic and family violence strategic framework*, as a step in the development of a new strategic framework (NSW Department of Premier and Cabinet 2008).

Queensland women, organised as the Queensland Domestic Violence Action Group, lobbied for government action in the 1980s. Subsequently, the Task Force on Domestic Violence was established. It produced a report, *Beyond These Walls*, in 1988, which led to the *Domestic Violence (Family Protection) Act 1989*, now the *Domestic and Family Violence Protection Act*. The Domestic Violence Council was established in 1990. The 1989 Act was amended in 2003 to extend coverage to a broad range of non-spousal relationships, including informal care relationships, intimate personal relationships and family relationships. Service providers were given training to equip them for the changes and were encouraged to develop networks and share knowledge and experiences. The Stop Violence against Women Campaign was launched in 1992 and, since then, Domestic and Family Violence Prevention Month has been an annual event.

Concern about violence against women during pregnancy led to the development of a domestic violence initiative in 1998 as a screening aid in antenatal clinics and emergency departments. In 2003, the Queensland Centre for the Prevention of Domestic and Family Violence was established to conduct research, provide education and evaluate initiatives. A domestic and family violence strategy, For Our Sons and Daughters, 2009–2014, was launched in 2009. Initiatives take place under an annual program of action (Government of Queensland 2009).

The Domestic Violence Council was established in South Australia in 1985. It produced a report in 1987 after which the Domestic Violence Prevention Unit was set up in the Office of the Women's Adviser to the Premier. Its purpose was to implement the reforms suggested by the council. In the early 1990s, South Australia promoted the formation of a network of domestic violence action groups across the State. The groups involve representatives of agencies and organisations working in domestic violence at the local level, including the police, housing authorities, community corrections, charity groups, regional health authorities and women's health agencies (Riverland Domestic Violence Action Group web site). Action groups include a non-English-speaking background domestic violence group and a lesbian domestic violence group. The Women's Safety Strategy, which is ongoing, was released in 2005. The Whole of Government Reference Group, involving eight departments, operates and has convened a number of working parties, including an Aboriginal family violence group, a culturally and linguistically diverse women's group and a women with disabilities group.

The Gray Liberal Government in Tasmania commissioned a report into domestic violence in 1984, prompted by the murder by her husband of Maureen Thompson, who had been beaten repeatedly and had eventually obtained a restraining order, which the police had refused to accept. The subsequent *Report on Domestic Violence in Tasmania* made a number of recommendations, some of which were implemented after intense campaigning by women. The Crisis Intervention Unit was established in the Department of Community Services in 1985. The *Family Violence Act* was passed in 2004, and, in the same year, the Safe at Home strategy began, as a whole-of-government response. The program, considered groundbreaking in terms of its focus on coordination, was introduced by then Attorney-General, Judy Jackson, who was passionately committed to reform (Australian Domestic and Family Violence Clearinghouse 2006:5–8). It combines 16 separate initiatives across four government departments. The aims are to improve safety for those experiencing violence, change the behaviour of offenders and focus on prevention. A consultant's review in 2009 found that these objectives were being partially achieved (Department of Justice 2009).

In Victoria, a domestic violence committee was convened by the Premier's Department in 1981, followed by a major report published by the Women's Policy Coordination Unit in 1985. The following year, a discussion paper on child sexual assault was released and the Domestic Violence Incest Resource Centre established. The *Crimes (Family Violence) Act* was passed in 1987, which initiated intervention orders. At the same time, Aboriginal and Torres Strait Islander and migrant and refugee women took action against violence in their communities (Weeks and Gilmore 1996:144–5). In 2002, the Victorian Law Reform Commission was asked to review the 1987 legislation. The Government responded with the Women's Safety Strategy (Government of Victoria 2002). A central aim was to develop a coordinated, integrated response. To this end, the Statewide Steering Committee was formed and it launched a report in 2005. Endorsed by 11 ministers, the strategy focused on four areas: protection and justice, options for women, violence prevention and education, and community action and coordination.

In 2004, then Police Commissioner, Christine Nixon, took the lead in developing the Code of Practice for the Investigation of Family Violence, one of the aims of which was to provide support for aggrieved family members to stay in their own homes. The new code resulted in a significant increase in the police issuance of intervention orders. It also encouraged partnerships between the police and the community. The following year, the Statewide Steering Committee to Reduce Family Violence produced a major reform framework, entitled *Reforming the Family Violence System in Victoria*. The Law Reform Commission reported on the 1987 legislation in 2006 and recommended new legislation, focusing on the safety of victims, with various measures to support those experiencing violence to stay in their own homes (McFerran 2007). The *Family Violence Protection Act* came into effect at the end of 2008 and replaces the 1987 legislation. The definition of family violence has been broadened to include economic and emotional abuse, police powers have been extended, tenancy arrangements have been made easier to adjust and measures to encourage increased reporting have been introduced (DVRCV 2009).

In Western Australia, awareness about the magnitude of violence against women began to emerge in government circles in the 1980s (Murray 1999:9). The first action in response to feminist claims was to set up the Task Force on Domestic Violence in 1985. The task force's report, *Break the Silence* (1986), made 103 recommendations. The Domestic Violence Coordinating Committee, representing key departments, was established to develop appropriate legislation. The ensuing policy changes included training projects and financial assistance for women escaping violence. In 1988, a community education campaign, *Freedom from Fear*, was launched, which challenged perpetrators to take responsibility for their actions.

The Domestic Violence Prevention Council was established by legislative means in the Australian Capital Territory in 1986, along with the office of Domestic Violence Project Coordinator. From that time onwards, the expectation has been that a person acting violently would be removed from the family home. The Domestic Violence Crisis Service (DVCS), with a 24-hour crisis line, began operation in 1988 and was subject to major review in 1997–98. In response to review findings that women wanted the service to support partners as well and did not necessarily want their relationships to end, the service changed the way it worked and the language it used, and found ways of 'engaging respectfully' with partners, piloting a DVCS Men's Line (Simpson 2003:6–8).

ACT community-based services have been leaders in developing coordinated responses to domestic violence, the value of which is now widely recognised. The Family Violence Intervention Program (FVIP) was established to facilitate cooperation between agencies in 1998, partly in response to perceptions that domestic violence was not being taken seriously in the criminal justice system. It relies on cooperation between 12 agencies, including police, the Office of the Director of Public Prosecutions, DVCS, Legal Aid and the Office of Family, Youth and Children's Services. The scheme is facilitated by a steering committee, data and evidence are presented to regular weekly meetings and protocols and practice principles are developed, along with support systems and perpetrator education programs. Evaluation shows the program to be highly successful and a national leader (Australian Domestic and Family Violence Clearinghouse 2007; McFerran 2007; Mulrony 2003b).

In response to pressure from activist women's groups, the Northern Territory Government produced the Northern Territory Domestic Violence Strategy in 1994, which was described as 'all paper, no infrastructure' (Edwards 1998:46) because few programs were put in place and those that were, were poorly resourced. Like other jurisdictions, the Northern Territory has legislated to specify conduct that constitutes domestic violence, the relationships covered and to regulate the issuance of domestic violence protection orders. The principal piece of legislation is the *Domestic and Family Violence Act 2007*, amended in 2009 to provide for mandatory reporting of serious physical harm by health workers—a requirement that is highly controversial. The Government's rationale is that a message is sent to the community that violence against women and children is unacceptable. Mandatory reporting has been criticised, however, on grounds that there is no evidence that it improves safety, that police lack the capacity to investigate all reported cases and that health workers might lack the expertise to meet their obligations. A significant number of women who experience violence oppose mandatory reporting and might therefore be deterred from seeking medical treatment (Marcus 2008).

In sum, despite differences in policies and programs, Australian jurisdictions have produced sets of legislative arrangements with shared features. In all jurisdictions, courts are empowered to make AVOs and to exclude from a shared residence the person against whom the order is made. The types of conduct that constitute domestic violence, the relationships covered and the penalties for breaching an AVO are all regulated and are all broadly similar. In all jurisdictions, temporary orders can be obtained quickly and stalking is now a criminal offence everywhere (Commonwealth of Australia 2009a). There are, however, still significant differences in the discourses in different jurisdictions, variations in levels of penalty and, in some places, differences in issue coverage. For example, emotional and financial abuse and forced social isolation are not offences in every jurisdiction (Murray and Powell 2009).

As in other areas of public policy, here, ideas frequently spread from jurisdiction to jurisdiction. In the 2000s, for example, the importance of coordinated, integrated responses, based on multidisciplinarity, has been recognised in most jurisdictions. Progress has not been striking and evidence suggests there are no easy solutions but shared approaches and frameworks do seem to be producing results (Mulrony 2003b; Willcox 2008:4–6). Another key focus in most jurisdictions in recent years has been on prevention (discussed further below), where work with young people is intended to foster respectful and non-coercive relationships (Mulrony 2003a).

Aboriginal women have continued to form their own organisations, such as Aboriginal women's councils (Flick 1990:66), and have continued to set up their own, often unique, services. Aboriginal Legal Services often provide specially tailored services in relation to violence. In addition, most jurisdictions have made some attempt to consult with Aboriginal women about their needs. For example, following consultations in New South Wales in the early 1990s, the Women Out West Project and the Aboriginal Women and the Law Project were put in place (Thomas and Selfe 1992). Similarly, some efforts have been made to better respond to the needs of women with disabilities who are at least twice as likely to be assaulted, raped and abused as women without a disability. In response to research undertaken by the Victorian Women with Disabilities Network in 2008, the Government funded a policy officer position for the network and Victorian Police have sought to use the evidence in their review of the Police Code of Practice (Healey 2009:8–9).For an indication of the multiplicity and variety of such programs, see the Australian Domestic and

Family Violence Clearinghouse web site database of good-practice programs by jurisdiction: <http://www.austdvclearinghouse.unsw.edu.au/au_resources.html>

Australia has been slow to act in relation to domestic homicide—an area where policy responses began more than a decade ago overseas. Fatality reviews were established in the United States in the 1990s, for example, with a view to finding patterns and commonalities. In Australia, intimate partner homicides have not declined and might be increasing (Oberin 2009:4). In response to the death toll, Victoria established Australia's first domestic violence review panel in 2008, led by the Coroner's Court. In May 2009, the Queensland Premier announced the establishment of the Domestic Violence Death Review Panel, following a four-year campaign by women. The panel will oversee research and provide advice to the Government. Towards the end of 2009, the New South Wales Government set up a permanent expert panel, chaired by the Coroner, to investigate all domestic violence-related deaths (Barrett Meyering 2010:9–11; Pollard 2009).

Sexual Assault Enters Public Policy

> Persistent efforts over the last 30 years (especially by feminists in western contexts) have aimed to render sexual violence a visible concern by challenging the idea that it is a private matter. (Carmody 2009:3).

After an early start and three decades of activism, sexual assault remained a marginalised issue (Carmody and Carrington 2000:142–3). Amanda Goldrick-Jones (2002:123) argues that Australian feminists began to campaign for rape law reform long before well-known American analyses of rape, such as Susan Brownmiller's book *Against Our Will* (1975), were written. Activism has included lobbying for law reform, public shaming, developing support services, mounting campaigns involving videos, films, pamphlets, stickers, posters and billboards, writing books, journal articles and conference papers, doing radio and television interviews, making community education announcements, training professional staff and students and direct action, including street marches and tree-planting ceremonies (Carmody 2009:3).

There are a number of reasons that feminists found it hard to keep this policy issue on the public agenda. First, service provision and legislation are State and Territory responsibilities, so there has been no national overview of the sector or the problems it faces. Further, victim-blaming justifications are strong and have persisted. Moira Carmody argues that the radical feminist analysis of the causes of rape had to be modified before governments were prepared to act; piecemeal reform was manageable, whereas structural transformation was not (Carmody 1990:304). Even in professional circles, rape was often left off agendas of crime-prevention conferences, for example, despite knowledge about the severe health and other problems caused. Similarly, rape is still left off homelessness agendas, although it is known to be a major reason for young women's, and possibly young men's, homelessness. It was also left off drug and alcohol agendas, although the majority of women clients at drug and alcohol agencies identified as sexual assault survivors (Doyle 1996:44).

Slowly and painstakingly, however, feminist activism produced policy responses. South Australia took the lead in establishing the first review of rape law and procedures in the mid-1970s. As a result, rape within marriage became an offence and the definition of rape was extended. In response to feminist agitation in New South Wales, the Premier set up a task force to inquire into sexual violence in 1978. WEL had put forward a draft Bill, Rape and Other Sexual Offences, written by Dr Jocelynne Scutt in 1976. The draft Bill eventually influenced legislation in New South Wales, the Australian Capital Territory, Tasmania, the Northern Territory, Victoria and New Zealand (WEL NSW 2005). A child sexual abuse task force was set up in Queensland in the mid-1980s. In Victoria, a regional network of sexual assault services is part of the women's health program initiated in 1987. At that time, seven centres were already operating and an additional three were approved (Women's Policy Coordination Unit 1987:69). By the 1990s, policy responses in the States and Territories included the provision of counselling servicesCounselling services are always in heavy demand and there are generally long queues. and medical services within hospitals (instead of being delivered by police surgeons), the development of protocols and guidelines for providing support to survivors and the development of training packages for professionals, including the police and court personnel. Legislative reforms included removal of the rape-in-marriage immunity and reform of the rules governing the conduct of trials, including a bar on cross-examination in relation to sexual history (Carmody 1990:305; Carmody and Carrington 2000:341; Australian Capital Territory 2005:4–6).

Persistent advocacy saw government efforts stepped up in the 1990s. The Queensland Government launched the Women's Health Sexual Assault Program, a pilot, in 1991, which provided rape crisis and sexual assault support services. Additional funding for existing and new support services was made available in 1993–94 through the Women's Health Prevention of Violence against Women Program. In New South Wales, the Department of Women commissioned a study of sexual assault trials in 1996; the ACT Law Reform Commission released a discussion paper on sexual assault in 1997 and produced a report in 2001; the 1998 Task Force on Sexual Assault and Rape reviewed Tasmanian policies; the Victorian Law Reform Commission completed a reference on sexual offences in 2004; and the Western Australian Government introduced reform legislation in the same year (Australian Capital Territory 2005:6).

While no jurisdiction has a specific policy on sexual assault and the issue is usually considered under violence and safety agendas (Keel 2005b:4), legislation has resulted in significant advances. Evidence about the complainant's sexual history is not allowed anywhere, except in the Northern Territory, where it is allowed with the permission of the court. There are exceptions, however, depending on relevance. Corroborative evidence is not required in any jurisdiction—that is, a conviction may be made on the evidence of a single witness. In practice, however, it is lawful for juries to be warned that witnesses might not be reliable. The power of a court to subpoena documents, including those that might have been produced in a confidential relationship between a complainant and a counsellor, has been restricted, except in Queensland. Provisions vary from State to State, however, and exceptions are made in particular circumstances. In terms of defining sexual intercourse, all jurisdictions have expanded 1970s definitions with considerable variation. Similarly, determinations of the meaning of 'consent' have been brought into law everywhere but provisions are not uniform. In some jurisdictions, the prosecution is not required to prove that the accused knew that the complainant was not, or might not be, consenting, whereas, in others, awareness and intention must be proven. In Victoria and New South Wales, accused persons must now demonstrate that consent was actively and consistently obtained. Provisions also vary in relation to incest but in every State and Territory, sexual intercourse between close relatives is a criminal offence (Carmody 2009:12; Heath 2005).

In terms of support for women and girls who have experienced sexual violence, a tapestry of services—some government, some non-government—is spread across the land. In New South Wales, major hospitals have sexual assault units, with trained personnel who provide forensic, support and counselling services. Evidence may be given to the police only with the complainant's consent. The work of the NSW Rape Crisis Centre has been discussed. There are 29 publicly funded sexual assault services in Queensland, 20 of which are NGOs, along with a State-wide helpline. Yarrow Place Rape and Sexual Assault Service in Adelaide offers a full range of crisis services for adults but, as it is the only agency in the State, country areas have limited services. Yarrow Place collaborates with other agencies in the criminal justice system, such as the Office of the Director of Public Prosecutions, and works in partnership with such agencies as the Victim Support Service. Tasmania's sexual assault support services (SASS) are community based and informed by feminist principles. They cover the three health system regions, offering comprehensive services, including support services for men. All engage in advocacy and lobbying. Galileo House offers services for children and young people up to the age of eighteen years. Victoria's network of 16 sexual assault centres (CASA), offers free, 24-hour emergency support services, including medical, legal and court support. The CASA Forum is a State-wide agency, providing training, community education and legal information. CASA also undertake advocacy work.

In Western Australia, the Sexual Assault Resource Centre (SARC) provides 24-hour crisis services for adults in the metropolitan area who have been affected by sexual violence within the previous two weeks. It has a State-wide mandate, and provides referrals, a telephone consultation service for regional professionals and education and training, including training to provide forensic services. It chairs the Sexual Assault Services Advisory Group, on which relevant agencies are represented. Regional services are located in the Goldfields, Albany, Geraldton, South Hedland and in the Kimberley. A number of regional hospitals also provide sexual assault services.

The community-based Canberra Rape Crisis Centre offers a 24-hour crisis line and comprehensive, culturally sensitive support services, including legal services. It meets regularly with a range of relevant agencies and engages in advocacy work. Its executive officer at the time, Veronica Wensing, was awarded the 2009 Telstra ACT Businesswoman of the Year. Finally, in the Northern Territory, SARC Darwin is a government centre that provides 24-hour medical services by female doctors. There are regional offices in Katherine, Tennant Creek and Alice Springs. Ruby Gaea Centre against Rape is run by a feminist collective and provides extensive support and referral services for women and children.

Sexual Assault Prevention

Sexual assault prevention is a complex and challenging area for policymakers, educators, researchers and service providers (Carmody 2009:1), but recent research and debate have produced 'a conceptually rich and empirically robust' set of ideas (Clark et al. 2009:7) that are now finding a place on policy agendas. Primary prevention aims to change the underlying causes of violence, modify attitudes, undermine myths and create new standards of acceptability. The notions of primary, secondary and tertiary prevention are similar to those used in primary healthcare discourse. Primary prevention takes place before problems occur; secondary prevention addresses groups at elevated risk or provides early intervention in the face of early signs of violent or victim behaviour; tertiary prevention aims to prevent a recurrence of sexual violence and/or alleviate ongoing effects (Carmody 2009:5).

A number of prevention research and pilot projects have been initiated recently. A sex and ethics research and violence prevention project was jointly undertaken by the University of Western Sydney and the NSW Rape Crisis Centre between 2005 and 2008. Young people from metropolitan and rural New South Wales were interviewed to find out what they thought about sexuality and sexual assault prevention education and how they negotiated sexual relationships. Findings were that education had not prepared them for the complexity of intimate relationships or given them positive skills. Subsequently, a sex and ethics education program was developed to help young people navigate relationships and develop non-violent skills. At the same time, the Violence Prevention, Intervention and Respectful Relationships Education in Victoria Secondary Schools Project was being conducted by VicHealth. The project mapped the prevention programs already in operation, identified and explored best practice in violence prevention and developed a capacity to contribute to policy making and program design. Its 2009 report, *Respectful Relationships Education*, found that some very good violence-prevention programs were operating in Victorian secondary schools but that most were short term, did not engage the whole school and had not been properly evaluated. An exception is the Sexual Assault Prevention Program for Secondary Schools, developed by CASA House. It involves a whole-of-school approach, delivers staff training, and peer education and programs are offered to all levels, rather than to selected groups. The aim is to promote sustainable, school-owned change (Government of Victoria 2009b:5, 59–71).

Various primary prevention programs are now being piloted with funding support from the Commonwealth, under its Respectful Relationships Program. The Sex and Ethics Program, which has been developed to operate in other settings as well as schools, has received funding to train educators and to run groups in three non-metropolitan New South Wales locations and through the AIDS Council of New South Wales. In Queensland, educators are being trained through the National Rugby League to run groups with young men. Pilot projects include the implementation of a prevention program in three ACT secondary schools by the Melbourne Royal Women's Hospital CASA and Canberra Rape Crisis Centre. Provisions include professional development for school staff, train-the-trainer peer education programs and a theatre production. The Northern Territory Department of Education and Training provides teacher-training programs, based on South Australia's Keeping Safe program. The Western Australian Departments of Health and Education are developing respectful relationships education programs for remote-area schools in partnership with SHine South Australia. In Victoria and Tasmania, La Trobe University is trialling and evaluating a Respectful Relationships program for people with intellectual and other cognitive disabilities. A variety of other State and Territory-funded preventive programs also operates (ACSSA web site). Another significant Commonwealth-funded project has been commissioned by the National Association of Services against Sexual Violence (NASASV) to develop standards for best practice in sexual assault prevention education. Six principles, regarded as 'relevant, achievable and inspirational', were produced as a set of guidelines (Evans et al. 2009:2–3).

The primary prevention programs aiming to reduce and eventually eliminate violence against women and girls are in their early stages and results from pilots are not yet available; however, the distance travelled is significant when we remember that an issue that could not be spoken about in public 40 years ago is now 'part of young people's education' (Keel 2005a:24).

Conclusion

The Australian women's health movement has succeeded in influencing policy in the States and Territories in many ways. Over the years, particularly in the 'golden' 1980s, all jurisdictions developed and adopted women's health policies or strategies. Women's health centres have continued to operate even when Commonwealth support has been withdrawn. Services for women and children experiencing violence have been publicly supported, although intense and time-consuming struggles have often been required to maintain funding. Measures to address the problems created by domestic and sexual violence have been developed and adopted. Whereas in the 1970s there was almost no support for women and children trying to escape from violence, many services, well coordinated in some jurisdictions, are now available, although there are never enough to meet demand. All jurisdictions have modernised their laws in a number of ways. Service providers in public agencies, such as the police force and the courts, have been trained in feminist approaches through feminist-devised training modules. Surveys show that community attitudes have changed positively in response to feminist arguments. Whereas women were once required to ensure their own safety, men are now increasingly expected to take responsibility for violence, including sexual violence. More recently, primary prevention initiatives have been expanded with the aim of promoting healthy attitudes and behaviours among the young—a project that has real prospects for reduced violence in the future.

On the negative side, discussed more fully in Chapter 10, women's health centres and services are not sufficiently resourced to meet demand. In the violence field, many projects have been one-off pilot programs, too localised to have a significant general impact. Moreover, they often raise expectations that cannot be fulfilled and leave a significant void when terminated. And a number of policies can be classified as symbolic gestures, giving the impression that action is under way but with no funded implementation plan and no follow-up.

In the 1970s, both domestic violence and sexual assault were buried in the private sector from whence they were extracted by feminist crusades. Yet, of the two issues, it has been much more difficult to keep sexual violence on policy agendas and to change attitudes towards it, even among professionals. A recent review of sentencing and judicial comments in 2008 Victorian judgments found that stranger rape and rape with violence were regarded as more serious than known-offender rape and attracted heavier sentences. There was also a disconnect between judicial comments about the enduring effects of rape by a known assailant and the sentences applied, leading researchers to suggest that 'judges are subject to influence by rape and sexual assault mythology' (Kennedy et al. 2009:19). In searching for explanations about why these myths are so strongly held, Australia's heavily masculinist culture, discussed in Chapter 2, comes to mind. So, too, do the infamous statements of certain judges in relation to acceptable sexual behaviour. Anecdotal evidence suggests that many Australian boys are taught that 'real men' do not hit women whereas less, if anything, is said about sexual violence. Perhaps part of the explanation is that 'rougher than usual handling' is tacitly accepted and has its roots deeply embedded in Australian culture.

8. Commonwealth Policy Responses

Commonwealth receptiveness to the claims of the women's health movement has waxed and waned, depending on the political leanings of the party in power. Support under the Whitlam Government was replaced with withdrawal of funding and abnegation of policy responsibility under the Fraser Government. Renewed support during the period of the Hawke and Keating Governments (1983–96) saw women's health again recognised as a legitimate national policy sphere. The next Commonwealth Government, the Liberal-National Coalition led by John Howard (1996–2007), was hostile to feminism and completely withdrew from a women's health policy role in 1997. Labor returned under the leadership of Kevin Rudd in 2007 and brought with it a commitment to a second NWHP, following calls from the movement for revision and revival since 1995. Thus, the two major parties have displayed very different attitudes to women's health. But while the contrasts are sharp, the case is not entirely black and white: non-Labor governments have supported occasional initiatives and Labor's support has sometimes been less than wholehearted. Moreover, no matter which of the parties has held power, the women's health sector has always been seriously under-funded. The launch of the NWHP in 1989 can be seen as the pinnacle of the movement's policy achievements at the national level.

Women's Health in a Changing Society

In September 1985, more than 700 women gathered in Adelaide for Australia's Second National Conference on Women's Health: Women's Health in a Changing Society. There they resolved that a national women's health policy should be developed, to be in accord with the World Health Organisation (WHO) strategy of 'Health for All by the Year 2000'. In particular, the policy was to be based on the social view of health, recognising that population health is improved if individuals and communities are able to participate in health policy decision making (Kerby-Eaton and Davies 1985:47). The processes of policy development, the conference suggested, should be a shared enterprise between Commonwealth, State and Territory governments, the women's health movement and community groups. The resolution called for the establishment of a working party to further the proposal. In passing this resolution, participants were returning to the first recommendation of the inaugural National Women's Health Conference in 1975, which had resolved 'that a separate policy be formulated on women's health needs and services' (Commonwealth Department of Health 1978:2).

The second resolution of the Adelaide conference called for the establishment of a parallel national women's health program, which would give effect to the aims of the policy and operate within its guidelines. The Commonwealth was asked to commit to ongoing funding.

Four years later, the world's first National Women's Health Policy was endorsed in principle by all Australian health ministers in Burnie, Tasmania, on 21 March 1989. It was launched by the Prime Minister, Bob Hawke, the Health Minister, Neal Blewett, and NSW Health Minister, Peter Collins, at Westmead Hospital, Sydney, on 20 April 1989. Policy development had been a lengthy but participatory process. Both the policy and the program were broadly consistent with the principles articulated in Adelaide. State and Territory governments had been involved in formulation and there had been extensive participation in decision making. Estimates have it that the representatives of more than one million women from diverse backgrounds and all parts of the country were consulted.

The Adelaide women's health movement members who organised the conference knew what they wanted from it: they wanted to put women's health firmly on the national political agenda and they wanted endorsement for a national policy. With that endorsement in hand, they were then able to persuade the then Deputy Secretary of the Commonwealth Department of Health, Ann Kern, of the validity of the proposal. Health Minister, Neal Blewett, was supportive and was not averse to the Commonwealth taking a leading role. The Secretary of the Commonwealth Department at the time, Bernie Mackay, previously Director-General of Health in New South Wales, was interested in health promotion.

The First National Women's Health Policy

In November 1985, two months after the conference, the Prime Minister announced that a national policy on women's health would be developed, which would partly fulfil Australia's international obligations following the Nairobi conference marking the end of the UN Decade for Women (Commonwealth of Australia 1989:1). At the same time, he outlined proposals for what later became known as the National Agenda for Women. As in so many previous consultative processes, women's health had emerged from the agenda consultations as a top priority.

Liza Newby, who had been Director of the Women's Interests Division of Premier and Cabinet in Western Australia, was appointed Special Adviser to Commonwealth Health Minister Blewett in 1987 to coordinate development of the new policy.[1] The following October, a subcommittee of the Australian Health Ministers Advisory Council (AHMAC) on Women and Health was created to assist with the process. The original subcommittee was broadly representative: Commonwealth representatives included the Medical Services Adviser, a representative from the office of the minister, a representative from the Office of the Status of Women (OSW) and a representative from the Australian Institute of Health and Welfare. Women's health advisers or, in some cases, directors of medical services, represented the States and Territories. Non-governmental membership included representatives of Aboriginal and non-English-speaking background women, the Consumers Health Forum, the ACTU, the Royal College of General Practitioners, the Australian Nursing Federation (ANF) and the Australian Women's Health Network. In policy machinery terms, a Commonwealth women's health unit had been set up by the Fraser Government in 1978 but had been abolished a couple of years later by the Lynch razor gang, a ministerial cost-cutting team. The new Commonwealth Women's Health Unit was set up in 1985.

Following informal discussions with a range of stakeholders, including service providers, women's groups and government representatives, Newby, with the AHMAC Subcommittee, wrote a preliminary paper, *Women's health: a framework for change*, a discussion paper for community comment and response. Minister Blewett, who had read a draft and contributed to the document, released it in February 1988. Commonwealth money was allocated for an extensive consultation process.

Responsibility for organising consultation meetings was delegated to women's health advisers in the States and Territories. Pre-consultation forums were sponsored in those jurisdictions that had little or no women's health infrastructure at the time—namely, the Northern Territory, Queensland and Tasmania. In some States, for example, South Australia, a coordinator, who worked with key groups and individuals, including femocrats, was employed to oversee consultation arrangements. Background papers were prepared for meetings so that when the Commonwealth team met with women, there was a level of familiarity with a range of issues. Consultations took place in both metropolitan and rural areas, including day-long workshops, and were well attended. More than 300 submissions were received from government and non-governmental agencies, unions, health professionals, professional organisations, groups of women and individuals (Commonwealth of Australia 1989:2–4).

A major effort was made to work with Aboriginal women's groups to facilitate participation. Special meetings were organised and, in a few cases, individual appointments were made. Large numbers of Aboriginal women took part in

1   The position had been advertised in 1986 but had not been filled.

the NT consultations. There was, however, a view that including Aboriginal women's concerns and preferences in the NWHP might detract from the work being undertaken at the same time to develop the National Aboriginal Health Strategy. In any case, many women thought that a separate, dedicated process was needed to properly capture the views of Aboriginal women. Immigrant women (or, as they were called at the time, NESB women) participated strongly and wanted their concerns included.

Consultation organisers remember that the women who attended were constructive and positive and put forward practical suggestions. They saw health from a social perspective, they knew what they wanted from the health system and they knew what was missing from the services on offer. On the basis of the consultations and submissions, the first NWHP was written in the second half of 1988 and in early 1989, largely by Laurie Gilbert, Director of the Commonwealth Women's Health Unit from 1987 until the end of 1989, in collaboration with the AHMAC Subcommittee. A steering committee was established to pilot the policy through departmental processes.

Obstacles Confronting Commonwealth Femocrats

A number of difficulties beset the femocrats charged with writing the policy and having it endorsed. The Women's Health Unit had a very heavy workload and it was short of staff. Many staff members were on short-term appointments and on very steep learning curves. Some positions were approved but never filled; even at the Commonwealth level, women in the bureaucracy are reported to have been 'very wary' of moving to an area with a feminist label, fearing that career advancement would be jeopardised. The result was that the team writing the NWHP was smaller than intended. Moreover, the unit had to deal with ordinary departmental work as well, which included responsibility for producing input to the women's budget statement, responding to ministerial questions and the requirements of interdepartmental committees and producing all the preliminary report documents that went to AHMAC.

Another problem was simple disruption. There were three reorganisations of Commonwealth government departments during the development and implementation of the policy. Having been called the Department of Health since its foundation in 1921, the department had three different names in the second half of the 1980s, there were three different departmental heads and the Women's Health Unit had four division heads and three different locations. These changes made the job of Commonwealth femocrats difficult. The continuity necessary to drive reform processes was difficult to achieve in rapidly changing circumstances.

Two of the policy's key supporters in the Commonwealth Department, the Secretary, Bernie McKay, and the Deputy Secretary, Ann Kern, both left in 1987, at the beginning of the development phase. As at the sub-national level, for many senior bureaucrats, women's health was not a high priority and was a contentious issue for others. Moreover, policy changes were being made on the basis of what women said (during consultations), which was a departure from standard practice that was not widely accepted. Traditionally, experts made policy, in what they knew to be in everyone's best interests, advised by organised medicine in processes that were generally secret. In addition, departmental officers were concerned about opposition from organised medicine and a real effort was made to get the support of medical unions. In this, Dr Cathy Mead, Chair of the Working Group of the AHMAC Subcommittee on Women and Health, played a crucial role. She is medically trained, understands the issues and, broadly, succeeded in containing medical opposition. Christine Giles, Manager of the Victorian Women's Health Policy and Programs Unit and also a member of the AHMAC Subcommittee Working Group, is said to have been able to persuade key Commonwealth bureaucrats to support the project. That Health Minister Blewett offered positive support was crucial to the outcome. The whole process was timed around elections in order to gain maximum political mileage for the Commonwealth. Completion was scheduled to be in time for the budget cycle preceding the 1990 election.

It is reported to have been touch and go whether Australia's health ministers would endorse the policy and there was uncertainty about whether meaningful sums of money would be allocated to the program. Budget decisions the previous year did not inspire confidence. Proposals had been made to fund projects identified as needed in NWHP consultations but none was successful (Szoke 1988:33). Femocrats and AHMAC Subcommittee members worked hard to generate support for funding. They held meetings with the Women's Caucus Committee of the Federal Parliamentary Labor Party. Labor women could then inform women in their constituencies of progress, maintaining momentum. A great deal of lobbying was done, which included discussions with State and Territory health ministers and senior departmental officers. This laborious process eventually brought about a significant change in attitudes.

The change, however, was not enough to transform women's health into a high-priority item; participants remember a budgetary allocation process that was completely ad hoc. The Women's Health Unit was required to put up costing proposals for the 1988–89 Budget, on the understanding that initiatives in all five action areas would be funded. The cost was to be $100 million over five years, to be shared between the Commonwealth and the States and Territories—a modest enough proposal. A women's health branch of the Commonwealth department was also to be established to implement the program. In the event, only the first three action areas were funded. Combined Commonwealth, State and Territory funding totalled only $33.72 million over four years or just under $8.5 million per year (Commonwealth of Australia 1993:6). Given that Australian health expenditure between 1989 and 1993 averaged $32.09 billion per year (AIHW 1997:2), this was a tiny sum of money.

The proposed Women's Health Branch was never established. An additional $6 million for alternative birthing services, $3 million for the provision of reproductive health services in rural areas and $1 million for breast and cervical screening programs were allocated. In States with relatively small populations, the amount of money for specific services was ridiculously small. For example, in Western Australia, the total Commonwealth funding for the alternative birthing services program was $35 000.

Infrastructure Established under the NWH Program

The NWH Program was initially funded for four years, following which funding of $59.512 million or just less than $15 million per year was approved for a second four years—a modest increase. The projects that were funded were enormously diverse and varied considerably from place to place, partly depending upon the infrastructure already established. As a cost-shared program, Commonwealth/State/Territory assessment committees were formed in each jurisdiction to recommend the funding of selected projects to ministers. Community support had to be demonstrated before funding would be approved. The terms of reference of the AHMAC Subcommittee were altered to allow it to take responsibility for monitoring and overseeing implementation.

A number of national projects were undertaken in the first four years, mainly in professional training and education. These included an education package for schools, focusing on the effects of sex-role stereotyping; an education kit for general practitioners, with fact sheets in 10 languages; a general practitioner education project, intended to improve knowledge of women's health issues; a continuing education package for nurses, focusing especially on rural and remote area work; and a distance learning package for midwives (Commonwealth of Australia 1993:23–7). During the second four years, the national effort consisted of small projects, including continuing education for general practitioners, the development of outcomes and performance indicators for women's health and a collaborative services project for older and isolated women (Commonwealth of Australia 1997:109–17).

Of the States and Territories, New South Wales had the most extensive women's health infrastructure. Instead of establishing new centres and services, a number of mainstream reforms were introduced, including the establishment of regional women's health coordinators, ethnic obstetric liaison programs, Aboriginal antenatal outreach, multicultural family planning and health services for older women. Twenty-eight of the 89 projects were directed towards the needs of rural women (Commonwealth of Australia 1993:28–32). During the second four years, funding was mainly allocated to continue the innovations of the first four years; however, a small number of NGO services were funded, including family planning and rape crisis services, information for immigrant and refugee women and services for Aboriginal women (Commonwealth of Australia 1997:19–20). One of the programs was the Aboriginal Maternity Service, located in the northern NSW town of Tamworth, providing antenatal, intrapartum and postnatal services for Aboriginal women and non-Aboriginal women with Aboriginal partners. Among its health-promotion activities were support for breastfeeding and information about good nutrition, exercise and the benefits of smoking cessation. An infant immunisation rate of 100 per cent was achieved. In keeping with tradition and grandmothers' stories, the message was that Aboriginal women are 'the best nurturing mothers in the world' (Nichols and Hurley 1999:24–8).

In Queensland, where the existing women's health infrastructure was limited, the focus was on funding separate women's health services, as discussed in Chapter 3. In addition, the Mobile Women's Health Service was funded, staffed by 15 women's health nurses trained to work as independent practitioners. Service provision included reproductive health services, together with counselling, stress management and preventive health education. A number of smaller projects were also funded (Commonwealth of Australia 1993:35–7). In the second four years, 97 per cent of the funding was allocated to Queensland's eight community-based women's health centres (Commonwealth of Australia 1997:22–3).

In South Australia, services for women living in non-metropolitan areas were identified as the top priority. The Country Women's Health Services Advisory Group was set up in 1990, replaced with the broader State Steering Committee in 1991, which met monthly to oversee proposal development and implementation. Clinical and health promotion services for rural and remote women were funded, community women's health nurses were employed and the Women's Health Business Project for Aboriginal women was undertaken. A '008' women's health information line was introduced, along with a newsletter,

Stating Women's Health (Commonwealth of Australia 1993:41–3). During the second four years, funding continued for services for women living in rural and remote areas, and, in all, 17 Country Women's Health Services were set up, all of which were integrated into existing services. Each service was required to have a Women's Health Advisory Committee, facilitating discussion and community participation. A number of respondents to the evaluation questionnaire rightly identified the low level of funding as a major obstacle to achieving program goals (Commonwealth of Australia 1997:23–5).

The first two years of the program in Tasmania focused on local research to identify needs, followed by seed funding for a range of one-off programs, intended to be innovative and participatory. A strategic planning document was produced, with identified priorities and plans for regional women's health programs. The Health for Women in the Workplace project, the Flinders Island Women's Health Project, the Centre for Excellence in the Middle Years Project and the Social Health Project were set up (Commonwealth of Australia 1993:43–6). Ongoing funding for the Hobart Women's Health Centre was provided in the second phase, along with the employment of three Regional Women's Health Coordinators whose responsibilities included service development, training, advocacy for mainstream sensitivity to women's needs, information provision, consultation, initiation of best-practice models and policy advice. Each region of the State developed a Women's Health Strategic Plan (Commonwealth of Australia 1997:26–8).

The NWH Program enabled Victoria's network of women's health services, set up under the Victorian Women's Health Program, to be expanded. The network of sexual assault services was also extended to provide after-hours cover and to cater for the needs of rural areas. The Multicultural Centre for Women's Health received additional funding for information services, along with Healthsharing Women. Other projects included support for Greek women who suffered mental illness, an older women's housing project, a service mapping project, an access and equity program for immigrant and refugee women needing to use sexual assault services, a good practices in mental health project and statistics and evaluation framework projects (Commonwealth of Australia 1993:32–5). Support for this network of services continued in the second four years.

Western Australia, as we have seen, did not come into the program until 1991. All the State's women's health centres except Perth's original centre and the Fremantle multicultural women's health centre were established with NWH Program funding. New regional sexual assault centres were also established and existing ones expanded. Women's health information services were set up and a variety of quality-assurance, research and data and service development and monitoring projects was introduced (Commonwealth of Australia 1993:38–40). In the second four years, support continued for women's health infrastructure so that by 1997 the program was funding five sexual assault referral centres in regional areas and 11 community-managed women's health centres in both metropolitan and rural locations (Commonwealth of Australia 1997:25–6).

Effectively, only one project, a community-controlled women's health centre, could be financed from the funding available to a small jurisdiction such as the Australian Capital Territory. Nevertheless, the opening of the centre was cause for jubilation among activists. Tiny amounts of money were provided for information provision, which included pamphlet and booklet production, translation of information material into languages other than English and a limited number of community workshops (Commonwealth of Australia 1993:49–50). Funding distribution in the second four years replicated that in the first. In the Northern Territory, there were few dedicated women's health services before the program and this situation was maintained. Program grants were advertised in 1991 and projects funded include the Aboriginal and Torres Strait Islander Women's Health Service in Darwin, with another in Tennant Creek, a cervical cancer screening program for Aboriginal women, the establishment of a carers' network and a project supporting the development of culturally appropriate health-promotion services by Aboriginal health workers. Family Planning NT received money to provide reproductive and sexual health education forums for young people. The AIDS Council of Central Australia was funded to employ a women's HIV/AIDS project officer, and the Wunara Aboriginal Corporation received money for the 'Beat the Grog Signs' project (Commonwealth of Australia 1993:9). In the second four years, a total of 39 projects were funded, approximately half of which were managed by community-based organisations and the other half by the Territory Health Service. As in the Australian Capital Territory, in the Northern Territory, the amount of money available was small (Commonwealth of Australia 1997:28–30).

Criticisms of the Policy and Program

Apart from criticisms of the inadequacy of program funding, some women felt that the NWHP and the NWH Program reflected the concerns of Anglo-Australian, middle-class women. Whatever the validity of the view, projects for a diversity of cultural groups were funded. It is true, however, that the concerns of Aboriginal women were largely left aside, as discussed. Regrettably, the National Aboriginal Health Strategy, which was meant to address Aboriginal women's health, was never sufficiently funded or effectively implemented. A 1994 evaluation found gross under-funding by all governments, lack of accountability and lack of political support for the National Council of Aboriginal Health, which had been established to oversee implementation. The evaluators recommended that the Commonwealth renew its commitment to the principles underpinning the strategy, that it accept the holistic Aboriginal view of health and that it recognise the importance of local community control (Commonwealth of Australia 1994:2–3).

Immigrant and refugee women were positioned differently but the long-term outcome was no more satisfactory. As part of the National Agenda for Women, the Commonwealth–State Council on NESB Women's Issues was established in 1989 (Commonwealth of Australia 1991:66). The council chose health as its first priority, not because the health of immigrant women was not addressed in the NWHP, but because it was felt that the special health problems faced by NESB women warranted a dedicated strategy. Thus, it produced the National Non-English Speaking Background Women's Health Strategy (NESBWHS) in 1991. The main concerns identified were high rates of workplace-related illnesses and injuries and a higher than normal incidence of poor mental and emotional health. The strategy was intended to complement the NWHP (Commonwealth of Australia 1992:xi–xxxiii). Like the NWHP, the strategy took a social view of health, offered a strong critique of conventional medical care and advocated inter-sectorality.

This strategy, too, failed to attract resources and became essentially 'an un-actioned information document' (Schofield 1996: 30–5). On the basis of major presentations, the Third AWHN National Women's Health Conference recommended that the strategy be updated and implemented (Davis et al. 1996:13–14). No action was taken, however, and soon afterwards, the Keating Labor Government lost office.

The Indirect Impact of the NWHP

The existence of a national policy, endorsed by all State and Territory health ministers, strengthened the position of local-level femocrats and the policymakers who supported them. They were able to argue that the principles and priorities of State and Territory women's health policies and strategies should be in line with those of the NWHP. The national policy also provided protection for women's health infrastructure. For example, one of the first acts of the newly elected, neo-liberal-leaning Greiner Government in New South Wales was to review Health Department-funded NGOs, which raised fears within the sector. Shortly afterwards, however, government statements endorsed the principles of the NWHP: national recognition of the claims of the women's health movement produced a stronger level of legitimation than would otherwise have existed. Jennifer Cashmore, former SA Minister for Health, who overcame opposition and secured agreement to begin work on a women's health policy, attested to the importance of the national policy's influence. In her view, her party's policy developed for the December 1993 SA election would have been unthinkable had it not been for the NWHP.

Perversely, however, the existence of the NWHP could be used to justify inaction when the political climate was unfavourable. For example, in 1996–97, femocrats in Western Australia who had developed proposals for a State women's health policy were told this was not a priority and, furthermore, that there was no need for a State policy since the national policy had been endorsed.

Domestic Violence and Sexual Assault Enter the Commonwealth Policy Agenda

The first Commonwealth policy directly addressing domestic violence was part of the National Agenda for Women. It was the three-year National Domestic Violence Education Campaign (NDVEC), run by OSW and judged 'very successful' by the Agenda Implementation Report. At the same time, a survey was run to plumb attitudes to domestic violence. A high level of social sanctioning was found: one in five people considered physical violence by a man against his wife to be acceptable sometimes, more than half thought it was okay to yell abuse and one-third still thought it a private matter (Laing 2000:4). The campaign raised community awareness of violence but because violence support services received no additional funding, service providers were 'stretched to the limit'. One set of evaluators argued that action as well as rhetoric was needed from the Commonwealth (Earle et al. 1990:4–6).

In 1990, the National Committee on Violence against Women was established by the Keating Government, with a budget of $1.35 million over three years, or $45 000 a year. The committee was charged with covering all forms of violence against women, initiating research and undertaking education work, with special emphasis on the requirements of groups with special needs, all with a few thousand dollars a year. A position paper was produced in 1991 (Commonwealth of Australia 1991:63–4) and the National Strategy on Violence against Women was introduced in 1992. Its aims were to share information and coordinate the policies, programs, law enforcement and legislation in the different jurisdictions. It had no programs of its own nor did it provide funding for the States and Territories, which were expected to continue to support their own programs and any new initiatives that might be proposed. Heads of government were asked to deliver annual statements on eliminating violence against women. The strategy, which, with so little funding, was more of a public relations exercise, ran until the Government lost office in 1996. The Women's Safety Survey conducted in

1996 by the Australian Bureau of Statistics (ABS) showed that 7.1 per cent of Australian women had experienced an act of violence in the previous 12 months (Commonwealth of Australia 1996).

The next Commonwealth initiative was the Howard Government's Partnerships against Domestic Violence (PADV), introduced in 1997; $50.3 million was committed over the six years to 2004. Again, one of the objectives was to encourage Commonwealth, State and Territory coordination, not that the Commonwealth had many activities of its own at this point. New project funding was provided, which was intended to be seed money for prevention research. An additional $25 million was committed, primarily to set up the Australian Domestic and Family Violence Clearinghouse, which publishes newsletters and papers on key issues and new initiatives. PADV was criticised both for its location within a conservative discourse and for the paucity of its funding (Chappell 2001:66–7). Ruth Phillips (2006) argues that the results of the 1996 Women's Safety Survey 'compelled' the Howard Government to maintain a policy on violence against women but that the terminology was changed to 'family violence', 'family dysfunction' and 'family breakdown', suggesting that violence was not primarily 'against women', thereby obscuring the links between gender and power.[2] This shift in terminology can be seen as an example of what Howe (2009:28) calls the act of 'disappearing' men's violence, in a context where 'it's still not permissible to name it as such'. Men and women, outside feminist forums, she argues, still engage in denials and disavowals. Nevertheless, funds were provided, including for projects in Aboriginal communities and for early intervention for children at risk. After three years, PADV is said to have run out of political steam and no major Commonwealth announcements were made between 1999 and 2003.

The next Commonwealth initiative was a community awareness campaign, 'Violence against Women, Australia Says No', launched in 2004, after delays during which the Prime Minister is reported to have altered the language. The campaign operated through TV, cinema and magazines. It provided a 24-hour helpline and resources in secondary schools (Carrington and Phillips 2006). Community education materials were also made available through the PADV web site. Phillips concludes that, while PADV acknowledged violence as a problem and funded some worthwhile projects, 'both the discourse and the practice' undermined the potential for the long-term structural and attitudinal change that is necessary to reduce violence against women (Phillips 2006:214).

Previous Commonwealth anti-violence strategies had included sexual assault but the Howard Government moved to address the two separately. It launched

---

2   Many Aboriginal women prefer the term 'family violence' because it covers the full range of traumas that individuals and families suffer, including domestic violence, rape, child abuse and spiritual and cultural abuse (Lester 1992:38).

the National Initiative to Combat Sexual Assault in 2001, under which the OSW commissioned consultants to undertake research on the criminal justice system and sexual assault, with a view to developing a framework for sexual assault prevention. An international literature review on assaults against females sixteen years of age and older was followed by analyses of existing research in Australia, the United Kingdom, Canada, New Zealand and the United States. The Australian Centre for the Study of Sexual Assault (ACSSA) was set up under this initiative. ACSSA provides information to assist policymakers and develops evidence-based, prevention-oriented strategies. All forms of sexual assault are investigated but there is a focus on women and girls over fifteen years of age and adult survivors of child sexual assault (Commonwealth of Australia 2004a; Carrington and Phillips 2006).

In 2005, the Commonwealth announced that PADV had concluded and would be replaced with the Women's Safety Agenda, which was to include both domestic violence and sexual assault. The program would have $75.7 million over four years and would build on the groundwork of PADV and the National Initiative to Combat Sexual Assault. Under the agenda, funding was continued for the Australian Domestic and Family Violence Clearinghouse (Carrington and Phillips 2006). Towards the end of its term of office, the Howard Government introduced significant changes to the *Family Law Act* that have implications for women and children experiencing violence. Said to be the result of lobbying by fathers' rights groups, the changes introduced shared parenting after separation and mandatory participation in dispute resolution. The changes have been heavily criticised for putting parental rights, particularly fathers' rights, ahead of the rights of children. Mediation is not required in cases involving violence or child abuse. However, because violence and abuse are often difficult to prove and the consequences of unproven accusations can be heavy, there is concern that many women refrain from speaking out (DVRCV 2008).

The Rudd Labor Government, elected in 2007, appointed the National Council to Reduce Violence against Women and their Children (hereinafter called the National Council), in May 2008, thereby fulfilling an election promise. The then Prime Minister, who had been involved in domestic violence policy development in Queensland in the early 1990s, was committed to action and in the early 2000s, he became a White Ribbon Ambassador. The Minister for the Status of Women, Tanya Plibersek, was equally committed, and the White Ribbon campaign had close ties with her office. The National Council was appointed for a year to provide advice on the development of an evidence-based national plan. It undertook research and consultations with approximately 2000 stakeholders. A five-part report, *Time for Action: The National Council's plans for Australia to reduce violence against women and their children, 2009–2021*, was released in April 2009. On the release of the report, the Government agreed to act on 18 of the 20 priority recommendations. It also agreed to develop a national plan through the Council of Australian Governments (COAG) because many of the council's recommendations require cooperative action between levels of government.

The new funding commitments were $12.5 million for a 24-hour, seven-day-a-week telephone and online crisis service, $26 million for primary prevention projects, including $9.1 million over five years for the respectful relationships program and $17 million for a public information campaign. Some $3 million was allocated for research on nationally consistent laws and perpetrator programs. These are not large funding commitments and WWDA has requested clarification about possible overlaps with previously announced funding (Parkinson 2009:6). The Australian Law Reform Commission has been asked to work with State and Territory law reform commissions to examine the interrelationship of relevant laws. The Violence against Women Advisory Group was appointed for two years from September 2009, to advise on issues raised in the council's report and to oversee the establishment of the National Centre of Excellence, which will evaluate the effectiveness of strategies, improve best practice and support workforce development.

The National Council's report and the Commonwealth's commitment to action have been welcomed by women's movement spokeswomen, who are cautiously optimistic about the potential for valuable outcomes. The council has been commended for the quality of its work. The personal commitment and statement of zero tolerance made by then Prime Minister Rudd were both well received. The reform project is seen as ambitious but Commonwealth leadership on violence against women and girls, including sexual assault, is regarded as well overdue. According to Julie Oberin, longstanding movement activist and Chair of WESNET, the Rudd Government's approach to domestic and family violence and homelessness 'has for the first time in history, the capacity to radically address decades of neglect in these fields' (Oberin 2009:2). She acknowledges, however, the enormity of the problems and the huge obstacles to be overcome.

In February 2011, the National Plan to Reduce Violence against Women and their Children was launched. It is intended to be a framework for a single, unified strategy for the next 12 years (Commonwealth of Australia 2011d). Six national outcomes have been formulated, which are that communities are safe from violence, that relationships are respectful, that Indigenous communities are strengthened, that services meet the needs of women and their children experiencing violence, that justice responses are effective and that perpetrators stop the violence and be held to account. The document incorporates the first three-year plan, which will focus on prevention. Proposed actions are support for local community work to reduce violence against women, commitment to the continuation of the respectful relationships education program in schools, telephone support for frontline workers, perpetrator programs with their own national standards, a national centre of excellence that will focus on evaluation, the continuation of Personal Safety and Community Attitudes Surveys to track the effectiveness of policies and an Australian Law Reform Commission inquiry into the impact of Commonwealth laws. There is also to be a national recognition scheme for domestic and family violence orders, including a national database. Outcome six proposed by the National Council—that systems be made to work together effectively, through coordinated, evidence-based responses—has been dropped from the national plan. It is much too early to evaluate the impact of the Plan which will depend on levels of political commitment and resources.

Responses to Violence in Aboriginal Communities

Violence in Aboriginal communities and the destructive impact of colonisation are well documented. Aboriginal women and members of their communities have continued to work in their own ways on what many, but not all, call 'family violence'. Larissa Behrendt has compared the characteristics of Aboriginal dispute-resolution mechanisms with those of the British legal system. She explains that Aboriginal approaches encourage the participation of all community members who feel they have an interest in either a dispute or its outcome and that resolution processes take place before the family and/or the community, acknowledging the social context of dispute resolution (Behrendt 2002). Thus, even if Aboriginal people trusted the criminal justice system, many would approach family violence quite differently. In general, the facilitation of community responses is preferred, with a focus on healing families, rather than punishing individuals. In some approaches, male perpetrators are integrated back into their communities after punishment, treatment and healing (Keel 2004; Memmott et al. 2006).

Among the initiatives that women have had a part in developing are night patrols, initiated in the Northern Territory as a self-policing mechanism and later adapted and modified in other places. Night patrols assist in ensuring social order, preventing potentially violent situations and assisting the vulnerable. By 2003, they were described as 'a distinctive feature of the community landscape in Indigenous Australia' (Blagg 2002:200; Blagg and Valuri 2003:7).

Other women-led responses include constructing family healing centres instead of refuges, establishing shelters on women's law principles, which render them out of bounds for men, and using sacred objects in women's spaces as a deterrent to male violence. Traditional women's business has been reinstated in some settings as a dynamic factor in community life, along with the reinforcement of grandmother law, under which senior women become involved in dispute resolution, sometimes through mediation (Blagg 2002:4).

While some projects are women-only initiatives, others involve both men and women. The *Aboriginal and Islander Health Worker Journal* has published annotated indexes of Indigenous health information, which provide an overview of health projects up to 2008. Other responses include mentoring schemes, worker gatherings for networking and sharing knowledge, theatre projects around family violence and community-controlled counselling projects oriented towards social and emotional health (Memmott et al. 2006).

All Australian governments have funded projects intended to address violence in Aboriginal communities. The main Commonwealth initiatives in recent years include the Family Violence Prevention Legal Service (FVPLS) program, first established as a pilot project and an initiative of the Aboriginal and Torres Strait Islander Commission (ATSIC) in 1998. The initial aim was to meet the legal needs of victims of family violence. The program provides assistance predominantly to women and children. In 2004–05, on the abolition of ATSIC, control passed to the Commonwealth Attorney-General's Department, after which the program was expanded, both in services and in functions. It was extended again in 2006–07, and since that time 31 community-controlled services have been funded. The Early Intervention and Prevention Program was added and the program now provides counselling, practical support and assistance, information regarding support services and referrals. Educational and community-awareness projects and early identification and prevention strategies have also been developed. In 2006, 5717 clients presented themselves to the Family Violence Prevention Legal Service (FVPLS) (Commonwealth of Australia n.d.).

Under PADV, there were new initiatives for Aboriginal people. The first was the National Indigenous Family Violence Grants Program (NIFVGP), which ran between 1999 and 2004 and provided funding for 74 community-based projects. The principles of cultural appropriateness, holism, intersectorality, local community control and leadership and community development were embedded in the design. Following this, FaHCSIA funded a number of programs including the Family Violence Partnership Program (FVPP) and the Family Violence Regional Activities Program (FVRAP). Under the FVPP, the Commonwealth contributed $37.3 million over four years, and through agreements with the States and Territories family violence and child-protection initiatives were put in place. Under FVRAP, support was provided for grassroots projects that had been identified in communities and operated through centres called Indigenous Coordination Centres. FaHCSIA also ran a number of other programs, including the Stronger Families and Communities Strategy and the Family and Community Networks Initiative. In addition, COAG ran trials in eight community locations in 2002 and 2003 (Memmott et al. 2006).

This is not the place to discuss the contentious NT National Emergency Response introduced by the Howard Government in 2007 and continued by the Rudd and Gillard Governments. As a top-down policy, however, there is wide concern that it ignores the demonstrated principles of best practice. Experts argue that the program flies in the face of evidence that successful programs are built from the ground up in collaboration with communities (Kelleher 2009:13–14). Evaluation of the NIFVGP, for example, showed that projects to address family violence are best developed, driven and nurtured by Aboriginal people at the community level (Memmott et al. 2006:22).

According to Hannah McGlade, a Perth-based Aboriginal human rights lawyer, the new national plan needs to go much further than the recommendations made in the council's report. She recommends three specific strategies: the establishment of a national research and capacity-building agency, specifically addressing violence against Aboriginal women, to be located within the proposed National Centre of Excellence; the placement of the victims of violence at the centre of proposed healing centres; and the funding of Aboriginal women's legal services in all Australian jurisdictions rather than relying on the erroneous notion that mainstream services can serve the needs of Aboriginal women and children. McGlade argues that the new national plan 'must unequivocally recognise and affirm that Aboriginal women play a central role in ending the violence' (McGlade 2010:4–5).

The national plan does recognise the centrality of Aboriginal women in reducing violence:

> The *National Plan* is focused on supporting Indigenous communities to develop local solutions to preventing violence. This includes encouraging Indigenous women to have a stronger voice as community leaders and supporting Indigenous men to reject violence. Improving economic outcomes and opportunities for Indigenous women are critical to reducing violence. (Commonwealth of Australia 2011d:20)

As mentioned, the third national outcome of the plan is that Indigenous communities are to be strengthened; however, as in so many other cases, results will hinge largely upon whether resources are made available to pursue these objectives.

The women's health movement has been able to influence a number of other Commonwealth policies, the most important of which are reviewed briefly below.

Better Health Policy

The movement succeeded in having the terms of reference of the 1985 Better Health Commission expanded. The commission was established to examine the health status of Australians and to recommend national goals for improvement. Originally, its terms of reference asked it to report on 'the major preventable health problems of women in their reproductive years'; however, the minister agreed to extend the terms of reference to include the 'health problems of women of all ages', after the 1985 National Women's Health Conference. Women on the commission, including Dr Janet Irwin, argued for a comprehensive, social view of women's (people's) health and women at the grassroots level were able to make contributions. Ultimately, the commission, which reported in 1986, endorsed the WHO 'Health for All by the Year 2000' initiative. When it came to addressing the question of 'why women's health should be given more consideration than men's health', it decided, however, that women's illnesses were not different from those of men but that women's health needed attention because it did not get proper consideration from a 'male dominated health care system' that excluded humane and caring values (Commonwealth of Australia 1986a:147–8)!

Women's Health Research

Research and data collection formed one of the five priority areas of the NWHP but, initially, no funding was provided. In 1989, however, the Commonwealth Department of Community Services and Health funded a workshop, which was asked to develop a list of research priorities as a guide to funding under the Health and Community Services Research and Development Grants (Broom 1990). Subsequently, and just before the 1993 election, Prime Minister, Paul Keating, announced that the Commonwealth would fund a major longitudinal study on women's health. Submissions were called and a contract awarded for the project, later renamed Women's Health Australia. It received its first resources in 1995 and is managed by a multidisciplinary team of researchers from the Research Centre for Gender, Health and Ageing at the University of Newcastle and from the University of Queensland (Lee et al. 2005). The aim is to collect data and evidence that can be used to inform policy.

The study involves three age cohorts and includes more than 40 000 women over 20 years. It examines attitudes and lifestyles, together with the biological, psychological, social, economic and lifestyle factors that influence health outcomes. Women's use of time is studied, including the impact of paid and unpaid work, family roles and leisure. It also identifies women's health-service needs and evaluates the adequacy of the services on offer. Findings are released regularly. The only new funding announced with the 2010 NWHP is $5.3 million to enable the project to recruit a cohort of younger women—an extension that AWHN and the movement had supported for some time.

Policy Responses to Trafficking

In 1999, the Howard Government introduced legislation amending criminal code provisions on slavery. The new legislation imposes penalties on people responsible for bringing women into Australia under 'slavery-like' conditions. Prosecutions under the new law were slow but, in 2008, the High Court found a brothel owner guilty of slavery. Further prosecutions followed in Victoria. The Howard Government replaced deportation with the offer of temporary visas for women willing to help police and made provision for some support services. Significant problems with the visa system remained, however, and, in 2009, the Commonwealth introduced further reforms. Project Respect has worked for all these changes and now advocates legislative reform that will allow trafficked women to receive compensation. It wants to see programs introduced to alter attitudes and for sex slavery to be incorporated into violence-prevention policies (Maltzahn 2009). The Victorian Parliament's Drug and Crime Prevention Committee held an inquiry into People Trafficking for Sex Work and tabled its final report in June 2010. It made some 30 recommendations, including that a whole-of-government Sex Industry Regulation, Policy and Coordination Unit be established in the Department of Justice.

Women with Disabilities and Public Policy

The influence of women with disabilities on Australian policy has been disappointing, despite the tenacity and professionalism of members of Women with Disabilities Australia (WWDA), which received one of four National Violence Prevention Awards in 1999. The association campaigns on an expanse of issues and produces valuable resources. It has worked extensively on violence against women with disabilities, for example, and has produced reports, action plans, model processes and national information kits. Spokeswomen draw attention to the fact that their concerns are regularly overlooked by the disability movement, the women's movement, the women's health movement and by governments at all levels (Howe 1999; Meekosha 1990, 2001; Tilley 2000). Meekosha (1990:36–7) argues that the uncritical acceptance of physical strength and self-reliance by feminism has had the effect of excluding some women while, at the same time, many doctors and others hold a view that women with severe disabilities should not be mothers. Margaret Cooper and Diane Temby (1995) point out that even under the first NWHP and Program, women with disabilities were 'relatively marginalised'.

Some commentators explain this situation by pointing to the low status generally accorded women with disabilities. Chenoweth (1997:26) has argued that this group of women is so devalued that they are denied even a sexual identity and exist in a state of 'extreme marginalisation'. WWDA works to undermine the multiple surrounding myths, many of which controvert basic human rights. Myths include the claim that women with intellectual disabilities are promiscuous, that they should not have children because they are not fit mothers and that sterilising women with disabilities will protect them from rape (Chenoweth 1993:4).

Recent research confirms that there are still major knowledge gaps about the experiences of women with disabilities, including the experiences of Aboriginal and immigrant and refugee women, and major gaps in policies and available services (Healey 2009:8). In terms of public policy responses, Tilley (2000) points out that although women with disabilities are often mentioned in the preambles of policy documents, they are nevertheless almost entirely ignored when it comes to developing and funding appropriate programs. Certainly, disability policies in Australia have consistently failed to apply a gender lens. Most have proceeded on the assumption that men and women experience disability in the same way and that there is therefore a common set of issues.

Governments have enacted legislation with the aim of benefiting people with disabilities. The national *Disability Discrimination Act* was passed in 1992, which provides protection for men and women against discrimination on the basis of disability. A set of standards specifying rights and responsibilities about equal access and opportunities for people with a disability accompanies the Act. Successive Commonwealth, State and Territory disability agreements have been hammered out, the first of which was signed in 1991. It provides a framework for the development, delivery and funding of specialised services. Through the agreements, governments share responsibility for the provision of programs and support services.

In 1994, the Commonwealth developed the 10-year Disability Strategy, which helped to meet its obligations under the *Disability Discrimination Act 1992*. The strategy aimed to enhance equal opportunity for Australians with disabilities and improve the accessibility of services, such as transport, telecommunications, education, health, housing and so on. Among a number of other national projects are the National Disability Advocacy Program, National Auslan Interpreter Booking and Payment Service, National Print Disability Services Program and the National Disability Conference Initiative. Australia ratified the UN Convention on the Rights of Persons with Disabilities in July 2008. The convention contains a stand-alone article on women with disabilities and the text is cognisant of gender throughout. Governments are therefore obliged to prioritise women with disabilities as a group warranting specific attention and to take positive action to ensure that women and girls with disabilities enjoy the full gamut of human rights and freedoms.

After advocacy by WWDA, the National Partnerships Against Domestic Violence Taskforce agreed to fund a national project to develop information resources for women with disabilities who experience violence. This was the first Commonwealth-funded project on women with disabilities and violence, and WWDA members participated on various committees. The national plan recognises that 'policy solutions to address domestic violence and sexual assault must take into account the diverse backgrounds and needs of women and their children' (Commonwealth of Australia 2011d:11). It argues that

> new perspectives and strategies are required by all Australian governments in the delivery of best responses, as early as possible to victims of violence. Women may require specialised support based on individual needs in recognition of issues such as age, English language proficiency, disability, sexuality and prior victimisation.

The plan does not, however, explore the way policy solutions might need to differ to respond appropriately to women with diverse needs.

Following on from the National Disability Agreement in 2008, the National Disability Strategy (Commonwealth of Australia 2011b) was developed and written by the Commonwealth, States and Territories, under the auspices of COAG. It will help to fulfil the country's obligations under the UN convention. The strategy is based on extensive consultations and 750 written submissions and was endorsed by COAG in February 2011. It sets out a national plan with the stated aim of improving life for Australians with a disability, their families and carers for a decade. In theory, at least, all Australian governments are now committed to a unified national approach. Implementation and evaluation plans are to be worked out in the first year, in what is envisaged as a participatory process. As part of the strategy, the Productivity Commission is undertaking a study of the costs, benefits and feasibility of a national long-term care and support scheme, including a national disability social insurance scheme. The commission is being assisted by an associate commissioner, an expert in disability issues and an independent panel of experts.

The influence of the women's movement is apparent in that this strategy which, unlike previous documents, employs a gender lens. It recognises that women and men have different needs, priorities and perspectives and that some experience multiple problems. It draws attention in several places to the disadvantages experienced by women with disabilities, such as high levels of violence, including sexual violence, lower levels of participation in paid work and poorer economic outcomes and discriminatory attitudes in relation to parenting. It discusses the need for a coordinated and comprehensive approach, in which governments work together and with the wider community, stressing that 'the views of people with disability are central to the design, funding, delivery and evaluation of policies, programs and services' (Commonwealth of Australia 2011b)—all familiar ideas for those who take a social perspective of health. This document argues explicitly that 'the Strategy is based on a social model of disability and recognises that attitudes, practices and structures are disabling and can prevent people from enjoying economic participation, social inclusion and equality' (p. 16).

It remains to be seen whether funds will be allocated to put appropriate policies and programs in place.

Neo-Liberalism Comes to Women's Health

Since the 1990s, a set of political ideas very different from that of the 1970s has increasingly dominated political discourse. As neo-liberalism gradually supplanted social liberalism,[3] health and social policy expansion gave way to attacks on the authority of government and attempts to dismantle and de-fund as many programs as politically possible. It is true that the Commonwealth committed itself to a further four years of funding for the NWH Program in 1992 and later to funding for the longitudinal study of women's health. Otherwise, however, little of an expansionary nature took place, even though Labor held office until 1996. At the State level, too, funding was tightened and the women's health policy machinery began to be dismantled.

The health and social policies of the Kennett Liberal Government (1992–99) in Victoria illustrate the influence of neo-liberalism and demonstrate the hardship and distress that follow the withdrawal of support from services that were under-funded and oversubscribed in the first place. Between 1992 and 1994, Victorian Government spending on health and community services was cut by 27 per cent. After 1994, instructions were given that 54 per cent of required government budget savings were to be found from the sector. The accommodation support program was cut by $7.5 million or 12 per cent. Large numbers of residential care units were closed, including refuges, respite care centres, centres for disabled people and drug and alcohol rehabilitation centres. Researcher Olga Bursian interviewed workers from family support,

---

3   Neo-liberalism can briefly (if not very accurately) be described as a view that envisages a small role for governments and a large role for markets in the distribution of material resources. An expanded role for government, such as that attempted by the social liberal Whitlam Government, is seen as an illegitimate foray into realms that should remain in private hands.

foster care, maternal and child health and residential care programs to find out about workloads, stress factors, morale, worker's relations with management, training opportunities, job security and the general impact on women's lives. She found that the cuts resulted in heavier workloads, more complex demands on workers, fewer services to refer people to and fewer preventive services. In foster care, workloads were found to be unmanageable. Autistic, violent and psychiatrically disturbed children were housed inappropriately with children with fewer problems. High to intolerable stress levels were reported among staff and management alike. Professionals found themselves acting against their best judgments, volunteers were asked to carry out complex tasks for which they had insufficient training and uncertainty about funding led to anxiety because positions could be de-funded without notice. Occupational health and safety problems emerged and pay and conditions were eroded (Bursian 1995).

It was in this atmosphere that the Howard Government set about formulating a range of health policies that had a deleterious impact on low-income groups, particularly women (Gray 1999, 2004). It divested itself of policy responsibility for women's health through the introduction in 1997–98 of the National Public Health Partnership, although it continued to provide Commonwealth funds. Under the so-called partnerships, funding was broadened into eight public health programs: the NWH Program, the Alternative Birthing Services Program, the National Education Program on Female Genital Mutilation, Breast Screen Australia, the National Cervical Screening Program, the National Childhood Immunisation Program and the National Drug Strategy. The women's health movement, through the AHMAC Subcommittee on Women and Health, resisted this change for a number of reasons, not least because the language of the discussion papers was the language of commodification, elitism and social control (Broom 1998c).

During the development of the bilateral Public Health Outcomes Funding Agreements (PHOFAs), it was suggested that a number of standards and safeguards should be incorporated but, in the event, few performance measures were developed and none related to women's health programs. There was no longer any legal requirement that the States and Territories should spend any proportion of the money that was channelled through the agreements on women's health. Initially, Commonwealth funding was guaranteed only until 1999, when the first set of agreements expired. The implementation of the Public Health Partnerships was a major defeat for the women's health movement.

A second set of agreements, negotiated in 1999, this time for a five-year period, did include certain outcome measures in relation to women's health, including that health departments should maintain community-based services for women and that they should foster partnership and collaborative arrangements between gender-specific health services and mainstream services. The sub-national jurisdictions were required to report yearly against the criteria.

In keeping with intentions to reduce the size of government, the AHMAC Subcommittee on Women and Health was disbanded in 1998. The chief reason cited was cost saving. The capacity of the women's health movement to contribute to policy and to obtain information from policymakers was thereby significantly weakened. Under the partnership, a steering group of chief health officers was established, with a representative from the Australian Institute of Health and Welfare (AIHW) and the National Health and Medical Research Council (NHMRC). There were no longer channels through which the views of consumers, trade unions, general practitioners, nurses and the women's health movement could flow.

The Commonwealth seemingly took no further interest in women's health until 2004 when the PHOFAs came up for renegotiation. During the process, information circulated that the draft agreements for the period 2004–09 contained no reference to women's health. Rumour had it that a draft clause explicitly stated that Commonwealth money was not to be spent on any program not stipulated in the new agreements.

The AWHN Management Committee went into crisis mode. Representatives from all States and Territories met in Melbourne to discuss and decide upon strategy. Press releases were written and released, a background paper was put together and disseminated and an explanatory letter was written, which was sent to all relevant parliamentarians in every jurisdiction. A lobbying strategy was worked out that would involve Commonwealth, State and Territory governments, because all would sign the new agreements. Members made appointments to meet with State and Territory politicians, especially women. At the national level, as Deputy Convenor of AWHN, I unsuccessfully sought an appointment with Health Minister, Tony Abbott. Instead, I met several times with ministerial staff in June 2004 and was assured that there was 'no hidden agenda' and that the Commonwealth was willing to consider an extra category to be included in the new agreements, called 'promoting women's health'. This category was a possibility, I was told, if it did not restrict the Government's aim of promoting as much 'flexibility' as possible in service delivery.

At the same time, small delegations of AWHN Committee members met with senators from the two minor parties, the Australian Democrats and the Greens, where the point was made that without intelligence from community groups, such as AWHN, they did not get to hear about proposed policy changes. As a result of discussions, Senator Lyn Allison asked a series of relevant questions on notice in the Parliament. These included asking whether a 2003 review had recommended a stronger Commonwealth role in women's health, whether the absence of mention of women's health in the draft PHOFAs indicated reduced Commonwealth commitment and whether the Commonwealth had any plans to review the NWHP. She also requested that a copy of the review of the previous year be made public. Senator Allison's questions brought the Commonwealth's attempt to deliver a deadly blow to women's health into the light of day whereas previously it had lurked in the mists of hearsay.

At the time, speculation about the date of the 2004 national election was being fuelled by the Prime Minister's refusal to comment (Bennett et al. 2005). Women's groups thus began to prepare, making arrangements to talk with key parliamentarians. WEL made several deputations, in which AWHN participated, including one to Shadow Health Minister, Nicola Roxon. At these meetings, the threat to women's health under the proposed PHOFAs and the need to review the NWHP were both discussed. An AWHN delegation made a presentation to the Labor Women's Caucus Committee in July 2004 where the same issues were raised. The delegation asked for an election commitment from the Labor Party to review and renew the NWHP. Although no commitments were given, support was promised and the view was expressed that review of the policy was a project to which Labor women might be able to secure agreement. When the 2004–09 agreements were finally signed, they retained reference to all existing women's health programs—a major achievement for the movement.

The Second National Women's Health Policy, 2010

The Third AWHN National Women's Health Conference passed a resolution that the NWHP should 'be updated and extended to take account of issues of increasing importance to women in the late 1990s' (Davis et al. 1996:14). Similarly, the Fourth AWHN National Women's Health Conference, in Adelaide in 2001, argued that Commonwealth leadership was necessary to ensure that funding and commitment for women's health were maintained across the nation (AWHN 2001:9).

During the PHOFA period, the States and Territories continued to support the existing women's health infrastructure and sometimes small advances were made. Nevertheless, after 10 years of neo-liberal Commonwealth government, the participants who met at the Fifth AWHN National Women's Health Conference, in Melbourne in 2005, were pessimistic about the prospects of a women's health revival. The only glimmer of light was the support for AWHN's proposals expressed by members of the Labor Women's Caucus Committee. At the conference, an inspiring address was delivered by Ilona Kickbusch, well known internationally as an innovator in public health, women's health, health promotion and global health. She suggested that women's health groups needed to build coalitions with like-minded groups, identify possible funding sources, stage women's health summits in all jurisdictions and develop an assemblage of strategies, including internet strategies, media strategies and 'get out the vote' strategies.

While such an agenda was daunting for the movement and the almost penniless AWHN, the speech was inspirational and ideas from it found their way onto AWHN planning agendas. Improved electronic communication strategies were developed, coalitions were built and the membership base was strengthened. Women's health summits were held in three States and in 2006 AWHN began planning a national summit. The first step was the development of a draft discussion paper, which set out a new national agenda for women's health. The paper was circulated widely for comment and feedback. In September 2007, a national summit was held at Parliament House, Canberra, to which approximately 120 representatives of national organisations with like interests were invited, along with Commonwealth parliamentarians. The AWHN position paper was presented, further feedback was requested and, after incorporation of the final contributions, the paper was published in March 2008 as *Women's Health: The new national agenda*. Hundreds of copies were distributed across the country to parliamentarians, key stakeholders and all relevant health and women's organisations.

Shortly after the summit, as part of a health policy package for the 2007 election, Shadow Health spokeswoman, Nicola Roxon, announced that, if elected, her party would develop a new national policy on women's health that would encourage specific services for women and would promote women's participation in health decision making and management. She also pledged that the focus of the health system would be shifted to achieve more preventive health care, enhanced health promotion and greater attention to managing and monitoring chronic disease. The women's health movement greeted the announcement with excitement; women's health had been missing from the national policy agenda for more than a decade.

Early in 2008, the AWHN committee met to devise a plan to influence the shape of the second NWHP. The strategy had two major elements. The first was to contact relevant Commonwealth, State and Territory politicians and bureaucrats to keep them informed of the movement's views and priorities. The second was to maintain regular communications with members and interested organisations, to let them know about developments and to gather views and contributions.

After Labor came to office, more than a year passed before the policy development process was launched with the publication of a background paper, *Developing a women's health policy for Australia: setting the scene.* The first consultation was held at Parliament House, Canberra, in March 2009. The meeting was chaired by Professor Sally Redman, Director of the Sax Institute. At the meeting, a consultation discussion paper, *Development of a new national women's health policy*, was launched, which was an expansion of the earlier document. Both recognised a social view of health as central and both recognised that there are significant health inequalities between different groups of women. The new policy, it was argued, needed to focus on those groups with the highest risk of poor health, including Aboriginal and Torres Strait Islander women.

The invited participants were from 14 groups, including AWHN. A woman from Congress Alukura was invited but was unable to attend. Minister Roxon was present in the morning. She said the Commonwealth was not afraid to make decisions that would not have a major impact for 10 to 20 years and was not afraid to work across Commonwealth, State and Territory boundaries. The minister acknowledged that many factors affecting women's health, such as economic and physical security, are located outside the health portfolio but she envisaged that the main thrust of the new policy would be within the portfolio. Among the issues raised in discussion were the paucity of services for rural women, the need for a greater understanding of difference and different patterns of health and illness, the OHS problems faced by immigrant and refugee women, violence against women, economic security, personal security and the need for a national sexual and reproductive health strategy. The importance of health education to teach practitioners about cultural and gender competence was stressed, together with the need for prevention and health-promotion programs.

In the second phase of the consultation process, March to June 2009, the organisations present at the round table were asked to consult with their constituencies and then make submissions to the Department of Health and Ageing (DOHA) by July 2009. The submission process was open to any group in Australia and AWHN developed a template to facilitate contributions. DOHA received almost 100 submissions by the middle of the year.

As discussed, AWHN and the Aboriginal Women's Talking Circle managed a project through which Aboriginal women were consulted and an Aboriginal women's submission was written, with funding support from FaHCSIA. From September to December 2009, DOHA held consultation forums in all capital cities, six regional cities and in Fitzroy Crossing in north-west Western Australia. The policy was released on 29 December 2010. There was no official launch.

The new policy covers key women's health issues, including many of the views and experiences put forward in consultations and submissions. Its stated purpose is to continue to improve the health and wellbeing of all Australian women, especially those at greatest risk of poor health. It is framed within a social health perspective and identifies the need to promote equity between groups of women through a focus on the social determinants. It acknowledges that women's access to resources, such as income, education, employment, social connections and safety and security, including freedom from violence, influences their health outcomes and their ability to access services. The policy recognises health inequities between groups, with certain groups, particularly Aboriginal and Torres Strait Islander women, having poorer outcomes (Commonwealth of Australia 2010b:7–8).

The social determinants of health are to be addressed through five policy goals: highlighting the significance of gender as a key determinant; acknowledging that women's health needs differ throughout their lives; prioritising the needs of women with the highest risk of poor health; ensuring that the health system responds to all women with a clear focus on illness prevention; and health promotion. Effective, collaborative research, data collection, monitoring and evaluation and knowledge transfer are to be supported. The short-term focus, however, is on the burden of disease in four priority areas: prevention of chronic disease and control of risk factors, mental health and wellbeing, sexual and reproductive health, and healthy ageing.

While the new policy expresses much that the movement endorses, it is extremely disappointing in a number of ways. First, the contribution of women's health centres and services over decades is not acknowledged which is also, in effect, a refusal to acknowledge the crucial importance of strong primary health care. Second, chronic disease is to be addressed through the control of risk factors, such as obesity, unhealthy eating and physical inactivity. Disappointingly, however, the policy does not explore the risk factors in the light of their social determinants. Third, and most importantly, any actions that are to be undertaken to address either social determinants or the burden of disease are vague and unclear. It is extremely important that the social determinants of illness be linked to specific actions that will reduce the impact of those determinants. Such actions, of course, require resources and it is disappointing that the only funding announced with the policy is for Women's Health Australia, a laudable project and one strongly endorsed by the movement but in itself insufficient as a national effort to address the social determinants of women's health.

Conclusion

On the whole, Commonwealth Labor governments have responded positively to the women's health movement, formulating a broad array of policies, strategies, programs, plans and initiatives. The high point of the movement's influence was in the 1980s and early 1990s when, as one commentator argued, feminist thought and action to improve women's health had a strong influence on reform debates (Dwyer 1992b:211). The NWHP was an international first and influenced policy overseas as well as in the various Australian jurisdictions. The NWH Program expanded specialised women's health centres and services and funded a variety of new projects. The separate women's health sector has produced best-practice models of service delivery, especially in the area of preventive health care, which have had an influence on mainstream discourse and practice. Physical and sexual violence against women and girls, OHS, the health needs of Aboriginal women and women with disabilities and immigrant women, best-practice cancer treatment, maternity-care reform, strong primary, preventive health care and a social view of health are all issues that the movement has succeeded in drawing to public attention.

It can be argued that viewed from one angle, the women's health movement has changed the face of national health policy discourse. We have a new national women's health policy, which captures many of the arguments feminists have made, a national plan against violence against women and the National Disability Strategy that recognises social determinants and employs a gender lens. The large and avoidable differences in health outcomes for people situated differently are recognised in public policy documents for everyone to read. It is unlikely that a commission set up to focus on better population health would now claim, as the Better Health Commission did in 1986, that the diseases suffered by men and women are the same. Moreover, it is no longer so easy to claim, brightly, that Australia has some of the best average health outcomes in the world while ignoring serious disparities between groups.

From another angle, however, much of the changed focus and language can be seen as symbolic. Symbolic politics, in the simple sense, is a surrogate for substantive political action. The symbols used carry political meaning that is an end in itself and distract from the reality that policies and programs are not being developed. In this case, the use of the language of the social determinants of health, preventive health care and gender analysis gives the impression of an appropriate policy response to contemporary evidence. At the level of actual decision making, however, the focus is still squarely on hospitals and medical services, and new investment in primary health care, for women or anyone else, is small. The second NWHP is an action-free zone at the time of writing, a classic attempt to appease the women's health movement without spending any money. Even at the pinnacle of achievement, the obstacles that femocrats and the movement encountered during the development of the first NWHP and the small amount of funding eventually allocated show that politicians perceived the need to be seen to be taking appropriate action while in reality making only a minimal investment.

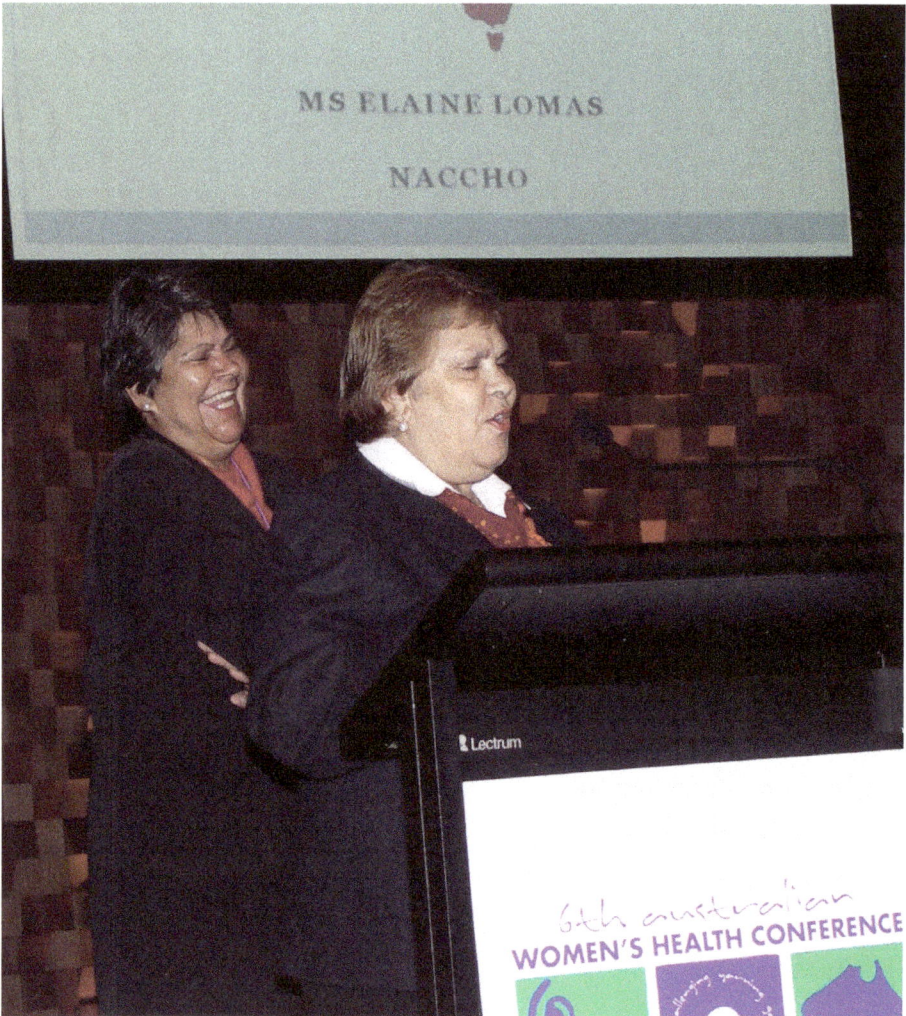

Elaine Lomas, Operations Manager, NACCHO, supported by Irene Peachey, entertains the Sixth AWHN National Women's Health Conference with an address entitled 'Cooperation and collaboration between NACCHO and AWHN and the Talking Circle'—not a hilarious topic in anyone else's hands!

Photo: Tracey Wing

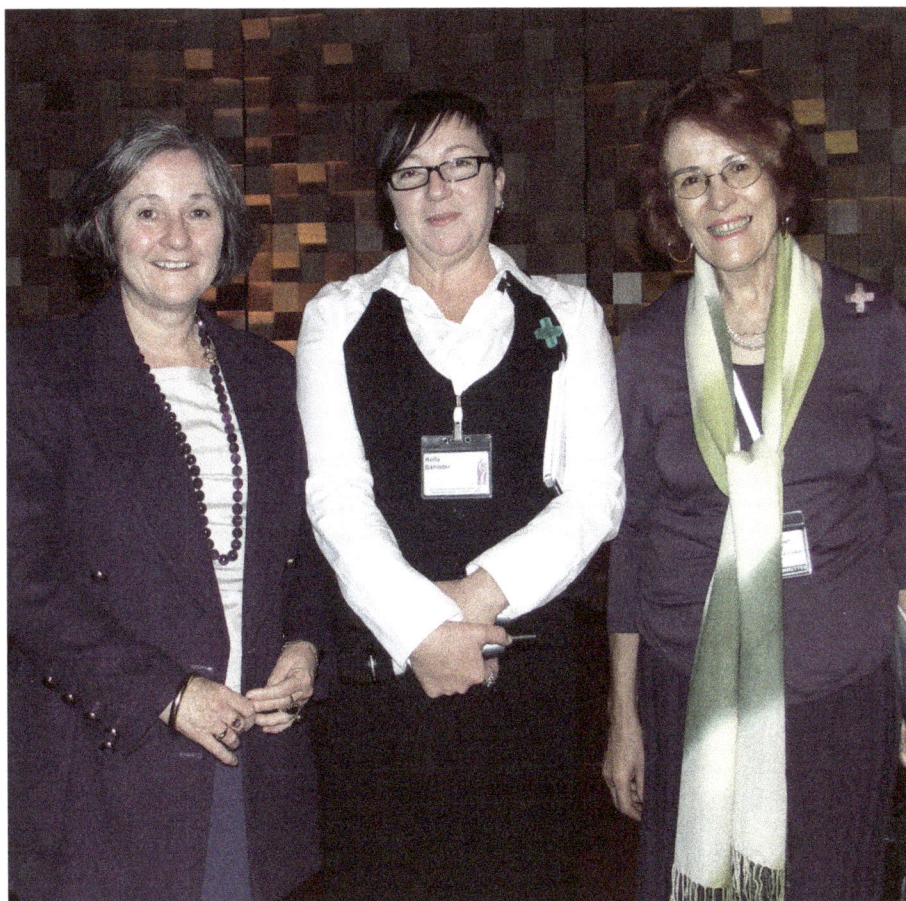

Senator Claire Moore, representing the Commonwealth Government, with Kelly Bannister, Conference Convener, and Gwen Gray, AWHN Convener, at the Sixth AWHN National Women's Health Conference, Hobart, 2010.

Photo: Tracey Wing

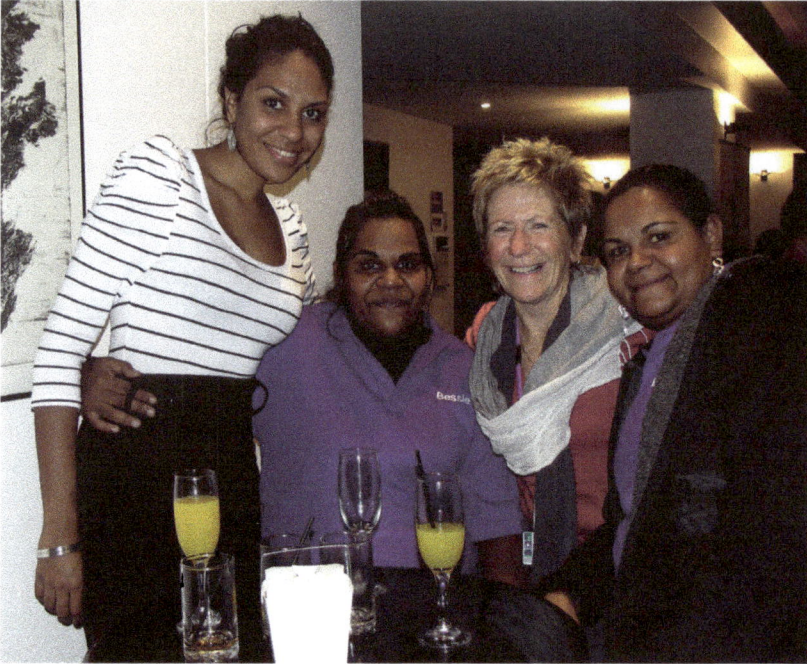

Raquel Kerdel and Bessie Rigney (SA Aboriginal Women's Committee), Carla Vicary (Murray Mallee Community Health Service) and Edie Carter (SA Aboriginal Women's Committee) at the Sixth National AWHN Women's Health Conference Party, Hobart, 2010.

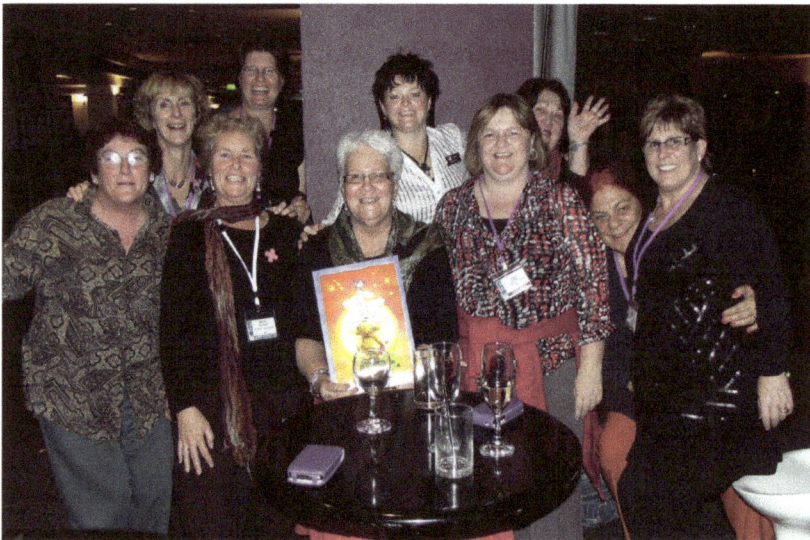

A Western Australian contingent at the Sixth AWHN National Women's Health Conference Party, Hobart, 2010.

Photo: Tracey Wing

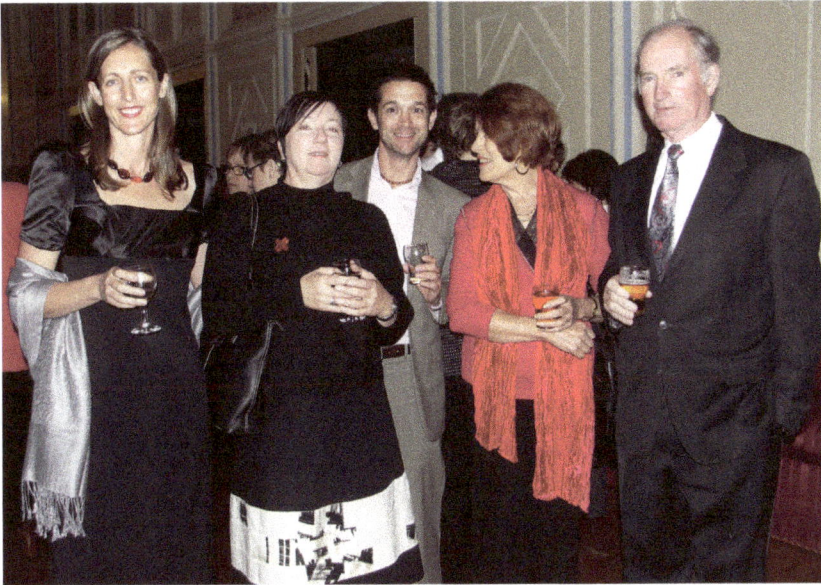

AWHN committee members and a couple of guests: Marion Hale, Kelly Bannister, Andrew Mitchell, Gwen Gray and Peter Howe at the pre-conference reception, Government House, Hobart, 2010.

Photo: Tracey Wing

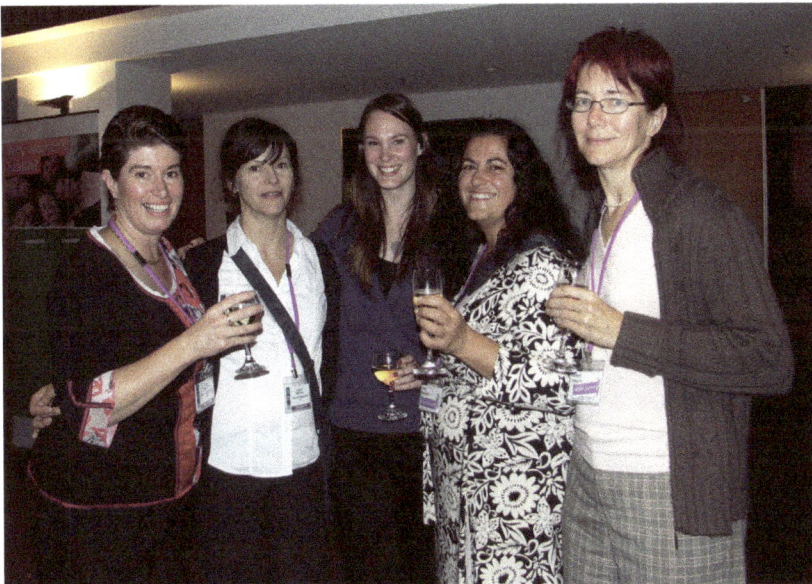

Women's Health West board members and staff at the Sixth AWHN National Women's Health Conference Party. From left: Karen Passey, Linda Memery, Georgie Hill, Sally Camileri and Dr Robyn Gregory, Executive Officer.

Photo: Tracey Wing

9. Explaining Australia's Policy Responses

Having surveyed the history of women's health policy development since the 1970s, it is now time to return to the questions posed in the introduction. Why is Australia the only country to have enacted two national women's health policies? Why is it also the only country to have attempted to establish a national network of community health centres? Why is it a leader, internationally, in developing public responses to domestic violence? And what are the conditions that have come together at different times to create windows of opportunity for structural health reform? As in most areas of public policy, the reasons for particular outcomes are multidimensional, directed and shaped by numerous pressures. As well as facilitating factors, there are almost always countervailing forces, particularly in a policy area such as health—the largest industry in all OECD countries. It is an area where ethical issues abound, where large incomes are at stake and where profits depend on the policies adopted. In the Australian federation, health is particularly complex, not just because nine governments share responsibility but also because of the peculiar Australian arrangements where most doctors operate as private businesspeople, outside the control of government, while drawing the lion's share of their income directly from the public purse, with virtually no conditions attached.

Before attempting to answer the questions posed, this chapter examines the main forces that came together to facilitate the policy uptake of women's health concerns. The last two questions, concerning the main obstacles to policy reform and the reasons that the structures of the health system remain intact despite strong evidence in favour of change, are addressed in the final chapter.

There is no question that the Australian women's health movement has been relatively successful in comparative terms. No other country has developed two national women's health policies and multiple sub-national policies and very few have national strategies or even women's health plans. Internationally, a few national women-specific health initiatives have been taken. The Irish Department of Health developed its Women's Health Plan in 1995, when the permanent Women's Health Council was established. In Canada, the first national women's health statement was released in 1990; however, because the Provinces have constitutional responsibility for health, there was no national policy. The Health Minister at the time, Mary Collins, was influenced by Australian developments and owned a copy of the NWHP. The Glasgow Women's Health Policy was launched in 1992 and updated and relaunched in 2002. WHO Europe has designated the Glasgow work, which was influenced by Australia's first

NWHP, an example of good practice. New Zealand, the United States and the United Kingdom all had strong women's health movements but none has made policy responses that compare with Australia's.

Moreover, Australia stands out in the area of direct service provision: no other country has a network of publicly funded, independent women's health centres and services. In the four other major English-speaking democracies, women did attempt to set up separate health centres but on a smaller scale and only a handful remains. Violence against women in its many forms has been put on policy agendas in many countries but research published in 2002 shows that the Australian effort compares well with other countries (Weldon 2002). The policy responses developed since Weldon's study mean that Australia is probably still among the leading nations.

Perhaps most importantly, the social view of health or socioeconomic-determinants perspective that has guided the movement's actions and advocacy since the 1970s is more widely understood and is now acknowledged regularly in major Australian health policy documents. The vexed question of why a social perspective is not more prominent in actual health policy decisions will be addressed in the final chapter.

Health policymaking is notoriously difficult and generally undertaken amid intense controversy. A leading Canadian economist has called it 'the issue from hell' (Evans 1993). Women's health policy fits into the same mould and movement members faced many obstacles when trying to get their concerns heard. In the early years, the ideas being put forward were unfamiliar and often seen as extremist. Women's groups lacked authority, status, legitimacy, political experience and resources. The men in the senior positions in the bureaucracies frequently resisted the new ideas and others were dubious about the wisdom of establishing separate services. Medical unions have always opposed any form of alternative services that might reduce the size of private medical markets by substituting for doctor-provided services. Since the rise of women's health activism, many women doctors appear to have taken the movement's criticisms personally. It took time, energy and considerable perseverance therefore to persuade policymakers of the validity of the claims. Even where acceptance emerged, it was often fragile and transitory.

A number of forces were, however, working in the opposite direction to facilitate policy expansion, as summarised below.

Factors Facilitating Policy Adoption

- A strong, grassroots movement able to put effective pressure on political parties.
- The first centres and services established in a radical change context.
- Women working for change, often behind the scenes, in political parties and trade unions.
- The Australian practice of employing feminists in advisory and policy development roles: the femocrat phenomenon.
- Women's policy machinery installed in all nine government bureaucracies.
- The election of responsive governments that believed they needed the women's vote.
- The underdevelopment of the Australian health and welfare system.
- The openness of Australian government, allowing activists access to decision makers.
- Programmatic Australian political parties.
- Federalism perhaps a facilitating factor, perhaps not.
- The strong strand of social liberalism in Australian political culture.

These influences are now examined in turn.

Grassroots Activism

The early Australian women's health movement comprised strong, broad-based grassroots groups. In her study of 36 democratic governments to explore the reasons for responsiveness to the problem of violence against women, Weldon found that the mobilisation of a strong, autonomous women's movement was a major factor in explaining successful outcomes. By 'autonomous', Weldon means independent of political parties and other organisations. She also suggests that a proliferation of groups is a sign of strength and, as we have seen, there has been a remarkable proliferation of women's health groups over the past 35 years. Self-governing women's movements are effective because they are able to articulate problems on their own terms and exert outside pressure on political parties to take up their issues. Women's movements that are organised mainly from within political parties, such as in Italy, have been less successful in having violence taken up as a political issue (Weldon 2002:79–86). The Australian women's health movement, being grassroots based, is quite independent in Weldon's sense, although some members belonged to political parties, unions and the like as well.

The achievements of the movement suggest a very strong commitment among grassroots women; some were health professionals and others had special skills but, on the whole, ordinary women mobilised in numbers to work for better health services and social change. In no other country did so many passionately committed women determine to set up their own health services. Australian women were prepared to take whatever forms of direct action seemed necessary to establish services where women's bodily integrity, views and decision-making rights would be respected. If, after testing conventional avenues, it was felt necessary to break the law, they did so. Nardine refuge workers in Perth, for example, squatted in an empty State-owned house with a woman and her children who had been waiting for months for public housing. The police were called, the family was evicted and several Nardine workers were found guilty of trespass and put on good behaviour bonds (Murray 1999:8). But women's housing problems were publicised.

Women went to extraordinary lengths to sustain the services they created, giving hours of their time and often their own money, working through all available channels to influence decision makers. As well as marches and other forms of direct action, they held forums and speak-outs, wrote letters and petitions, circulated policy papers, made appointments with politicians and bureaucrats and sought media coverage. As services became established, an institutional base from which to work became available and action tended to take more conventional forms; however, street marches and demonstrations, such as the 'Mother of All Rallies' staged by homebirth advocates in 2009, are still held in support of reproductive rights. Such visible activism, especially when it is electorally close to home, is not easy for politicians to ignore. A strong women's movement alone, however, is not sufficient to shape public policy, as periods of government inaction and regression demonstrate. It was necessary for a number of other influences to be operating simultaneously.

Favourable Political Opportunity Structures

The policy context in which the early movement operated was extraordinarily favourable for the introduction of new policies, especially those that would benefit the least advantaged. Radical equality-seeking social movements were active across the OECD, calling for everything from minority rights, industrial democracy and environmental protection to disarmament and a new world economic order. In Australia, community health, public health and Aboriginal health movements were emerging, buttressed by accumulating evidence that a biomedical model of health care was unnecessarily and dangerously limited. Extensive disquiet about Australian health and welfare services grew as research showed that people, especially the elderly, were living in dire poverty and were unable to access basic services, despite the impact of one of the longest economic booms in Australian history. The publicly subsidised private health insurance system, of most benefit to the well-off, came under heavy attack. In this context, a Labor government was elected in 1972, after 23 years in opposition, on a platform of extensive social policy reform. The political climate of the day was conducive to sweeping policy change—an opportunity as radical as it is rare—and its impact continued well into the 1980s. The converse, of course, is the steady emergence of neo-liberalism as the dominant discourse, which supplanted the social justice emphasis of the preceding period. The support of the Whitlam Government at a formative stage was fundamental to the women's health project because it established an institutional foundation for the movement. The institutional base was expanded and consolidated under supportive sub-national governments and the Commonwealth in the 1980s and early 1990s but the early support was crucial.

Women in Political Parties and Trade Unions

Women in political parties and trade unions frequently cooperated with grassroots health groups and worked hard within their organisations to create the conditions where women's health concerns would be reflected in policy. Arguments have been made that a greater proportion of women in legislatures facilitates policy advancement. In Australia, however, the movement's greatest policy successes were in the 'golden' 1980s before women entered legislatures in large numbers. As more women entered parliaments at both sub-national and national levels, women's health slipped rather than advanced as a policy priority, suggesting other, more powerful forces at work, such as the advent of neo-liberalism. This finding is consistent with that of Weldon in her cross-national study of policymaking on violence. She found no relationship between the percentage of women in legislatures and government responsiveness to violence (Weldon 2002:87–104).

This finding does not, however, negate the very important role that numbers of women played within parties and trade unions in the pursuit of women's health concerns. Nor does it negate the role that women parliamentarians still play on selected issues. In the early days, women set about educating party and union men concerning feminist perspectives—a process that involved hard work and often required written papers. Political party women had to explain the meaning of a women's health perspective. In trade unions, women worked to change the ambit and the meaning of OHS and to promote the principles of industrial democracy. The influence that they were able to exert sometimes did depend on their numbers: more women in unions meant that 'new' issues such as workplace sexual harassment were able to be raised and pursued. For women in political parties, their low numbers were perceived as a barrier to change. According to one party member, women's issues often placed women parliamentarians in an uncomfortable position of opposition to their male colleagues. Moreover, the few women who were elected were contacted about everything feminist, which was a heavy load. On issues other than abortion, however, male politicians were generally prepared to accept women's perspectives in the 1970s and 1980s. But this was not always the case and the role of women parliamentarians, working collaboratively, was sometimes crucial. For example, in Victoria, a small group of women parliamentarians, in close connection with outside groups, women in the bureaucracy and women in ministers' offices, pushed hard against very strong male opposition to have the Women's Health Program adopted in the mid-1980s. In Queensland, it was very difficult for women to persuade male members of the Goss Government to participate in the NWH Program because women's health was so closely associated with abortion in many minds.

From the mid-1970s until the early 1990s, there was a strong perception among members of both major political parties that the women's vote had to be courted (Auer 2003), a perception at least partly created by the findings of opinion polls. The ability to persuade male party members that electoral advantage would follow from women's health innovations was crucial to success. As a New South Wales female parliamentarian told me in the early 1990s, the men in the party were aware that the women in the party could deliver the women's vote. But where men were not so convinced, the political battle was harder.

Party structures through which women might have worked had existed within the major parties for decades but the role that women played had been largely auxiliary (Sawer and Simms 1984:131–40). Women were instrumental in having new committees and caucuses established in State and Territory ALP branches in the 1970s and 1980s, which facilitated issue articulation. The National Labor Women's Conference and National Status of Women Policy Committee were established in 1981. In the Liberal Party (LPA), a number of feminist groups were established in the early 1980s, including the Liberal Feminist Network in Victoria, with counterparts in New South Wales, South Australia and Queensland. The first National Liberal Women's Conference was held in 1986. The National Country Party, now The Nationals, similarly made changes to increase the representation of women in party structures. In some jurisdictions, women were able to ensure that they were represented on policy committees, including health committees. Labor women tried to push policies through at every level: at national conferences, State and Territory conferences and at national women's conferences. Many LPA women supported women's health issues within their parties but often faced strong opposition from men. For example, the LPA had been in power in South Australia for almost three years before Health Minister, Jennifer Adamson, was able to announce that a women's health policy would be developed, fulfilling an election commitment. Women from the conservative parties were sometimes able to prevail, however. One such instance occurred when female members actively opposed National Party government efforts to tighten, rather than liberalise, abortion laws in Queensland in the 1980s. Party women were able to garner enough support to defeat the proposed legislation.

In unions, as in political parties, women worked to ensure that they were represented on committees and elected as officials. As we saw in Chapter 5, women in unions created networks with women's organisations, community organisations and political parties. In many cases, union women were also Labor Party members and sometimes members of the women's health movement as well. Women in unions constituted part of a health movement that succeeded in having workers' health and working women's centres established.

Opportunities to progress women's health varied from jurisdiction to jurisdiction, depending, in part, on political culture. Queensland was widely viewed as 'a bit of a backwater' until the 1990s. In Western Australia, the sections of the ALP platform that dealt specifically with women were only an outline of principles until the mid-1980s, when they were rewritten to include feminist concerns. The difficulties of achieving attitudinal change were immense in a State such as Tasmania, where the entire health system had centred on hospitals for decades. Tasmanian political party women struggled to gain legitimacy for the unfamiliar concept of a social view of health. In some cases, the appointment of party women to key health positions produced results. For example, Anne O'Byrne was appointed Chair of the Tasmanian Northern Region Health Board in the mid-1990s and was able to establish a women's health issues subcommittee, which was given responsibility for administration of women's health financing.

Many women in political parties worked closely with grassroots women. Senators such as Patricia Giles (1981–93), Margaret Reynolds (1983–99) and Dr Rosemary Crowley (1983–2002) worked extensively with women's groups on a wide range of feminist issues, including women's health. Particularly in small jurisdictions such as South Australia, women politicians from all parties invited women's health movement members to contact them and sometimes offered to speak on their behalf. Political party women were sometimes willing to collaborate with NGOs when shaping the questions to be asked in parliament. Where minor parties have been a significant political force, women's health generally gained active allies, both at the Commonwealth and the State and Territory levels. For example, Christine Milne was able to influence a review of the Tasmanian Department of Health in the late 1990s in ways that would support women's health. Greens Senators Christabel Chamarette and Dee Margetts facilitated a number of Health Policy Think Tanks at Parliament House in the mid-1990s, at which a social view of health was explored and endorsed. Senator Kerry Nettle (2002–08) was a strong supporter of women's health and worked with the movement wherever possible to promote issues and perspectives. The predominantly female parliamentarians of the Australian Democrats were generally strong movement allies. Senators Natasha Stott Despoja and Lyn Allison supported women's health perspectives throughout their time in the Senate from the mid-1990s until 2008. Senator Stott Despoja put forward a number of health-related Private Member's Bills, including legislation intended to regulate pregnancy counselling services and ensure the provision of full information about options, a Bill in support of stem-cell research and a Bill with significant women's health implications intended to prevent patent law from applying to naturally occurring genes.

Marian Sawer (2011) suggests that the increasing numbers of women in legislatures and in high office have often 'had to leave feminist values at the door', due to the changing political context where equal opportunity and social justice issues have been steadily pushed off political agendas. The women's health experience bears this out at the national level in view of its lost salience after the mid-1990s. Women are, however, still playing an important role. At the national level, female parliamentarians, regardless of party, have been far more likely than their male colleagues to support health-related reform legislation where a conscience vote has been allowed. Between 1996 and 2006, conscience votes were taken on five pieces of legislation, relating to four issue areas: euthanasia, research involving embryos, human cloning and the importation of RU-486. The most striking feature of voting was the extent to which women supported the Bills in both Houses. On average, 86 per cent of women in the Senate and 80 per cent in the House of Representatives voted in favour, compared with 44 and 61 per cent of men, respectively. In the case of LPA senators, 87 per cent of women supported the Bills, compared with 32 per cent of men (McKeown and Lundie 2009).

An infrequent but nonetheless productive development has been the emergence of cross-party political action by women in the national Parliament. In 1983, LPA Senator Kathy Martin, Democrats Senator Janine Haines and ALP Senators Patricia Giles and Susan Ryan banded together to support ratification of the UN Convention on the Elimination of All Forms of Discrimination against Women (CEDAW). The Pregnancy Counselling (Truth in Advertising) Bill 2006 was co-sponsored by Senators Stott Despoja, Judith Troeth (LPA), Carol Brown (ALP) and Kerry Nettle (Greens). Party collaboration is a regular feature of the operation of the Parliamentary Group on Population and Development (PGPD), formed in 1995, which raises awareness about international population and development issues, especially sexual and reproductive health issues. It works with the United Nations and with NGOs, such as the Australian Reproductive Health Alliance (ARHA), Sexual Health and Family Planning Australia (SH&FPA) and the International Planned Parenthood Federation. Membership includes representatives from all parties, including men. The most celebrated instance of cross-party collaboration between women, discussed in Chapter 5, took place in 2006 in relation to the removal of the Harradine amendment, which had restricted the importation of RU-486. In this instance, political party women worked extensively with NGOs, particularly the many groups represented by Reproductive Choice Australia (RCA).

To summarise, in the early years when a feminist health perspective was being articulated and disseminated in organisational structures and beyond, small numbers of women in legislatures and trade unions, in cooperation with femocrats and grassroots women, played a crucial pioneering role. At a time when feminist issues have been driven off agendas, the role that women parliamentarians have been able to play is more limited, despite their increasing numbers. As in all areas of public policy, multiple influences are at work and the proportion of women in legislatures is but one.

The Work of Femocrats

There is general agreement in the literature that femocrats—feminists who took positions in bureaucracies and worked for reform from inside rather than outside government—succeeded as agents of policy change (see, for example, Eisenstein 1996; Sawer 1990). The evidence of women's health experience supports such a view. Neither feminist critiques of bureaucracy[1] nor the difficulties of working in less than friendly structures prevented Australian feminists from entering the public service in increasing numbers from the 1970s onwards. Following the lead of the Commonwealth, which appointed the first adviser on women's affairs, Elizabeth Reid, in 1973, all jurisdictions appointed women's affairs specialists during the next two decades and all, at some time, appointed women's health advisers. Most of these women had experience in the women's movement, the the women's health movement, or both. And while this phenomenon facilitated policy advancement in one sense, it deprived the movement of some of its energies (Lynch 1984:38).

The first women's health adviser was Liz Furler, appointed Ministerial Adviser in South Australia in 1984. She later worked as a femocrat in Tasmania before being appointed to the Commonwealth Health Department. Carla Cranny was the first Women's Health Adviser in New South Wales, appointed in 1985. A women's health advisory position was created in the Australian Capital Territory in the mid-1980s, filled by Marilyn Hatton. In Victoria, Christine Giles was appointed to manage a new women's health unit, set up in 1987, and Thea

---

1   Discussed in Chapter 1.

Mendelsohn took a similar position in Western Australia in the same year. The position of Senior Policy Officer, Women's Health, was established in Tasmania in 1989, with Vicki Pearce the first incumbent. Jude Abbs became Queensland's first Women's Health Adviser in 1991, and Jen Roberts was appointed to head the single-position Women's Health Strategy Unit established in the Northern Territory in 1992. Feminist ministerial advisers were also key players in policy advancement in some jurisdictions, operating in much the same ways and within the same set of opportunities and constraints as femocrats.

Given that key stakeholders compete for position in policymaking processes, feminists in senior bureaucratic roles are in a position to advance a women's agenda. Femocrats played crucial roles on numerous occasions in promoting women's health issues. In New South Wales, for example, feminists working in the bureaucracy are held to have been invaluable to the early women's health centres, especially when Commonwealth funding was slashed and the State was being asked to pick up the shortfall. Femocrats were crucial to the passage of the first NWHP through policy development processes in the Commonwealth bureaucracy and important in gaining support for it at the State and Territory level. In New South Wales and Victoria, at least, femocrats cooperated with maternity consumer groups and offered them increased access to policymaking in the 1990s. Members of the Australian Midwifery Action Lobby Group (SA) and Mothers and Midwives Action (Victoria) were in 'regular contact' with women in the bureaucracy and the politicians who supported reform (Reiger 2006:333).

Even where femocrats were unsuccessful in achieving immediate gains, as in women's health in Western Australia in the mid-1980s, their work can be seen as having advanced issues and paved the way for future policy expansion. In women's health units, women were in a good position to choose the most appropriate strategies for the situation. For example, during lean times in Western Australia, femocrats decided to focus on one or two issues rather than try to advance the whole women's health agenda. They put themselves in a position to take advantage of opportunities, major and minor, that presented themselves. One women's health service is said to have been established because a femocrat inserted its announcement into a minister's speech.

One of the recurring themes in the scholarly literature (see, for example, Dowse 1984; Eisenstein 1996; Sawer 1990; Summers 1986) is that femocrats faced serious dilemmas. Their working environments were often hostile to feminism but at the same time they were expected to maintain close connections with 'sisters' outside—a relationship considered conspiratorial in some quarters. It is generally thought that to be successful, the trust of key people had to be gained, inside and outside government, which was an objective not always achieved. In the early days, in particular, many community women were suspicious of the role of femocrats, while at the same time seeing them as a possible buffer between themselves and male politicians (Smith 1984:5). At the same time, the femocrats in the Commonwealth Women's Health Unit were viewed with suspicion in their own workplace during the formulation of the NWHP. There was a belief in the department that they were in league with community women and that far too much money would be expected for the project. Another concern was that the unit did not have the confidence of medical unions.

Some femocrats report having been fortunate enough to find mentors who encouraged, supported and advised on how best to pursue their aims. Senior personnel in finance were considered to be crucial allies since, ultimately, their approval or at least acquiescence was needed. One strategy devised in one State to promote trust was to take key departmental men out to lunch, where they were introduced to feminist friends and colleagues, thus demonstrating that feminists were real people!

Femocrats had different views about the appropriateness and usefulness of relationships with grassroots groups. Some experienced women regarded themselves as accountable to the women's movement and thought grassroots support was essential to pressure policymakers. Other femocrats found it difficult to keep contact with the movement outside and believed it was impossible to maintain friendships. They feared being isolated from departmental information if they were seen to be too close to community women. Responses tended to vary from jurisdiction to jurisdiction. In some places, it was felt that no hint of a connection with outside groups was acceptable. Elsewhere inside/outside relationships could be maintained in a state of delicate balance. One femocrat told me she never openly acknowledged outside groups although she worked with them extensively. While some information could never be divulged, ways could be found of releasing information without breaking rules or betraying ministers, including participation in public seminars and forums. Femocrats in the Commonwealth Women's Health Unit were in frequent touch with the media, giving out information about policy developments. Articles were also supplied for magazines, including medical journals.

Networking was an important element of the work of most femocrats, who report enhanced effectiveness through links both inside and outside the bureaucracy. Inside, femocrats established ongoing links with each other and with key people in other departments. For example, staff of the Commonwealth Women's Health Policy Unit worked closely with the OSW and other relevant departments, including social security and finance. In the health sector at the State and Territory level, femocrats often attended women's health network and health service provider meetings. Interaction was also facilitated by overlapping organisational membership: some femocrats were also members of political parties, NGOs and so on.

Other constraints within which femocrats worked were the inability to speak out publicly and the requirement that policy proposals be moderate. They also found it difficult to work in the face of frequent departmental restructures that occurred, for example, during the development of the NWHP and in New South Wales in the 1980s. Frequent restructuring also made life difficult for community women because working relations were disrupted. As neo-liberalism became more prominent and feminist ideas lost some of their salience, organisational changes resulted in women's health units being located far from the top levels of policymaking, whereas initially they had been considerably closer.

While there is general agreement within the movement that women's health femocrats played a positive role, occasional criticisms were expressed, illustrating the contradictions of the role. In one jurisdiction, community women felt that the women's health unit had achieved little, and it has been argued that towards the end of the 1980s the feminist bureaucracy in New South Wales appeared to be 'less of an interpreter for the grassroots and more of a publicist for the Labor government' (McFerran 1990:203). McFerran also acknowledges, however, the contributions made, especially to the refuge program, and she argues that 'turning the state back on itself' is 'an artful game' in which the relationships between femocrats and community groups are crucial (McFerran 1990:191).

Women's Policy Machinery

The influence of femocrats is closely related to the impact of the policy units in which many of them worked. As discussed, women's health units or dedicated policy positions were established in all jurisdictions in the 1980s and 1990s. This type of machinery was more extensively developed in Australia than in comparable countries, with perhaps the exception of Canada (Sawer 1989:427, 1990:xv–xvii). The original proposals to set up special institutional structures came from the women's movement itself. In 1974, ACT WEL wrote a submission to the Royal Commission on Australian Government Administration, suggesting that permanent task forces on women's issues, staffed by senior officers, be established in government departments. Functions were to monitor activity and policy and program development, to initiate research and to liaise with target groups, interdepartmental committees and advisory councils. The royal commission accepted the proposal and recommended that departments be 'encouraged to develop women's units on an experimental basis' (Sawer 1990:28–9). Thus, the machinery itself resulted from feminist advocacy.

In her 36-country study of policy responses to violence, Weldon found that women's policy machinery was an important factor in making political institutions more responsive to women's claims. Policy units had introduced the category 'women' as a policy priority and had provided a basis for policy administration, research and review that would have otherwise been lost in the spaces between government departments. Women's policy machinery, Weldon found, 'partially corrects for the organisation of government around the priorities of historically dominant groups of men' (Weldon 2002:135). The general assessment of the women interviewed was that women's health policy machinery had performed an extremely useful role.

A major piece of women's health policy machinery was the Australian Health Ministers Subcommittee on Women and Health, set up to help coordinate the development of the NWHP. As a Commonwealth, State and Territory body, with NGO and professional representation, it operated as a forum where women's health experts from across the country could meet, bring ideas from their constituencies, learn from each other, formulate new ideas and develop strategies. During the implementation of the NWH Program, it reviewed and monitored progress and accepted references from AHMAC. Other roles were to produce and disseminate information and monitor and evaluate mainstream health policy for its impact on women (Commonwealth of Australia 1993). An effective body for advancing women's health policy, it was disbanded in 1998 by the Howard Government.

Women interviewed for this book also remarked upon the difficulties that emerged from not having sufficiently strong women's health policy machinery. In one jurisdiction, having only two women's health positions devoted to policy development, implementation, contract management and evaluation of services was a serious constraint. The arguments from this study support the findings of others that special units facilitated the development of women-friendly policies and contributed to positive attitudinal and behavioural change (Sawer 1990). Some of the examples discussed by Eisenstein include rape law reform, the positioning of violence against women on the national policy agenda, the establishment of women's health centres and services and the development of the NWHP (Eisenstein 1996:43–64). Only in one jurisdiction was it felt that women's health policy machinery had not been particularly useful.

Responsive Governments

The election of sympathetic governments stands out above all others as the key factor facilitating the progress of the movement's aims. This finding is contrary to that of Weldon, who found that office-holding by parties 'on the left' could not explain policy variation. Weldon does find, however, that it is interaction between a strong women's movement on the outside and sympathetic policymakers on the inside that has produced the most robust policy responses,

responses that were strengthened further where women's policy machinery was in place. To partly reconcile the two positions, it could be argued that the sympathetic policymakers that Weldon found to be crucial have been more often found in the Australian case in the ALP (and the minor parties). Moreover, 'sympathetic' insiders have been more numerous under Labor governments, which appointed most of the femocrats. In any case, Weldon's study is narrower than this one in the sense that it covers only one policy area, violence, whereas we have been able to observe the approaches of the two main parties across the gamut of women's health concerns. Whether it be at the State, Territory or national level, it is clear that Labor regimes have been more interested in introducing policies in response to women's health concerns.

The orientation of government is one of the central features of 'political opportunity structure' as identified by social movement theorists (Gray 2008). Favourable political opportunity structures operated in most jurisdictions at some point during the first 15 years of the movement, which was a crucial time for getting ideas accepted and services established. At the national level, the ALP supported women's health each time it held office after 1972. Although supportive of refuges, the Fraser Coalition Government cut funding for women's health centres, the Community Health Program and for feminist refuges between 1975 and 1981. The Howard Coalition Government was openly hostile to women's health, resiling from any policy role and passing program responsibility to the sub-national level. An example of its intransigent opposition to feminism is its attempt to suppress the Access Economics report that showed that domestic violence cost the Australian economy $8 billion per annum. The report was not released until *The Australian* newspaper filed a successful freedom-of-information application. The previous year the Government had taken money from the violence and sexual assault budgets to pay for the postage of anti-terrorism fridge magnets (Sawer 2008a:7).

A similar pattern is evident in the States and Territories, where ALP governments have taken a more positive stance than their Liberal or Coalition counterparts. Queensland provides a clear example. After 32 years of non-Labor government,[2] which had opposed all policies on women's health, including OHS reform, the Goss Labor Government was elected in 1989. In quick succession, a women's health policy unit, a domestic violence policy unit, a gender equity unit, a women's safety program in the Queensland Police Service and a women's policy unit in the Office of Cabinet were established. A women's health policy and a violence against women policy were developed in 1993 and a range of special women's health projects was funded, including a secretariat for the Queensland

---

2   Variously Country/National Party/Liberal Coalition governments and, after 1983, a National Party government.

Women's Health Network (Mason 1994). These efforts might have been less expansive than feminists had hoped but they stand in sharp contrast with the record of preceding governments.

This is not to argue that all Labor governments have enthusiastically supported women's health reform or that all non-Labor governments resisted. Occasional innovations were made by non-Labor governments, such as the decision to develop a women's health policy in South Australia in 1982. The Greiner Government in New South Wales in the late 1980s and early 1990s, neo-liberal in orientation, saw no need to expand women's health services but continued to support them at existing levels. And while the Greiner Government began to dismantle the women's policy machinery, the incoming Labor Government completed the process. In one jurisdiction, women reported that non-Labor governments very quickly realised the political and service provision value of cheap and popular women's health services. It was also realised that a political backlash would follow any attempt to dismantle them.

Some Labor governments have resisted reform. The Dunstan Labor Government in South Australia was reluctant in the 1970s to 'buy into' Commonwealth programs, such as community health centres and women's health centres. Some members of the Western Australian Labor Government in the late 1980s and early 1990s approached the women's health project with either hostility or indifference. And, as discussed, Labor governments have engaged in symbolic politics, giving the impression of substantive action, as in the case of a second NWHP. After 1986, it took six years of intense daily struggle for the movement in Adelaide to persuade a Labor government to support the Pregnancy Advisory Centre. Reproductive rights are always controversial but the press was supportive, there was strong support from women in the Liberal Party and committed feminist bureaucrats were working on the case, yet progress was very slow. Notwithstanding exceptions, the majority of key Australian women's health initiatives have been taken under Labor regimes.

The electoral success of the ALP in the 1970s and 1980s was crucial in setting women's health services on a relatively strong foundation. The level of commitment that the Whitlam Commonwealth Government displayed has not been seen since. Addressing the First National Women's Health Conference in Brisbane in 1975, Prime Minister Whitlam said:

> The basic problem…resides in the attitudes which individuals and institutions within our society have towards women, their health and their bodies…the aim of this conference must be to understand, challenge and change these attitudes…Good health care for women…must be based on adequate and sensitive research into causes and methods of

treatment but ultimately it can only come from a correct understanding of how women feel about their bodies and a correct understanding of the lives they live. (Commonwealth Department of Health 1978:18)

One of the femocrats of the early years takes the view that without the Whitlam Government and supporters in the Health and Hospitals Services Commission (HHSC), the women's health movement might have quietly faded away.

The steady decline in the salience of women's issues can be seen in the reduced support for national women's health conferences since the 1970s. Prime Minister Whitlam opened the first conference in 1975, which was organised and funded by the Commonwealth as its 'special contribution to International Women's Year'. The call for papers prompted 'a massive response' and 950 women and men attended (Commonwealth Department of Health 1978). Five volumes of proceedings were produced and published by the Commonwealth, producing a valuable resource. A senior Commonwealth Health Department official worked with the organising committee for the second conference in 1985, together with several officials from the South Australian Government. The Commonwealth and South Australian governments, both Labor, provided financial support. The conference was opened and closed by Senator Pat Giles, who conveyed apologies from Health Minister, Neal Blewett (Kirby-Eaton and Davies 1986:3–7). Senator Giles also opened the third conference, in Canberra in 1995, which was closed by Health Minister, Carmen Lawrence, whose department provided financial support (Broom 2001:100–1). The Howard Commonwealth Government refused to contribute financially to either the fourth or the fifth conferences and chose not to send representatives. All senior Commonwealth politicians, including senior Labor women and the Prime Minister, declined AWHN's invitation to attend the Sixth National Women's Health Conference in 2010; however, the Commonwealth made a financial contribution of $50 000 and was represented by Senator Claire Moore. Nevertheless, since the early 1990s, Commonwealth interest has fallen steeply. This decline is not so apparent at the sub-national level where, in some cases, good working relationships are in place.

Labor held power for a considerable part of the 1970s in New South Wales, South Australia and Tasmania. In the 1980s, the years of significant policy advance, Labor held office for most of the decade in all States except Queensland. From the sub-national level, momentum steadily percolated upwards to culminate in the first NWHP and Program under the Hawke Commonwealth Government. This period of Labor Party dominance was not only unusual in Australia; it was also counter to international trends at the time. In other large English-speaking democracies, except New Zealand, the 1980s was a period of conservative party dominance. The Conservative Party was in power in Britain from 1979 until 1997, in Canada from 1984 until 1993 and, in the United States, Republican administrations ruled from 1981 until 1993. Women's health policy did not advance markedly under the Lange Labour Government in New Zealand, which became an adherent of neo-liberal ideas and seriously alienated traditional supporters, particularly women. Thus, when national and sub-national women's health policies were being advanced in the 1980s, Australia was the only OECD country with a strong women's health movement as well as a preponderance of responsive governments, which is a situation that can be classified as a very favourable political opportunity structure.

The Australian Party System

The Australian party system is another factor that seems to have contributed to the achievement of women's health policy objectives. Political parties that have reasonably well-developed sets of policies, as in Australia, play a key role in policy advancement. In the predominantly two-party system, politicians use policies to differentiate themselves from their opponents and to compete with each other for electoral support. In this process, a level of consensus is reached within parties and relatively detailed policies are produced and presented to the electorate. There is considerable exposure of issues and policy alternatives, which are scrutinised by the media and promoted and defended by leaders.

Britain, Canada and New Zealand, like Australia, all have strong, programmatic political parties, with the result that different experiences in these countries cannot be attributed to the nature of parties. The absence of this type of party system in the United States, however, helps to explain why that country, despite its strong women's health movement and the early focus on separate services, did not develop women's health policies. Parties in the United States exist primarily to choose candidates and facilitate their election, not to be agencies of policy advancement. Further, party structures are decentralised and non-hierarchical, making agreement on policy unlikely (Herrnson 1994:83).

Australian parties, particularly at the sub-national level, have regularly announced advances in women's health policy as part of their election strategies, as did the Rudd Government when it promised a second NWHP and a focus on violence against women during its 2007 election campaign.

The Women's Health Movement and the Australian Health and Welfare System

One of the reasons for the relative strength of the Australian women's health movement, I suggest, was uncertainty of access to publicly provided services, including hospital, medical and social services. The publicly subsidised system of private health insurance left approximately 20 per cent of the population with no insurance and another group of similar size with serious underinsurance in the early 1970s. A study in South Australia in 1973–74 found that the main reason for imprisonment for debt was unpaid hospital bills (Scotton 1978:130). National health insurance was introduced in 1975 but the system was steadily dismantled by the incoming Coalition Government, which reintroduced user charges and reinstated private health insurance (Gray 1984). Uncertainty about access prevailed again until 1984 when national health insurance was reintroduced.[3]

Strong women's health movements emerged in Britain, New Zealand, the United States, Australia and, a little later, in Canada. When measured in expenditure terms, the English-speaking democracies all have relatively weak welfare systems. It might be that women in continental European and Scandinavian countries felt less disadvantaged because they had more secure access to health and social services. Further, it is plausible that a social view of health is more likely to develop in the context of welfare state weakness, where, when all other things are equal, the poorer conditions of women's lives lead to poorer health outcomes.

The connection between welfare state development and the strength of women's health movements is speculative[4] and needs further study; however, some corroborative evidence exists. Although there has been an active women's health movement in Britain, women set up few separate services. An exception is the Women's Therapy Centre in London, which was established because psychotherapy was difficult to obtain under the National Health Service (NHS) (Broom 1991:63). Otherwise, women in Britain were reluctant to set up separate services for fear of appearing to promote private medicine at a time when the NHS was under threat from conservative forces (Doyal 1983:23; Elston 1981:203). The situation is entirely different in Australia where women from low socioeconomic groups—the main users of services provided free in feminist health centres—have always been less likely to hold private health insurance.

Relatively good access to hospital, medical and other services might be part of the reason New Zealand and Canadian women also set up fewer separate services. In the United States, women did set up their own services in the early years; however, public funding was not available as it was in Australia, so maintaining the services was more difficult.

---

3   National health insurance has lowered financial barriers to access; however, because successive governments of both persuasions have allowed out-of-pocket expenses to increase, serious obstacles to access have developed again.
4   Other factors could be differences in the degree to which medical attitudes are patronising, better access to reproductive health services, greater economic security through access to well-paid work and so on.

Access to Government

Australian political institutions have a reputation for being relatively accessible,[5] which has contributed to policy advancement. A former femocrat expressed the view that a person does not have to be an Oxbridge graduate to get access to senior levels of government. This might be related to the relative youth of Australian political institutions and the relative weakness of perceptions of social class. Professor Lesley Doyal, a British women's health expert who is familiar with Australian experience, is of the opinion that the relative openness of Australian government is an important factor in explaining different policy outcomes in Australia and Britain. In her assessment, members of the movement in Britain do not expect to have access to senior politicians and public servants, nor do they expect the creation of special women's policy machinery. And they certainly do not expect to be recruited to fill positions at senior levels of the bureaucracy.

Access to policymakers is particularly open in smaller jurisdictions, where people sometimes wear more than one hat and often know each other personally. Movement members in South Australia and Tasmania reported generally being able to arrange meetings with politicians and bureaucrats when they wanted them. Access depends partly on the political persuasion of the government in power. A government generally responsive to equality-seeking movements is more likely to permit access for women's groups. And none of the factors that impact on policymaking operates independently. Rather, they interact together so that the presence of femocrats working in women's policy institutions facilitates access for outside groups in a political culture that endorses consultation and some level of citizen engagement with government.

Relatively easy access to policymakers might help explain why the Australian women's health movement has been more successful than its British counterpart but further study is needed to answer the question of whether Australian government has been significantly more open to women's groups than governments in other English-speaking countries.

---

5   Evidence shows that different groups have very different access, both formal and informal, to Australian government. Matthews (1976) found that there was a massive over-representation of producer groups in Australian government institutions, such as advisory committees, and a serious under-representation of other groups, particularly disadvantaged minorities, including women, Aborigines, welfare recipients and immigrants.

The Role of Australian Federalism

In other studies of the impact of federalism on public policy, including women's policies, I have found that federal institutions can be both an asset and an obstacle. My argument has been that the way federalism works depends on its interaction with a range of other forces in the policy development environment and that its operation changes from time to time and from place to place (Gray 1991, 2006, 2010). Evidence from this historical study supports my earlier conclusions.

It has been argued by some that federalism impedes the development of public policy. The system, it is said, fragments the power of government, gives rise to conflict and controversy between levels, allows interest groups greater opportunities to obstruct policy processes, creates overlap and duplication and generally results in weak, conservative government (reviewed in Gray 1991:9–10).

Federalism does increase policy complexity. In the case of the first NWHP, activities that fed into the policy process took place in nine jurisdictions over nearly two decades. Activists had formed a multitude of groups, organisations, networks and centres at the community level and worked for reform in all jurisdictions. In each place, governments responded differently and each had their own policy agendas, sometimes innovative, sometimes not. Before the NWHP could be launched, endorsement was required from all nine Australian health ministers, advised as they were by nine different sets of bureaucrats. Until the last minute, health movement members, national and sub-national officials and Commonwealth and State and Territory femocrats had reason to fear that the policy would not be endorsed.

Institutional arrangements can have a different impact at different times depending on the other forces operating. For example, Australia is noted for its federal financial imbalance, which gives the Commonwealth control of the purse strings. This is a decided advantage for women's policies, including women's health, when a sympathetic government holds power at the national level. Conversely, it can be an enormous disadvantage, as when the Fraser Government slashed its funding for women's health centres, community health centres and feminist refuges. Generalisations therefore are likely to be fragile; however, one generalisation that can be made for the Australian federation—but not for all federations—is that the federal financial imbalance restricts the capacity of State and Territory governments to make policy innovations, especially where large outlays are required.

Complexity notwithstanding, a federal division of power can, at times, facilitate the maintenance and/or advancement of policy. When the Northern Territory Government was unwilling to support the establishment of the Central Australian

Aboriginal Congress health centre in the mid-1970s, funding was obtained from the Commonwealth. Similarly, when the Commonwealth reduced funding for the Community Health Program and women's health centres, women were able to appeal to the State level for assistance. In unitary systems, such options might not be available.[6] The States eventually agreed, after a struggle, to support the centres from their own coffers. Another example of federal arrangements working well for women took place between 1996 and 2007 when women's health centres, services and policies continued to be maintained or advanced in all jurisdictions, despite an antagonistic Commonwealth. These arguments are consistent with those of Louise Chappell (2001) who found that federal arrangements had allowed policy in relation to domestic violence to continue to develop at the sub-national level during the Howard years. Chappell reviews a number of studies that suggest a similar situation in relation to HIV/AIDS policy and policies for Aborigines.

The election of supportive governments at the same time in a number of jurisdictions can generate interest and create a favourable policy context, as in the 1980s. British observer Lesley Doyal is of the opinion that Australia's federal institutional structure is another of the reasons that women's health policy is far more developed than in Britain: it facilitated experimentation and innovation in a number of jurisdictions.[7]

As well as creating opportunities, federalism can create obstacles to policy expansion. During the second half of the 1970s and in the 1980s, when the non-Labor government in Queensland refused to support women's health, activists applied for Commonwealth funding through various avenues but were ineligible for national support because they were not national organisations. An example of sub-national obstruction took place during the Whitlam Government period when South Australia was governed by the Dunstan Labor Government, which was generally assumed to be reformist. For whatever reason, the South Australian Health Commission was allowed to strenuously oppose the Commonwealth proposal to fund the Hindmarsh Women's Health Centre. As discussed in Chapter 1, the approach of the Victorian health bureaucracy was similar. Indeed, one of the major obstacles facing the Whitlam Government's health reform program was created by federalism: its constitutional power to fund many of the projects it wished to support was limited.

---

6   In unitary systems where regional and local governments have a measure of financial independence, however, the options are similar.
7   We need to be cautious, though, about such generalisations: federalism could equally provide an unfavourable opportunity structure depending on the stance of governments towards a particular issue. Moreover, in practice, very few nations have only one level of government. Experimentation and innovation are features of local government activity under favourable institutional arrangements.

While it allows for innovation and experimentation in different jurisdictions when conditions are favourable, federalism also contributes to an unevenness of services across jurisdictions. The Northern Territory has no women's health centres in 2011, for example, and Tasmania has only one. There is also considerable variation in the sexual assault services across the country and in levels of funding commitment. New South Wales has many more agencies per capita than any other State. By 1990, it had 33 sexual assault services, one incest centre and one rape crisis centre, all of which received at least some public funding. At the same time, Western Australia, with almost one-third of the population, had only three publicly funded services. Queensland, which had more than half the population of New South Wales, had only two centres. There was no national policy overview at that time, with its potential to lead to more uniformity (Carmody 1990:304–8). Perhaps more seriously for the women's health project, without the policy impetus and the money that came with the NWHP, it is safe to argue that the women's health sectors in some States, notably Queensland, Western Australia and Tasmania, would be very much smaller than they are. By this point, they might even have disappeared. Thus, different political cultures in different parts of a federation generate unevenness in policy development, which also arises from experimentation and innovation. This is a problem if the dominant ethos is that citizens should have equal access to services, which tends to be the case in Australia and is certainly the position taken by the women's movement.

Federalism, then, has shaped women's health policies in different ways at different times. Like any other system of government, its operation depends upon the policy environment of the time and the impact of other interacting policy influences. A detailed examination of federalism is outside the scope of this book; however, many of the advantages and disadvantages so commonly claimed to emanate from federal institutions are features of unitary systems that have strong, relatively independent local or county government, such as in Scandinavia and many European countries. Moreover, all governmental systems create divisions of power when they divide responsibilities into separate portfolio areas. Such divisions might cause deadlocks and delays, as in the 1980s when the Commonwealth Department of Health approved and supported the establishment of Congress Alukura but the Department of Aboriginal Affairs tarried for some three years before committing the necessary funds (Carter et al. 1987). Departmental divisions certainly set up barriers to a comprehensive, whole-of-government response to problems such as violence against women. In summary, federalism is far from the only set of institutional arrangements that divides the power to govern. The way it operates depends on the interaction of many other policy influences so that it is very difficult to make firm generalisations about its impact even in a single federation.

Social Liberalism in Australia

A strong strand of social liberalism runs through Australian political culture. In contrast with its distant cousin, market or neo-liberalism, social liberalism is sympathetic to extensive government intervention in economic and social life and underpins the Australian practice of looking to government rather than to individuals or the private sector to help solve problems. A positive view of the role of the democratic state might be expected in a nation where white settlement was established by government, where extensive government intervention was necessary if settlements were to grow and where all the early institutions, such as hospitals, were government institutions. Since the nineteenth century, social liberalism has been an important force in Australia, and the policy responses called for by the women's health movement fit comfortably within that philosophical perspective.

Social liberal ideas in Australia derive from the work of English thinkers, including T. H. Green, L. T. Hobhouse, J. A. Hobson and J. M. Keynes, who developed a sustained critique in the late nineteenth and early twentieth centuries of laissez-faire or market liberalism.[8] Their work provides a philosophical foundation for the welfare state. These thinkers held that the role of government should be expanded to ensure a decent standard of living for all citizens and to provide the conditions under which individuals could reach their maximum potential. Rather than the minimal government role of laissez-faire liberalism, the democratic state, it was argued, has a moral duty to create the conditions for equality of opportunity and freedom from insecurity and deprivation.

Over the past century, many observers of political life have remarked on the extensive use that is made of the Australian state (government). 'Australian democracy has come to look upon the state as a vast public utility, whose duty is to provide the greatest good for the greatest number', wrote historian W. K. Hancock in 1930 (Hancock 1961:55). More recently, A. F. Davies (1964:4–5) argued that 'Australians have a characteristic talent for bureaucracy…[which] is exercised on a massive scale in government, economy and social institutions'. As Marian Sawer has shown, strong social liberal ideas have influenced Australian public policy for more than a century. Australian feminists, for example, have never trusted free markets and have espoused social liberal ideas and supported state intervention since the first wave of the movement (Sawer 2003). The calls that second-wave feminists made upon the state, then, are in keeping with an established and important seam in Australian political thought.

---

8   Neo-liberalism is the modern manifestation of laissez-faire or classical liberalism.

The deeply embedded support for social liberal ideas helps to explain, first, the relative success of the Australian women's health movement, especially in the early years, and, second, why the movement's approach has differed from that in countries where more individualistic, market-liberal ideas are stronger. Marian Sawer (1994:162) has drawn attention to an important difference between the Australian and US women's movements:

> Because of the tradition of seeking reform through political action rather than litigation, the language of Australian feminism has drawn upon shared value systems (the dominant social liberalism) both to mobilise supporters and to persuade power-holders. Australian feminism has not split like the American women's movement over issues of equal rights versus issues of special needs or individual autonomy versus the ethic of care because social liberalism contained all these elements. The Australian women's movement has been able to draw upon them as required for the political purposes of the day.

Social liberal ideas are embedded in the political cultures of other countries, including Britain, Canada and New Zealand. As discussed, however, when women's health movements were at the peak of their strength, political opportunity structures were unfavourable in those countries because conservative governments held power.

Despite the strength of the tradition, social liberal ideas have been strongly challenged by neo-liberalism in recent years, which is a large part of the reason that the commitment to social justice and feminist objectives has visibly weakened. The popularity of neo-liberal ideas among politicians and other opinion leaders in Australia over the past three decades might suggest that social liberalism is no longer an important political force. Australian opinion polling, however, consistently shows support for high levels of public spending on health, age pensions and education. A 2004 review of major polls found that in the previous 15 years, when faced with a choice between tax reductions and increased spending on social services, Australians increasingly favour the latter. One of the conclusions was that 'a government which cuts taxation while eroding the standard of health, aged care and education services is unlikely to have the support of public opinion' (Grant 2004:26). An explanation for this paradoxical situation is not attempted here, except to say that the interests with the resources to place their views on political agendas and to make contributions to the campaign funds of political parties appear to be the voices that are being heard. There is still strong support for women's health policies and programs, which the Commonwealth is currently choosing to ignore, except at a symbolic level. Present-day neo-liberal leanings aside, a majority of citizens consistently supports well-funded health and education services.

Conclusion

A combination of forces and influences interacted together to put women's health on Australian policy agendas and to induce governments to act. The strength and tenacity of the grassroots movement were very important factors, together with the dedication and commitment of women working in women's services over almost four decades. The context of a strong reform environment in which the early movement worked was important, as were related factors such as the relative weakness of Australian social policies and programs, which meant that there was significant community support for general social policy reform. The relative openness of Australian government helped the movement to put its claims before senior personnel and, once issues found their way into party platforms, at least some of them were implemented when a party came to power. Women in political parties and unions worked hard to persuade the men in their organisations to accept women's health ideas. The early and extensive establishment of Australian women's policy machinery and the appointment of femocrats in key positions were distinctive Australian developments that promoted policy uptake. The strong relationship that often existed between feminists in the bureaucracy and feminists outside was often used to promote policy advancement. Although it is impossible to measure the independent impact of separate influences, the strength of the Australian women's health movement, the election of supportive governments and a political culture that endorses social liberalism were key factors. Moreover, all these influences interacted together in various ways, sometimes reinforcing each other and constituting a countervailing force to opposing interests.

To return to the questions posed in the introduction, a complex array of interacting influences is the reason that Australia is the only country to have enacted two national women's health policies and to have attempted to establish a strong national network of community health centres. Policy development was supported by a community health movement and an Aboriginal health movement and led by strong exponents of structural reform—the same policymakers who supported women's health. And, of course, the women's health movement and the community health movement provided support and legitimacy for each other. One difference between the two areas is that health policy experts led developments in community health whereas women at the grassroots led the charge in women's health, as they did in the Aboriginal health movement. A similar set of policy forces has placed Australia among the leading countries in its response to violence against women.

Finally, what are the conditions that came together at different times to create windows of opportunity for structural health reform? In the case of the introduction of national health insurance and the Community Health Program in the 1970s, the first facilitating factor was that the Commonwealth Government was strongly committed to policy action and actively led public debate. That is, the ALP had formulated relatively detailed, evidence-based policies and had explained them to the community over several years. Because the proposals were controversial, debate had been long and intense and party members had worked hard to articulate the policies. By the time the party came to office, significant numbers of Australians understood and supported the proposals. Second, the activism and support of the health reform movement, including the women's health movement and the Aboriginal health movement and mobilised general women's and welfare reform groups, made it easier for the Commonwealth to pursue major change and harder for the Opposition to oppose, although oppose it did very strongly. Outside support, national and international, helps to shore up the political determination necessary to succeed against powerful opposing medical unions and other interests, such as the insurance industry. Thus, a reform-oriented policy environment, featuring strong support for social liberal rather than neo-liberal policy responses, strongly mobilised community support groups, evidence-based policies with supporters and a political party with strong political will, prepared to take the role of opinion leader, were crucial elements of policy opportunities. The planets in the policy universe rarely line up so well.

10. A Glass Half Full...

Australian women's health activists, in their long quest for the changes that will improve women's health—and the health of the whole population—have reason to feel both gratification and disappointment. For although they can lay claim to remarkable achievements, some of the most important goals are yet to be achieved. Moreover, along the way, crucially important opportunities for structural health reform have been missed. In the early days, movement members identified a set of problems, many of them rarely discussed in public, and then worked persistently until community attitudes shifted, decision makers took notice and policy responses were made. As a result, new laws and new programs to advance women's health were devised and funded across the country. The movement itself set up an infrastructure of community-based healthcare centres and services to support women in their daily lives and at times of distress and crisis. This infrastructure serves as an institutional base for the movement, supporting intelligence gathering, information sharing, policy development and advocacy work. Taking up the health reform ideas of the 1970s and applying a gender lens, the concept of a social health perspective was developed and disseminated. Arguably, wider understanding and acceptance of the social view of health is the movement's most important accomplishment. Unfamiliar in the early 1970s when the comprehensiveness of hospital and medical services was rarely questioned, the social perspective now explicitly informs most Commonwealth, State and Territory health policy documents.

On the other side of the ledger, the women's health sector has always been seriously under-funded, which has restricted its capacity to meet immediate needs and to develop innovative and collaborative health-promoting strategies. It also restricts its capacity to expand its constituency because, being thinly scattered, only a few women can have access to the services it provides. While the mainstream health system has responded to some aspects of the feminist critique, it remains heavily centred on the medical model, with its focus on treatment services. The best-practice models of preventive health care developed in the community sector have not yet had a system-wide impact, mostly because structural incentives steer provision in the direction of high-turnover treatment services. Health reform has been high on the national agenda since 2007, where policy documents recognise social determinants and talk about the importance of prevention. Yet proposals to strengthen primary health care—the locus of any significant preventative effort—have so far been restricted to supporting the services provided in general practitioners' surgeries on a fee-for-service basis. The 1970s vision of a holistic, prevention-focused, primary healthcare system is still the stuff of dreams.

Nevertheless, innovative models of practice continue to be developed in the small community-based worlds of women's health, Aboriginal health and community health. The States and Territories, within the limited finance available to them, are generating innovative approaches to primary health care through partnerships and collaborations with the community sector and others. And after a small injection of extra funding that came with the Emergency Response, policymakers in the Northern Territory's Aboriginal medical services are leading the way in Australian health reform, as the Aboriginal health movement led the way in the 1970s.

This concluding chapter looks at the achievements of the women's health movement and the goals that are still to be reached. It then examines the reasons that structural reform has been so hard to achieve, returning to the last question posed in the introduction: why, despite the wealth of evidence and the advocacy of women and other public health reformers, have the key structures of the health system remained virtually unchanged since the 1970s?

Two Steps Forward

At the local level, in female-run centres and services, women participate in health decision making, which is held to be the gold standard by health experts. The services provided are highly valued by those who use them, particularly by disadvantaged and marginalised women. Primary prevention undertakings, infrequently available in the hospital and medical systems, are tailored to meet local needs. Self-help is supported, health literacy is promoted and group programs are developed. Support and referral services and community-development projects are part of everyday practice, along with interaction and collaboration with local service providers.

Currently, 65 community-based, feminist women's health centres are providing services nationally, along with almost 400 refuges, shelters, safe houses and information and referral services for women escaping violence. Sexual assault services have been established in all States and Territories. Some are still independent and community based, others are government run, sometimes informed by feminist principles, sometimes with community representatives on their boards. There are approximately 150 community-controlled Aboriginal health centres, in which women play important roles. In addition, there are specialist centres, such as Children by Choice in Queensland, the Multicultural Centre for Women's Health in Victoria and Aboriginal women's health centres. Informed by a social perspective of health and illness, these organisations provide an extensive range of medical and non-medical services, tailored to respond to the expressed needs of the communities in which they are located.

In women's health centres, participation in health decision making is a daily reality. Clients are familiar with the concept of participation and they feel a sense of involvement with the centres they attend and a capacity to influence what happens there. Community women are often involved in centre management, and participation in the many group programs on offer opens the way for health development, empowerment, companionship, and the giving and receiving of support (Broom 1996:24–5, 1997:278). This is all the more valuable because women's health centres serve a clientele that is markedly disadvantaged compared with the female population overall. Clients are significantly more likely to have been born overseas, to identify as being Aboriginal or Torres Strait Islander, to have lower education levels and below-average incomes, to have been unemployed in the past year, to be lone mothers and not to be buying their own homes (Broom 1997:277). These are the women who are least likely to participate in civil society and most likely to have poor health outcomes. Women's health centres also undertake outreach work enabling them to make contact with women who might otherwise be excluded and whose needs often go unrecognised. Workers in women's health centres are caring for women while at the same time assisting them to gain skills to care for themselves. And judging by the popularity of the centres, they are doing these jobs well.

The number of women's health advocacy groups continues to grow, supporting more women and drawing attention to an ever-broadening sweep of health issues. Professionals, including legal, law enforcement, allied health and medical professionals, have received training in feminist health perspectives and cultural competence. The latter now appears in the curriculums of some medical schools (Ambanpola 2005).

Influenced by other social changes as well, the way women experience encounters with medical and hospital systems has shifted in response to the feminist critique. Professional attitudes are less patronising and judgmental and women's health concerns are less likely to be trivialised. Finding a woman doctor, particularly a general practitioner, is likely to be easier, as women now enter medical training in much the same numbers as men. Raising public awareness of problems, such as the over-prescription of tranquillisers and the dangers of certain drugs, has resulted in increased health literacy and more careful practice. Following earlier overseas developments, moves are at last being initiated in Australia to ensure that appropriate numbers of women are included in research projects.

The hundreds of refuges scattered across the country provide essential services for women and children, where previously there were almost none. Since the early days, when volunteers responded as best they could to the needs of the women and children landing on their doorsteps, feminist refuges have undertaken political advocacy as well as providing support services and crisis accommodation. As the expertise and professionalism of workers increased, the range of services was broadened and became increasingly sophisticated. Where budgets allow, refuges provide child care, children's programs, child-protection services and programs to enhance parenting skills. They assist with legal and financial matters and with access to long-term housing. Counselling services are provided and families are assisted to deal with health issues. As well as advocacy and community education, refuges provide outreach and training. Staff regularly contribute to policy development and interact with a plethora of government and non-governmental agencies as part of efforts to coordinate complex sets of services (Gander and Champion 2009).

Peak bodies, at both the sub-national and the national levels, support the sectors and act as a conduit to government. WESNET, the national peak body representing almost 400 agencies, identifies areas of unmet need, draws attention to new and emerging issues and stimulates debate within the sector through its newsletter and through forums and conferences. It lobbies governments to improve policies and expand services and undertakes research, including research on needs in rural and remote communities. The links between homelessness and violence have been explored and publicised and model national domestic violence laws have been drawn up (WESNET web site). State and Territory peak bodies also play crucial roles. In New South Wales, for example, the Women's Refuge Movement has operated for more than 30 years, advocating for the needs of the sector and the clients of the 57 refuges it represents.

Since the first faltering efforts of volunteers to respond appropriately to the often desperate women who contacted them, sexual assault centres have been slowly transformed into highly professional agencies in all jurisdictions, although there is considerable variation from place to place. Victoria, for example, has a statewide network of hybrid services that are government run but have community boards, while New South Wales has a mix of government and non-governmental agencies.

Significant attitudinal changes to violence and sexual violence against women and children have been realised, largely through the efforts of the movement and the policies formulated in response. A large national survey undertaken by VicHealth in 2009 found that 98 per cent of respondents recognised domestic violence as a crime—an increase of 5 per cent from a 1995 benchmark survey. People were also more likely to understand that domestic violence takes a variety of forms. As well as actual physical harm, it includes threats of harm and psychological, verbal and economic abuse. In 1995, one in seven respondents thought that women who are raped 'ask for it'. By 2009, however, only one in 20 people took this view (VicHealth 2010:8, 37, 42). Thus, as Alexandra Neame argues: 'Historical explanations of the causes, characteristics and prevalence of sexual assault have changed dramatically over the past three decades, primarily in response to effective campaigning by feminists to challenge the many myths surrounding rape and other forms of sexual violence' (Neame 2003:6).

The movement can count among its achievements Australia's two national women's health policies, the NWH Program, the National Plan to Reduce Violence against Women and their Children, the National Disability Strategy and the many crucial State and Territory policies and strategies. Since 2007, violence against women has been a priority item on the Commonwealth's policy agenda. Of developments in this area, Leslie Laing wrote in 2000:

> Within a quarter of a century, a subject once shrouded in secrecy has assumed a prominent place on the agenda of all State and Territory governments, and the Federal government. It is salutary to recall that, less than a century before the first feminist actions to place domestic violence on the political and social agenda, it was lawful for a man to beat his wife; women could not own property, nor could they have the custody of children. Clearly much has been achieved. (Laing 2000:5)

Since 2007, the profile of gender-based violence as a women's health issue has been raised by the leadership of the Commonwealth Labor Government and the report of the National Council. A national plan is now in place that offers the possibility of sustained action across jurisdictions.

A social view of health, promoted consistently by the movement for 40 years, has now entered the health policy lexicon. For example, the National Health and Hospitals Reform Commission (NHHRC) report commends the work of WHO's Commission on the Social Determinants of Health and supports its call for governments to take action in addressing those determinants. Some of the objectives identified by the NHHRC, such as strengthening consumer engagement and voice through increased health literacy, fostering community participation and empowering consumers, follow women's health principles and are well established in practice in the women's health and Aboriginal community-based sectors (Commonwealth of Australia 2009c: 7, 96).

The gains of the past 40 years are all the more impressive because pioneering women had so few resources, so little knowledge about the operation of government and policymaking and were novices when it came to submission writing and advocacy work. What has been said of the women's health movement in the United States can equally be said of the Australian movement:

> Few other recent social movements have addressed questions of health and medical care so directly, and few have contributed a practice so relevant to changing health beliefs, health practices and health care

institutions...the totality of the feminist contribution to public health practice is greater than the sum of its individual parts. (Freudenberg 1986:30)

Yet the precious opportunities to achieve population-health gain opened up by the movement and its allies have been largely wasted. Funding for the women's health sector has always been niggardly, crushing its potential to make a greater contribution to population health. Most importantly, the structural reforms needed to redress the imbalance between medical and hospital services and community-based primary health care have been absent from the Commonwealth agenda for decades, except for a brief moment when it was raised by the Rudd Government only to fade into oblivion as vested interests in health took up their battle positions. Moreover, as well as failure to invest in primary health care (as opposed to primary medical care), successive Commonwealth governments have presided over glaring structural impediments to the accessibility of conventional hospital and medical services, undermining the universal access that Medicare is supposed to provide.

One Step Backwards: Under-funding

The women's health sector has always been run on a shoestring. The needs of even the small number of women who have a service located nearby and want information, advice and care have never been adequately met, even under the Whitlam Government. Since then, no government has been prepared to provide funding at more than a minimal level. For clients, frustration, unnecessary suffering, traumatised children and avoidable ill health are some of the penalties being paid. For the Australian public purse, the costs are high. Medicare foots a large bill for avoidable illness and unnecessary hospitalisation. In the violence area alone, Access Economics calculated the cost at $8.1 billion per year in 2004 (Commonwealth of Australia 2004a:64–8).

Under-funding of the women's health sector results in high levels of frustration among women working at the coalface because they cannot provide the services that are patently needed. Managing in straitened circumstances contributes to poor morale and cynicism. Professional development is thwarted and recruitment is always a problem because the pay on offer is unattractive. Forward planning is impossible without financial security and even simple matters, such as leasing premises, can become a major stumbling block. Policies, especially pilot programs, are often largely symbolic and leave a local vacuum when they terminate. In some jurisdictions, women (both inside and outside government) feel that the women's health movement has been 'used' by political parties and bought off cheaply. At the sub-national level, political mileage has been gained from the announcement of new but minimally funded services in marginal seats. At the national level after more than a decade of hostility, the movement has no choice but to settle for the 2010 NWHP, released in the dead of night, which does not acknowledge the contribution of the community-based sector, much less provide funds to sustain it.

The situation of the Hunter Women's Centre in New South Wales illustrates the dilemmas that accompany financial parsimony. The centre has been unable to attract a doctor since 2003 and therefore cannot provide medical services, despite high demand. The absence of medical staff also means that the centre is unable to employ nurse practitioners, who are permitted to work only with the backup of a doctor. Moreover, because rates of pay are low, it cannot attract allied health professionals, such as dieticians. In 2008, the waiting list for counselling services was approximately six months. The centre was forced to reduce the length of appointments and refer women elsewhere. Another strategy is to try to promote more self-help skills. Only a partial response can be made to expressed need and only a minimal response to requests for outreach services in surrounding regional areas. The planning question is always which services can be cut, rather than how services can be organised to meet client needs.

A similar situation prevails at Leichhardt Women's Community Health Centre and most other centres, including those that provide crisis services, such as family violence outreach. At Leichhardt, waiting lists are not kept because there are no resources to manage them. Appointments are given on a first-come, first-served basis. The centre would like to employ a domestic violence counsellor and a counsellor familiar with the needs of adult survivors of childhood sexual assault but has no money to do so. Salaries are based on the social and community services (SACS) award, which results in lower pay rates than in either the government or the private sectors, so it is difficult to attract skilled professionals. The centre survives because older, experienced staff members are strongly committed to its philosophy. Staff members report, however, that a partner earning a good income is an essential support mechanism.

Funding to support women and children who have experienced violence remains inadequate. If it was shocking that there were virtually no services for women escaping violence in the 1970s even when their children were being sexually assaulted, it is a national disgrace that almost 40 years later women and children are still turned away because services are not funded to cope with demand. In rural and remote areas, there are very few support services. Unable to access crisis accommodation, women and children often return to violent situations, with all the painful and wasteful health problems that follow. The best available data indicate that *one in every two* women escaping violence and looking for accommodation in domestic violence homelessness services is turned away (Gander and Champion 2009:25). Nor, amazingly, do refuges receive funding to cover the cost of accompanying children, although governments acknowledge the value of investing in young people. Accommodation shortages result in many women and children being referred to motels and caravans, sleeping in cars, staying temporarily in overcrowded housing and/or returning home to perpetrators (Commonwealth of Australia 2009a:76).

Moreover, homelessness policies do not take sufficient account of violence against women. Crisis service providers still struggle to persuade governments at all levels that domestic violence is *the* major cause of homelessness in Australia (Gander and Champion 2009:25). There are very few crisis services for older women, so that older homeless, single women are in no better position in 2011 than they were in the 1970s (McFerran 2009:5–7). In addition, acute shortages of affordable housing nationwide mean that bottlenecks develop and extreme pressure is put on refuges with the result that client recovery is delayed. The National Council's finding that refuges, shelters and outreach services are inadequately funded has not so far resulted in any significant increase in resources. Staff shortages are such that there is often only one domestic and family violence 'safe at home' worker to cover a whole rural region or only two workers for an entire metropolitan area.[1] The connections between homelessness, domestic violence and sexual assault are not sufficiently recognised in policies. The incidence of sexual assault amongst homeless people is high, especially for women and young people, but there are no specialist services to meet their needs. Indeed, while policies generally note the position of groups that experience higher levels of violence, including women with disabilities, Aboriginal and Torres Strait Islander women, women in rural and remote areas and so on, the women's services sector cannot respond appropriately to clients with complex needs.

Sexual assault services have developed priority criteria to help manage heavy demand with the result that women categorised as non-urgent might have to wait months for counselling. In some jurisdictions, rape crisis facilities have been asked to provide services for men without additional funding. Some services are forced to close on one or more days a week and many have difficulty offering adequate after-hours services, court support, legal advice, services for children, preventive resources, community-development initiatives and advocacy in relation to issues such as child protection. The capacity to collaborate effectively with other organisations is reduced, finding time to offer student placements is difficult and staff training is limited due to resource constraints. In some places, there are even long waiting lists for support group programs. In such circumstances, the capacity to undertake prevention work is limited. As Carmody (2009:16) argues, if primary prevention is to be taken seriously, 'we need a skilled and adequately remunerated workforce that not

---

1   These issues are discussed in Barrett Meyering (2009); Braaf (2008); Morrison (2009); Oberin (2009).

only understands the content of the programs they are delivering but have a clearly articulated theoretical stance to the work they do and understand why they do it'. The inability to obtain post-violence accommodation, counselling and support and the lack of well-funded prevention programs lead to high and avoidable ill health, which extends into old age. Community-sector workers continually operate at the limits of their capacity—a workplace situation that is not health enhancing.

There is strong agreement that services in the violence sector need to be coordinated and integrated. The National Council (Commonwealth of Australia 2009a:7,187) argues that integrated strategies and action plans need to be developed at both sub-national and local levels. Plans should reflect input from the police and justice systems, and from education, community, health and human services, it is argued, and should include performance indicators, targets and time lines. Currently, only Victoria, Tasmania and the Australian Capital Territory are attempting to coordinate their responses (Willcox 2008:5). The National Council's recommendation that mechanisms be put in place to ensure that systems work effectively together has been omitted from the new National Plan to Reduce Violence against Women and their Children.

Inadequate funding limits the extent to which services can carry out prevention work. There is agreement that educational efforts need to include school students, university students, community leaders and service providers and they need to be expanded. The present Commonwealth Government recognises this problem and is currently supporting 'Respectful Relationships' programs. As with so many past efforts, however, the present projects are pilots—they might not continue and are unevenly spread across the country. Only $9.1 million over four years has been allocated to cover projects in various settings (Plibersek 2009). The new national plan envisages that prevention programs will be continued but no announcement has been made about funding allocations at the time of writing.

In terms of appropriate training, a 2009 consultation in New South Wales found that the police and general practitioners still lacked important knowledge about domestic violence, healthy relationships and women's rights (Peters 2009:3). Existing services are not adequately funded to do the training, protocol development and integration work that is required to ensure that the mainstream and community agencies respond appropriately to violence against women and children. Experts argue that training for judges, magistrates, registrars, court volunteers and the like must be made compulsory (Oberin 2009:6).

Another problem is that research has been so under-funded that information about violence against women and the services they seek is limited. We are not even sure whether levels are lower, stable or increasing (Commonwealth of

Australia 2009a:15–21). Oberin (2009:4) argues that intimate partner homicide might be increasing. Information is not collected consistently across the country and the data that exist have serious limitations. National data are currently too poor to be used to measure and evaluate the effectiveness of interventions.

At a time when violence against women occupies an important place on policy agendas, women's services workers report feeling sidelined and undervalued (Gander and Champion 2009:26). Refuge workers are experts in the complex needs of women and children who have experienced violence and in the strengths and weaknesses of service systems. They have a long history of contribution to policy, legislation and research. But this expertise is not utilised: leading advocates argue that there is still a lack of systematic and meaningful consultation. They point out that neither WESNET nor Homelessness Australia is represented on the Prime Minister's Council on Homelessness (Oberin 2009:10). As Gander and Champion conclude: 'It appears that the breadth and depth of our interventions, and the multilayered nature of our work, is not worth mentioning, building upon, or even maintaining with adequate funding' (2009:26).

This argument is underscored by the lack of reference to the work of the women's health sector in the 2010 NWHP. Given that dozens of submissions from the sector were received, the oversight cannot be unintentional.

Because primary prevention efforts in the violence sector have been weak and sporadic, it is not surprising that many old myths and beliefs remain strong, despite positive attitudinal change. Moreover, some attitudes are shifting in directions that are not supported by evidence. Almost half (49 per cent) of Australians in the VicHealth survey cited above still believe that women could leave violent relationships if they really wanted to and 80 per cent said they found it difficult to understand why women would remain. Twenty per cent of men and 17 per cent of women believe that domestic violence is excusable when perpetrators get so angry they temporarily lose control and 27 per cent of men and 18 per cent of women would excuse domestic violence where perpetrators are genuinely sorry afterwards. Thirteen per cent of people still agree that women 'often say no when they mean yes' and more than one-third of Australians believe that rape results from men being unable to control their sexual urges! Further, the belief that women lie about violence is still strong: 49 per cent agreed that women make false statements in order to improve their chances in custody cases. Only 61 per cent of respondents agreed that women rarely make false claims about rape, with men and boys more likely to support or excuse violence than women and girls (VicHealth 2009:7–9).

In relation to attitudes that persist despite significant social changes, it appears that many doctors still approach women in a disrespectful manner. The major finding of a 2011 health survey undertaken by Equality Rights Alliance is that women, especially young women, experience the services they receive as poor in terms of the negative way they are treated by medical professionals. Open, non-judgemental communication, respect and willingness to listen were identified as positive elements of medical encounters that were often missing. 55.3 per cent of the women surveyed would not recommend their general practitioners to other people! Women were also concerned about financial, geographical and physical barriers that reduced access to services.[2]

Sexual assault remains one of the most under-reported crimes in Australia, with an estimated reporting rate of less than one in five (Commonwealth of Australia 2009a:19). Social stigma, which flows from longstanding myths and the perception that legal processes are overly concerned with the rights of the accused, operate to deter reporting. Other problems include non-supportive environments for complainants, lack of expertise amongst relevant professionals and the unpredictability of judicial discretion. Women whose first language is other than English, Aboriginal women and women with disabilities experience even greater barriers (Neame 2003).

In summary, then, the National Council (Commonwealth of Australia 2009a; 2009b) confirmed what the women's services sector has been saying for many years: serious problems arise from under-resourcing, including difficulties accessing crisis and emergency services. There are long waiting lists for all kinds of services and support, including housing, and difficulties accessing legal advice and timely forensic examinations. Moreover, resource constraints prevent women's health workers from developing innovative responses to the needs that women living in their areas express. All of which is very bad not only for women's health but also for everyone's health. As a recent WHO report on women's health argues, 'improving women's health matters to women, their families, communities and societies at large. Improve women's health—improve the world' (WHO 2009:6).

Explaining the Half-Full Glass: Constraints on policy advancement

How do we explain the less than full support of successive Australian governments, national and sub-national, for the women's health enterprise? How do we explain the lack of progress towards the structural changes necessary to create a more comprehensive health system when the evidence so clearly

---

2 The survey report can be found on the Equality Rights Alliance website at <http://equalityrightsalliance. org.au/projects/stronger-policies-and-programs-womens-health>

supports such a direction? In answering the first question, it is hard to escape the conclusion that women's health is still not seen as fully legitimate. Indeed, at times, suggestions are made that separate women's health services are no longer needed. Having usefully blazed a trail in the early years, the argument goes, these relics of a bygone era should be incorporated into the wider health system. If the mainstream health system had embedded 'prevention and early intervention into every aspect' of the system, as suggested by the NHHRC (Commonwealth of Australia 2009c:95), the argument mighthave some validity. The community-based sector and the hospital and medical sectors, however, still provide very different sets of services, as we have seen. And even where secondary and tertiary prevention are practised, there is enormous variation across the country. For example, a few divisions of general practice have been innovative, improving the comprehensiveness of their services, as have a few group practices. For the most part, however, the mainstream operates firmly within a medical, individual treatment model.

Second, the under-funding of the sector means that it has been unable to expand its support base, which, in turn, limits its political relevance. While extremely popular with clients, the spread of services is too small to reach more than a tiny proportion of Australian women, so limiting the number of women supporters. Moreover, because many clients are disadvantaged, they are less able than advantaged women to exercise their political voice. The women's health sector therefore is a political lightweight, dependent on government largesse and struggling to lobby effectively for its own expansion.

Third, while some sub-national jurisdictions have shown considerable support for women's health, the financial centralisation of the Australian federation renders them unlikely to be generous funders, even under buoyant conditions. Moreover, the Commonwealth can, and does, manipulate the federal financial balance at will: the Howard Government, for example, reduced the national share of hospital funding from 44.3 per cent in 1998–99 to 38.6 per cent in 2006–07 (AIHW 2010c:ix), leaving the States and Territories seriously short of discretionary spending capacity. Fiscal centralisation, then, is a large part of the reason that the States and Territories have kept a tight rein on women's health funding.

In summary, less than complete legitimacy, low political resources and the Australian federal financial imbalance combine to undermine opportunities for policy expansion. The advance of neo-liberal ideas and the relatively new phenomenon where both major political parties seem able to ignore voters' preferences for well-funded public health and education systems have resulted in to a poorly funded sector that struggles to meet even urgent needs. Turning to probe the second question concerning the slow progress towards a more comprehensive health system, we find a somewhat different set of forces at work.

Structural Barriers to Improved Population Health

As well as political barriers to greater government investment in primary health care, there are also entrenched structural barriers that impede full access to treatment in the hospital and medical systems. While treatment systems are only part of what it takes to improve population health, they are nevertheless a key element of any health system. Structural barriers include (but are not limited to) the fee-for-service system of doctor remuneration, the Australian preference for small medical practices, increasing user charges and imbalance in the geographical spread of services. Financial barriers also inhibit access to allied health services, including dentistry, physiotherapy, dietary advice and the like. Further, there is still excessive emphasis on a medical model of care in medical and nursing education with insufficient emphasis on training to increase awareness of cultural, sexuality and gender differences. Culturally inappropriate services are a barrier to access.

Barriers to Accessing Medical Services

The fee-for-service method of payment works as an economic incentive for doctors to see as many patients as possible, as quickly as possible, producing high turnover, curative medicine. It discourages the longer appointments necessary for thorough check-ups, for the management of complex and chronic conditions and to engage in primary prevention work. Internationally, fee-for-service remuneration has come under heavy criticism. One OECD assessment argues that it gives physicians 'full discretion' over the level and mix of services and creates incentives 'to expand the volume and price of the services they provide' (OECD 2003). Policy in a number of European countries is moving away from fee-for-service towards other forms of payment and it has been replaced completely with contract and salaried payment in New Zealand. Recent research shows that the percentage of New Zealanders who go without care because of cost has fallen since 2004 when this change came into operation (Schoen et al. 2010:2327).

Although Medicare is a type of national health insurance, it provides only partial coverage against the cost of medical services outside hospitals. Australian user charges—that part of the cost of a service paid for by the user—have been allowed to increase steadily and are now among the highest in the world (Schoen et al. 2010:2327). There is a large international literature showing that user charges constitute a serious financial barrier to access, especially for low-income people (reviewed in Gray 2004:65–77). In 2009, 22 per cent of Australians went without care because of cost, 21 per cent paid user charges of $1000 or more and 8 per cent reported being unable to pay medical bills or having serious problems paying (The Commonwealth Fund 2010). Moreover, the cost of accessing the services of allied health professionals, including dieticians, physiotherapists, psychologists, counsellors, podiatrists, dentists, midwives and alternative therapists, is beyond the financial capacity of a great many Australians and is especially difficult for low-income women. These structural impediments mean that those lower down on the social gradient are often missed by conventional medical systems, bringing to mind 'the inverse care law' coined by Welsh doctor Julian Tudor Hart some 40 years ago. 'The availability of good medical care', Hart argued, 'tends to vary inversely with the need of the population served' in systems where market forces are allowed to operate (Hart 1971:405).

Some people are deterred from accessing services because health professionals are not trained in cultural or gender competence or trained to understand the health problems faced by those with non-heterosexual orientations. Aboriginal people report experiencing racism when using mainstream services, while people from backgrounds other than Anglo-Australian often find that the circumstances of their lives are misunderstood. For similar reasons, GLBTIQ people identify appropriate health services as a priority.

The inverse-care law operates strongly in relation to residents of rural and remote areas. There, services of all types are in short supply, despite evidence that rural people suffer poorer health than people living in metropolitan areas.[3] If we were to take population health seriously, reforms would need to be implemented to modify and, in an ideal world, eventually eliminate, all of these structural barriers. Australian health policy has failed to deal with the overt barriers that impact adversely on access to hospital and medical treatment, which does not augur well for the prospect of introducing the structural changes needed to strengthen the primary health care system.

Structural Barriers to a Stronger Primary Health Care System

The important barriers weighing against the development of a more comprehensive healthcare system include cultural factors, financial forces and the stake that powerful medical unions and other groups have in preserving the system as it stands. Ideas about what is appropriate and necessary in a health system take a long time to change. The century-old idea that a health system

---

3   We do not have problems of such magnitude in education because educators do not operate as private business entrepreneurs.

provides hospital and medical services and not much else is taking a long time to fade. Because there are so few comprehensive primary healthcare centres in Australia, most people have no experience of the care on offer and are probably unfamiliar with what is done in the name of holistic primary health care. What we do know, however, is that when people have an opportunity to access such services, they are prepared to line up on the pavement outside to do so.

In the 1970s, government members and committed bureaucrats 'talked up' the value of primary health care, whereas in the twenty-first century most health debate centres on hospitals and their waiting lists—a situation that vested interests find easy to manipulate. Despite passing discussion of preventive health care, recently focusing narrowly on chronic disease and 'lifestyle factors', opinion leaders are not promoting the value of community health care. When it comes to taking concrete, funded action, most policymakers, it seems, still see health policy as predominantly about hospital and medical services. Cultural factors are important as well, especially in maternity care: Australian women have become accustomed to having their babies in hospitals since there are so few alternatives. Perhaps they are about to become accustomed to having their babies by caesarean section. While RANZCOG defends Australian levels of caesarean section, these rates are high by international standards. Indeed all the English-speaking industrialised countries have high rates, except for New Zealand, which is now placed about the middle. The OECD country with by far the lowest caesarean section rate is the Netherlands, where medicalisation is less than anywhere else and where approximately one-third of babies are born at home (OECD 2011).

A preference for solo or small group practice, supported by the financing system, is another structural barrier to comprehensive, primary health care. Evidence shows that teams of health professionals are necessary to deliver an integrated range of preventive, educational, counselling, caring and social advocacy services, as well as conventional medical services, as the NHHRC recognised. Another problem with solo or small group practice is lack of accountability. Peer review of work is uncommon and the sharing of ideas and collegiality that comes with teamwork is not available. Health teams have been introduced in some European countries and in New Zealand and Canada.

Money is another factor militating against investment in primary health care. Even for the Commonwealth, the cost of hospital and medical services, which has increased faster than other prices for decades, is a large budget item. Containing hospital and medical costs is a major objective in all OECD countries and has not been fully achieved. Under these circumstances, it is difficult for governments to find new money to invest in community-based services. Delaying investment, however, ensures the continuation of a destructive spiral: low spending on primary health care results in avoidable illness and unnecessary hospitalisation, which leads to unnecessarily high cost to the public purse and, in turn, results in low spending on primary health care. The NHHRC drew attention to this dilemma, commenting on the lack of any nationally coordinated mechanism to deliver preventive health care. In relation to chronic disease, it argued that Australia spends less than 2 per cent of the health budget on 'a problem which consumes a major proportion of health expenditure' (Commonwealth of Australia 2009c:51). The Commonwealth responded by setting up the National Preventive Health Agency in 2010 with the aim of driving the Australian prevention agenda. It is too early to see if it will have an impact.

Finally, powerful interests vehemently resist structural reform. Health is an area where there exist exceptionally powerful vested interests. Medical professionals are respected, influential and have abundant resources to devote to political campaigns. Doctors' trade unions regularly and consistently attack governments that want to make changes that might undermine medical interests. In the Australian case, this is any policy that might threaten or even encroach upon private, fee-for-service medical practice. In addition, the private insurance industry, pharmaceutical companies and makers of high-tech medical equipment, like doctors, want to see continued high investment in curative medical care; investment in primary health care is not in their interests. At the Commonwealth level, what passes for health policy—and what is sometimes even called health reform—is mostly about the supply of hospital and medical services, about how they will be paid for (from the Treasury or from private pockets) and how much medical professionals will be paid for providing them.

Although the Commonwealth decides policy about hospital and medical services, the States and Territories do make health policy.[4] All jurisdictions provide at least some community health services, including early childhood health centres, community nursing and the like. Some have a network of community health centres, preserved since the 1970s, as in Victoria. Constitutional power for community health primarily rests at the sub-national level, so, in theory at least, the States and Territories should be the innovators in primary health care. The fiscal imbalance in the Australian federal system is, however, a strong disincentive to infrastructure expansion.

4 They also run the hospitals, of course, but even though they pay for more than half of the costs of hospitals, it is the Commonwealth that sets the parameters of both the financing system and overall policy.

The Rudd/Gillard Governments and Health Reform

The election of the Rudd Commonwealth Government in 2007 on a platform of health reform held considerable promise. As well as a second national women's health policy and a men's health policy, the Government committed itself to 'Closing the Gap' between the health outcomes of Aboriginal and Torres Strait Islander people and other Australians. In an important respect, present-day Australian governments wishing to strengthen the primary healthcare system have an advantage over the pioneers of the 1970s because there are now many successful models in the community sector. In addition, epidemiological evidence is much more robust and we now know more than ever before about 'the causes of the causes' of poor health outcomes. Evidence supporting reform is available in abundance: the Australian Institute of Health and Welfare (AIHW 2010b), for example, argues that cardiovascular disease, which it calculates is suffered by two million Australian women, is highly preventable and treatable.[5] The institute has also identified 'potentially preventable hospitalisations'—hospitalisations that would probably have been unnecessary if timely and appropriate non-hospital care had been available. In 2008–09, there were approximately 690 000 potentially preventable hospitalisations, which represent 8.5 per cent of all admissions. Apart from pain, suffering and death, unnecessary hospitalisation is enormously expensive, given that in 2008–09, Australian spending on hospitalisation totalled $31.3 billion.

In pursuit of its health reform agenda, the Rudd Government established the National Health and Hospitals Reform Commission (NHHRC) in 2008, with terms of reference that included 'a greater focus on prevention'. The commission's final report, *A healthier future for all Australians* (Commonwealth of Australia 2009c), drew attention to growing inequalities in access to services, particularly for Aboriginal and Torres Strait Islander people, rural dwellers and those needing dental, mental health and aged-care services. It emphasised the need for wide-ranging reforms, including stronger preventive health care and the need to embed preventive health services in hospital and medical systems. It argues that we have a 'health system skewed to managing sickness rather than encouraging wellness' and that 'when it comes to funding community-based activities, allied health care and preventive activities compared with funding pharmaceuticals... and medical services', the playing field is not level. It recommends 'significant investment in primary health care infrastructure' through, among other things, the establishment of multidisciplinary, comprehensive primary healthcare centres and services (Commonwealth of Australia 2009c:51, 102–4).

---

5   Some 17.6 per cent of women suffered from cardiovascular disease compared with 15.3 per cent of men, both mostly in older age groups.

The National Primary Health Care Strategy and the National Preventive Health Taskforce were also established. The National Preventive Health Taskforce emphasises the importance of strengthening Australia's primary healthcare system and expanding community-based preventive and outreach services, particularly in low socioeconomic communities. It argued that 'action and leadership on preventive health is urgent and long overdue' (Commonwealth of Australia 2009d:6). Stephanie Bell, Chair of the Aboriginal Medical Services Alliance, NT, remarked that the task force had drawn 'strongly on 30 years of work by Aboriginal community-controlled health services' (Bell 2010:4).

The recommendations of these reviews, at a time when the Commonwealth was committed to reform, created a favourable political opportunity structure for investment in health, as well as in hospital and medical services. Many of the initial proposals, however, including the key undertaking that the Commonwealth would assume responsibility for all primary health care, have been modified or abandoned in response to political manoeuvrings. The assumption of responsibility for primary health care by the Commonwealth had the potential to promote structural change since a single level of government would be steering policy. Moreover, the machinations of fiscal federalism would have been eliminated, although it would still be possible to shift costs, this time onto consumers, by increasing user charges or allowing them to creep upwards as the Commonwealth has done for many years.

Members of the health research community who are committed to structural reform have been highly critical of the Rudd/Gillard reform package. For example, Armstrong (2010) argues that

> [t]here has been an unnerving willingness to ignore the advice of countless experts regarding the need for substantial investment in primary health care and prevention and early intervention in mental health and dental health and to address underpinning issues, such as the social determinants of health to reduce demand for hospital care.

The major spending decisions announced in 2010 and 2011 support such an analysis, since most of them are directed towards strengthening hospital and medical services. There were no new allocations for community health or for the women's health sector.

Two areas, in particular, of the reform proposals attracted vociferous criticism for their omission: mental health and Aboriginal health. Current research shows that only one of every three Australians with mental health problems receives treatment. Fifty-four per cent of people who have been homeless and 41 per cent of people who have been in prison have a mental health disorder. In Victoria, one-third of the people shot by police had been diagnosed previously with mental illness. Estimates show that mental ill health costs the economy $20 billion per year. Australian of the Year in 2010, Patrick McGorry, a mental health expert, claimed the sector had been locked out of the health reform processes and the head of the National Advisory Council on Mental Health, John Mendoza, resigned in June 2010, arguing that Commonwealth parsimony was incomprehensible, given that 1200 people are turned away from public and private psychiatric units every day. Eventually, the Commonwealth responded positively to this blistering criticism: it allocated $1.5 billion over *five* years to mental health in the 2011 Budget—a modest enough sum considering the shortcomings that have been allowed to build up for more than half a century.

Commonwealth policy has been criticised on two main counts in relation to Aboriginal and Torres Strait Islander health. First, the continuation of the NT Emergency Response has been condemned by a range of bodies and individuals for its human rights violations and lack of effectiveness. Critics include Aboriginal leaders, the United Nations, Amnesty International, the Australian Indigenous Doctors' Association and the AMA. Second, the funding commitments announced as part of 'closing the gap' have been deemed inadequate and misleading. And although almost half of Australia's Aboriginal people live in cities and suffer avoidable health problems, no new spending has been allocated (Russell 2009).

The political exigencies of Labor's health reform efforts since 2008 are too complex to relate here. In relation to primary care, the Commonwealth is establishing two new sets of institutions: GP Super Clinics and Medicare Locals. Both *sound* as though they might be authentic primary health care organisations. Theoretically, both entities have the potential to operate as such. Under the right sets of rules and with the right leadership, both might adopt a population-health focus and develop innovative, participatory, health-promoting programs for their local areas. Fee-for-service medical practitioners providing fee-for-service medical services have, however, been positioned at the centre of both organisations, which does not augur well for the adoption of a social health perspective unless we conceive of change in terms of geological time.

Significant structural changes are required if the Australian health system is to be made more effective and more equitable and if it is to devote more energy and resources to improving population health. Population-health strategies need to be planned over the long term, which is a requirement that is difficult to achieve if governments are listing from crisis to crisis in treatment services provision, real or perceived. As the WHO reminds us, health systems do not automatically 'gravitate towards the goals of health for all through primary health care'. Rather, without planning, trends are towards a disproportionate focus on specialised curative care, fragmentation and commercialisation (WHO 2008b:xiii).

Meanwhile, in the Northern Territory, primary health care reform in the Aboriginal community-controlled health sector is proceeding apace on the basis of the additional $50 million per year allocated under the Emergency Response. While condemning the loss of identity and the disempowerment that flows from many aspects of the Response, especially from lack of community ownership, a group of doctors and administrators quickly saw a window of opportunity to strengthen primary healthcare services (Boffa et al. 2007). Because well-developed structures and relationships were already in place, the increased funding could be managed within the existing system. Under the scheme, the health workforce has been increased by 251 full-time equivalent positions. A 2011 evaluation found that despite ongoing challenges, the new initiatives are proving to be extremely successful (Commonwealth of Australia 2011a). Watch this space!

Conclusion

While experience shows that major health system change is difficult in Australia, as elsewhere, it also shows that it is not impossible: major structural changes were introduced in the 1970s and at several points since. The women's health movement, the Aboriginal health movement, the community health movement and key policymakers recognised 40 years ago that treatment services are only a part of what a good health system should provide. Therefore, women's health, community health and Aboriginal health infrastructure was established. The 1970s left a positive legacy for the Australian health system: the infrastructure might have been preserved and expanded incrementally without undue political fuss or financial cost. Having structures already in place is a major political advantage because the fiercest battles generally take place around new ventures.

It has been open to any Commonwealth government since the 1970s to make incremental investments in the community health sector, including the women's health sector. Small but regular funding increases would have become substantial over time. Before it came to office, the Hawke Government made a commitment to restore the Community Health Program funding that the Fraser Government had withdrawn. In government, however, it restored funding only to 1975 levels, which meant a large shortfall since the interim period had been one of very high inflation. Moreover, no adjustment was made for population increases. Political exigencies did not pressure that government to go back on its commitment and it could have supported growth in the community-based sector without undue budgetary stress. Aboriginal community-based health services could have been expanded incrementally, as is happening in the Northern Territory at present. The women's health sector need not be so short of money that it has to stretch to meet the most urgent needs of the women who queue up outside. It may be a long-term process to change community attitudes and to realise the benefits of violence-prevention programs but refuges should not be forced to turn away women and children who need shelter and support. This only adds to the burden of ill health, with all the unnecessary pain and expense that that involves. In the scheme of total health expenditure, spending on community health is tiny. Even small funding increases over the years would have made a significant difference and would almost certainly have reduced overall health expenditure by preventing unnecessary illness. The pity is that leadership, commitment and political will have been wanting.

So while the Australian women's health movement has some remarkable achievements of which it can be justly proud, opportunities have been created to achieve a great deal more. The movement remains strongly committed to a social view of health and will continue to insist that the 1970s vision of a health system providing comprehensive, community-based primary health care as well as hospital and medical services is not beyond the capacity of Australian governments. The survival of a strong, activist women's health movement in a 'post-feminist' era demonstrates the priority that Australian women place on health. It also demonstrates the inability of hospital-based systems to respond appropriately to the need for strong primary health care. The women's health movement, along with like-minded activists in Aboriginal health and public health, is carrying forward the struggle to have a social determinants perspective take its place beside a biomedical perspective in mainstream health policy. The health of all Australians stands to gain.

Appendix 1:
Time line of key events, 1960–2011

1960

- Australian Labor Party developed plans for comprehensive health reform.
- Critique of curative medicine developed, particularly well articulated in Canada.

1961

- Childbirth Education Association established.

1964

- Australian Breastfeeding Association set up, originally named Nursing Mothers Association.

1966

- Council for Aboriginal Women of South Australia set up.

1967

- *Castonguay Report* released in Quebec recommending community health centres.

1969

- Boston Women's Health Collective formed.

1970

- National Council of Aboriginal and Islander Women established.
- Women's Liberation (WL) formed.

1971

- Aboriginal Medical Service established in Redfern, Sydney.
- Abortion Law Reform Associations set up in all States and the Australian Capital Territory.

- Australian feminists wrote sex information pamphlet, branded obscene by newspapers.
- First edition of *Our Bodies, Ourselves* published.
- Quebec began to set up Province-wide network of community health centres.

1972

- Children by Choice, Brisbane, family planning and abortion information service set up.
- Election of the Whitlam Labor Government.
- *Health Commission Act* (NSW) paved the way for community health centres.
- Joint Women's Action set up in Canberra (Aboriginal and non-Aboriginal women).
- The Body Politic formed in Adelaide.
- Women's Electoral Lobby (WEL) established in Melbourne.
- Women's Abortion Action Coalition set up in Sydney.

1973

- Control formed in Sydney; began abortion referral service.
- Migrant Women's Association established in Sydney.
- Murawina Aboriginal Preschool and Women's Hostel set up in Sydney.
- WL organised speak-outs in Sydney and Melbourne; health emerged as major issue.
- Women's Abortion Action Campaign set up in Brisbane and Adelaide.
- Women against Rape formed in Melbourne.
- Women's Commission held in Sydney; health emerged as a major issue.
- Women's Health Collective formed in Melbourne.

1974

- Abortion Information service opened in Perth.
- Adelaide Women's Shelter opened, also known as Naomi Women's Shelter.
- Blacktown Community Cottage opened in Sydney.
- Bonnie Women's Shelter opened in Western Sydney.
- Brisbane Rape Crisis Centre opened.
- Brisbane Women's House Health Centre opened.
- Canberra Rape Crisis Centre opened.
- Canberra Women's Refuge opened.

- Collingwood Women's Health Centre opened in Melbourne.
- Elsie Women's Refuge opened in Sydney.
- Hobart Women's Shelter opened.
- Hunter Region Working Women's Centre opened; now Hunter Women's Centre.
- *Lalonde Report* released in Canada.
- Launceston Women's Shelter opened in Tasmania.
- Leichhardt Women's Community Health Centre established in Sydney.
- Liverpool Women's Health Centre opened in Sydney; later participated in establishing Rosebank Sexual Assault Service, Dympna House, incest counselling service and others.
- Nardine Women's Shelter opened in Perth.
- Sydney Rape Crisis Centre opened; now NSW Rape Crisis Centre.
- Women's Health and Community Centre opened in Perth.
- Women's Liberation Halfway House opened in Melbourne.

1975

- Aboriginal Women's Centre set up in Darwin.
- Alice Springs Women's Centre, primarily a refuge, opened in Northern Territory.
- Darwin Women's Health Centre opened.
- Dismissal of the Whitlam Labor Government; election of the Fraser Coalition Government.
- First National Women's Health Conference held in Australia in Brisbane.
- Hindmarsh Women's Health Centre opened in Adelaide.
- Industrial Health Group formed at Liverpool Women's Health Centre.
- Women's Health and Community Centre Rape Crisis Centre opened in Perth.
- Women's House Health Centre opened in Brisbane.
- Working Women's Centre set up in Melbourne.

1976

- Adelaide Rape Crisis Centre opened.
- Central Coast Women's Health Centre opened in Gosford, New South Wales.
- Christies Beach Women's Shelter opened in South Australia.
- Draft Bill on Rape and Other Sexual Offences, written by Dr Jocelynne Scutt for WEL, influenced State legislation.

- Marrickville Women's Refuge opened in Sydney.
- Marty House opened in Sydney for women with substance abuse issues.
- Sexual Assault Resource Centre opened in Perth.
- Foundation of Rehabilitation with Aboriginal Alcohol Related Difficulties set up by Aboriginal women.

1977

- Australian Council of Trade Unions (ACTU) adopted Working Women's Charter.
- Alice Springs Women's Health Centre opened in the Northern Territory.
- Bankstown Women's Health Centre opened in Sydney.
- Bessie Smyth feminist abortion clinic opened in Sydney.
- Bringa Women's Refuge opened in Dee Why, Sydney.
- Cawarra Women's Refuge Aboriginal Corporation established in New South Wales.
- Powell Street Clinic set up in Homebush, Sydney.
- Women in Industry, Contraception and Health (now Multicultural Women's Health Centre) established in Melbourne.
- Women's Committee established within ACTU.
- Women's Coordination Unit established in NSW Premier's Department.
- Women's Health Care House opened in Perth.
- Women's Pregnancy Advisory and Abortion Referral Service set up in Brisbane.
- Workers Health Action Groups formed from this year onwards.
- Workers Health Centre, Lidcombe, Sydney, established.

1978

- ACTU sponsored Working Women's Charter Conference.
- Anne Women's Shelter opened in South Australia.
- Geelong Rape Crisis Centre opened in Victoria.
- Task Force to Inquire into Sexual Violence set up in New South Wales.
- Warrina Women's Refuge opened in Coffs Harbour, NSW.
- Migrant Women's Refuge established in Melbourne.

1979

- Cawarra Aboriginal Refuge opened in Sydney.
- Elizabeth Hoffman House emergency accommodation and support for Aboriginal women and their children opened in Melbourne.
- Sexual Assault Service, Queen Victoria Medical Centre, opened in Melbourne.
- Wagga Wagga Women's Health and Support Centre opened in New South Wales.
- Working Women's Centre established in South Australia.
- Working Women's Centre opened in Adelaide.

1980

- Adelaide Women's Community Health Centre opened.
- Dawn House, providing accommodation and support services, opened in Darwin.
- Ngaanyatjarra Pitjantjatjara Yankunytjatjara Women's Council established in Central Australia to provide health and human services.

1981

- ACTU decision to support women's right to free, safe, legal abortion.
- Alice Springs Women's Shelter opened in Northern Territory.
- Blue Mountains Women's Health Centre opened in New South Wales.
- Domestic Violence Committee convened by Premier's Department of Victoria.
- Women's Health and Information Resource and Crisis Centres Association (WHIRCCA) established.
- Wirraway Women's Housing Co-Operative opened in Moree, New South Wales.
- Women's Community House opened in Alice Springs, Northern Territory.
- Women's Place, for homeless or intoxicated women, opened in Sydney.
- Refuge Ethnic Workers Program set up in Melbourne.

1982

- Federation for Aboriginal Women set up in Victoria.
- Louisa Lawson House opened in Sydney.
- Right to Choose Coalition set up by WEL.
- Women's Health Resource Collective, later Women's Health Information Resource Collective, opened in Melbourne.

- Working party established to develop women's health policy.
- Brisbane Women's Community Health Centre opened.

1983

- Election of the Hawke Labor Government.
- Elizabeth Women's Health Centre opened in South Australia.
- First woman elected to the ACTU Executive; Working Women's Policy developed.
- Health in the Workforce Factory Project set up in Sydney.
- The Women's Cottage set up, Hawkesbury District, Sydney.
- Toora Single Women's Shelter, now Toora Women, opened in the Australian Capital Territory.
- Women's Advisory Council established in Western Australia with a focus on health.
- Mookai Rosie Bi-Bayan, Aunty Rosie's Place, providing services for rural and remote Aboriginal women and children, opened in Cairns, Queensland.

1984

- Western Women's Council set up in Wilcannia, New South Wales.
- Jilimi, now Waminda Aboriginal Women's Health Centre, opened in Nowra, New South Wales.
- Immigrant Women's Support Service opened in Brisbane.
- Migrant Women's Lobby Group established in Adelaide.
- Illawarra Women's Health Centre opened in New South Wales.
- Elisabeth Women's Community Health Centre opened in South Australia.
- Southern Women's Health and Community Centre opened in South Australia.
- Dale Street Women's Community Health Centre opened in South Australia.
- Refuge Ethnic Workers Program opened in Victoria.
- SA Coalition for Workers Health Action established.
- First Australian Women's Health Adviser, Liz Furler, appointed in South Australia.
- Women's Health Policy Review Committee set up in New South Wales.
- Report of the Working Party on Women's Health Policy released in South Australia.
- Report on domestic violence in Tasmania released.
- Domestic Violence Incest Resource Centre established in Victoria.

1985

- Second National Women's Health Conference held in Adelaide.
- Crisis Intervention Unit set up in Department of Community Services, Tasmania.
- Darwin Counselling Group established to provide sexual assault services.
- Domestic Violence Council established in South Australia.
- Immigrant Women's Resource Centre opened in Sydney.
- Immigrant Women's Speakout Association formed in Sydney.
- Migrant Women's Support and Accommodation Service opened in Adelaide.
- Multicultural Women's Health Centre opened in Fremantle, Western Australia.
- Shoalhaven Women's Health Centre opened in New South Wales.
- Southwest Women's Child Sexual Assault Resource Centre, later Rosebank, opened in Sydney.
- Task Force on Domestic Violence established in Western Australia.
- Women in Trade Unions Network formed in Brisbane.
- Women's health 'policy in action' commenced.
- Women's Health Unit established in New South Wales and, thereafter, in most jurisdictions.

1986

- Albury–Wodonga Women's Health Centre opened in Albury, New South Wales.
- Australian Women's Health Network established.
- Break the Silence, task force report on domestic violence, released in Western Australia.
- Central West Women's Health Centre opens in Bathurst, New South Wales.
- Coffs Harbour Women's Health Centre opened in New South Wales.
- Domestic Violence Prevention Council set up in the Australian Capital Territory.
- Dympna Accommodation Program opened in Sydney.
- Goldfields Women's Health Centre opened in Western Australia.
- Migrant Women against Incest Network established in New South Wales.
- Ministerial Women's Health Working Party established in Victoria.
- Multicultural Women's Resource Centre set up in Broken Hill, New South Wales.

- NHMRC Working Party on Homebirths and Alternative Birth Centres established.
- NSW Women's Refuge Resource Centre established.
- Queensland Women's Health Network established.
- Sexual Assault Referral Centre opened in Darwin.
- Sexual Assault Support Service opened in Hobart.
- Women's Centre opened in Cairns, Queensland, to provide sexual assault crisis services.
- Working Party on Women's Health established in Western Australia.

1987

- Australian Health Ministers Advisory Council (AHMAC) Subcommittee on Women and Health created.
- Australian College of Midwives Incorporated established.
- Blacktown Women's and Girls' Health Centre opened in Sydney.
- Campbelltown Women's Health Centre, also known as WILMA, opened in Sydney.
- CASA House Centre against Sexual Assault opened at Royal Women's Hospital, Melbourne.
- Congress Alukura women's health, maternal and child health centre opened in Alice Springs, Northern Territory.
- Domestic Violence Prevention Unit set up in South Australia.
- Hobart Women's Health Centre opened.
- Immigrant Women's Health Service opened in Fairfield and Cabramatta, Sydney.
- Lismore and District Women's Health Centre opened in New South Wales.
- National Domestic Violence Education Campaign undertaken by the Office of the Status of Women (OSW).
- Penrith Women's Health Centre opened in Western Sydney.
- Regional network of sexual assault services set up in Victoria.
- Ruby Gaea, providing sexual assault services, opened in Darwin.
- Special Adviser to the Commonwealth Health Minister, Liza Newby, appointed.
- *Why Women's Health*, Victorian Women Respond working party report released.

1988

- Beyond These Walls, report of the Task Force on Domestic Violence, Queensland, released.
- Domestic Violence Crisis Service set up in the Australian Capital Territory.
- Domestic Violence Resource Centre opened in Queensland.
- Freedom from Fear, community education campaign on domestic violence, conducted in Western Australia.
- Geraldton Sexual Assault Referral Centre opened in Western Australia.
- Gloria Brennan ATSI Women's Centre opened in East Perth.
- Healthsharing Women established in Victoria.
- Key Centre for Women's Health in Society, now the Centre for Women's Health Gender and Society, founded at Melbourne University.
- Sexual Assault Counselling Service opened in Alice Springs, Northern Territory.
- Waratah Support Centre for sexual assault and domestic violence opened in Bunbury, Western Australia.
- Women's Health Service for the West opened in Victoria.

1989

- Alternative Birthing Services Program commenced.
- *Domestic Violence (Family Protection) Act* (Qld) enacted.
- First National Women's Health Policy and National Women's Health Program launched.
- Integrated Family Violence Networks established in Victoria.
- Laurel House opened in Launceston, Tasmania.
- Maternity Coalition established.
- Patricia Giles Centre, offering services for GLBTIQ people, opened in Perth.
- Whitfords Women's Health Centre, now Women's Healthworks, opened in Western Australia.

1990

- Canberra Women's Health Centre, now Women's Centre for Health Matters, opened.
- Cumberland Women's Health Centre opened in Sydney.
- Domestic Violence Council established in Queensland.
- National Committee on Violence against Women established.

- Perth Women's Centre opened.
- Townsville Women's Community Health Centre opened in Queensland.
- *Women's Health Development in the ACT* released in draft form.

1991

- Domestic Violence Strategic Plan released in New South Wales.
- Geraldton Women's Health Centre opened in Western Australia.
- Rockhampton Women's Health Centre opened in Queensland.
- Wide Bay Women's Health Centre opened in Queensland.

1992

- Brisbane Rape and Incest Survivors Support Centre opened.
- Edith Edwards Women's Centre, refuge, opened in Bourke, New South Wales.
- Ipswich Women's Health Service opened in Queensland.
- Logan Women's Health Centre opened in Queensland.
- National Strategy on Violence against Women introduced.
- North-East Women's Health Service opened in Victoria.
- Northern Territory Women's Health Policy released.
- Women's Health Strategy Unit established in Northern Territory.

1993

- Eastern Goldfields Sexual Assault Research Centre opened in Western Australia.
- Hedland Women's Health Service opened in Western Australia.
- Goulburn North-Eastern Victoria Women's Health Service opened.
- Mirrabooka Multicultural Women's Health Centre opened in Western Australia.
- Non-English Cultural Background Women's Health Reference Group formed in Queensland.
- Queensland Women's Health Policy launched.
- Rockingham Women's Health Service opened in Western Australia.
- Women's Health Prevention of Violence against Women Program set up in Queensland.
- Women's Health Victoria formed through amalgamation of Healthsharing Women and the Women's Health Information Resource Collective.
- Yarrow Place, incorporating the Adelaide Rape Crisis Centre, opened.
- Yorgam Aboriginal Corporation, providing support services for people who have experienced violence, opened in East Perth.

1994

- Gladstone Women's Health Centre opened in Queensland.
- Gosnells Women's Health Service opened in Western Australia.
- Gympie and District Women's Health Centre opened in Queensland.
- Northern Territory Domestic Violence Strategy released.
- South Australian women's health centres lost their independence.
- Tasmanian Women's Health Policy launched.
- Working Women's Centres set up in Queensland and Tasmania.

1995

- Third AWHN National Women's Health Conference, Canberra.
- Women's Health Australia longitudinal study on women's health commenced.
- Working Women's Centre set up in Northern Territory.

1996

- Election of the Howard Coalition Government.
- *New Directions in Reducing Violence against Women* released in New South Wales.

1997

- Immigrant and Refugee Women's Coalition opened in Victoria.
- Partnerships against Domestic Violence introduced.

1998

- Abortion removed from the Criminal Code of Western Australia, replaced with small section making it illegal for anyone other than a medical practitioner to perform an abortion.
- *A Strategic Framework to Advance Women's Health* released in New South Wales.
- Family Violence Intervention Program commenced in the Australian Capital Territory.
- Family Violence Prevention Legal Service initiated by ATSIC.
- Task Force on Sexual Assault and Rape set up in Tasmania.

1999

- National Indigenous Family Violence Grants Program introduced.

2000

- Women's Health NSW established (formerly WHIRCCA).

2001

- Australian Centre for the Study of Sexual Assault established.
- Fourth AWHN National Women's Health Conference, Adelaide.
- National Initiative to Combat Sexual Assault introduced.
- Women's Health and Well-Being initiatives paper released in South Australia.

2002

- Abortion removed completely from the Criminal Code of the Australian Capital Territory.
- Aboriginal Family Violence Prevention and Legal Service opened in Victoria.
- Four-year Women's Health and Well-Being Strategy released in Victoria.
- National Maternity Action Plan developed, led by Maternity Coalition.
- *Women's Health Outcomes Framework* released in New South Wales.
- Women's Safety Strategy introduced in Victoria.

2003

- BreaCan established in Victoria.
- Queensland Centre for the Prevention of Domestic and Family Violence established.

2004

- *Family Violence Act* (Tasmania) enacted.
- Safe at Home strategy commenced in Tasmania.
- Violence against Women, Australia Says No campaign commenced.
- Howard Government attempted to exclude women's health from Public Health Outcomes Funding Agreements (PHOFAs).

2005

- Fifth AWHN National Women's Health Conference, Melbourne.
- New Women's Health Policy launched in South Australia.

- *Reforming the Family Violence System in Victoria* released.
- *The Health and Well-Being of Northern Territory Women: From the desert to the sea* released.
- Women's Health Services formed from the amalgamation of Women's Health Care House and Women's Health Services, Perth.
- Women's Safety Strategy released in South Australia.
- Yinganeh Aboriginal Women's Refuge opened in Lismore, New South Wales.

2006

- Northern Territory Emergency Response introduced.
- Reproductive Choice Australia, a coalition of 20 NGOs, established.

2007

- *Domestic and Family Violence Act* (Northern Territory) passed.
- Rudd Labor Government elected.
- Partners in Prevention set up in Victoria, funded by VicHealth.
- Australian Labor Party announces commitment to develop Second National Women's Health Policy.

2008

- Abortion removed completely from the Criminal Code of Victoria.
- Construction of a new ACT community health centre announced.
- Construction of a new ACT Women's and Children's Hospital announced.
- *Family Violence Protection Act* (Victoria) passed.
- National Council to Reduce Violence against Women and their Children appointed.
- National Health and Hospitals Reform Commission established.
- National Maternity Services Review established.
- National Preventive Health Taskforce established.
- New South Wales Domestic and Family Violence Strategic Framework released.
- WHO Social Determinants of Health Report released.
- Women's Health Services Plan developed in the Australian Capital Territory.
- *Women's Health: The new national agenda* published by AWHN.

2009

- *A healthier future for all Australians*, report of NHHRC, released.
- *Australia: The healthiest country by 2020*, report of National Preventive Health Taskforce, released.
- Domestic Violence Death Panel, chaired by Coroner, set up in New South Wales.
- Domestic Violence Death Review Panel established in Queensland.
- For Our Sons and Daughters, 2009–2014, domestic violence strategy, Queensland, released.
- Pro-Choice Queensland established.
- Review report, *Improving Maternity Services in Australia,* released.
- *Time for Action: The National Council's plans for Australia to reduce violence against women and their children, 2009-2021*

2010

- Interim Women's Health Plan, 2009–2011, released in New South Wales.
- Modified maternity care arrangements began operation.
- National Maternity Services Plan endorsed by Australian health ministers.
- Second National Women's Health Policy released.
- Sixth AWHN National Women's Health Conference, Hobart.

2011

- National Disability Strategy developed after consultations.
- National Plan to Reduce Violence against Women and their Children launched.

Appendix 2:
Women interviewed for this book

Adele Thomas
Ann Hodge
Anne Deanus
Anne Warner
Belinda Whitworth
Bon Hull
Carmel O'Loughlin
Carolyn Mason
Cathy Miller
Chloe Mason
Christine Giles
Cynthia Croft
Di Jones
Else Franks
Fran Bladel
Helen Abrahams
Ilse O'Farrel
Jane Dunsford
Janette Gay
Jen Roberts
Jo Parish
Joyce Stevens
Judith Dwyer
Judith Watson
Judy Wotherspoon
June van der Klashorst
Kay Anastassiadis
Laurie Gilbert
Lisa Gardiner
Liza Newby
Lyn Reid
Lynnley McGrath
Mary Draper

Ali Sinclair
Ann Levy
Anne O'Byrne
Annie Zafer
Bernadette Callaghan
Cait Calcutt
Carol Cragg
Carolyn Pickles
Cathy North
Chris Brown
Claire Shuttleworth
Deborah Gough
Di Sergey
Fiona Owen
Gloria Garton
Helen Creed
Iris Ritt
Janet Irwin
Janine Combes
Jennifer Cashmore
Jocelyn Auer
Judith Blake
Judith Elsham
Judy Edwards
Julie Byles
Kas Eaton
Kay Setches
Lee Barker
Liz Ahearn
Lois Gatley
Lyndall Ryan
Margaret Reynolds
Megan Halbert

Andrea Shoebridge
Anna Moynahan
Anne Sinclair
Bebe Loft
Bernadette O'Connell
Carla Cranny
Carol Lowe
Cath James
Cheryl Davenport
Chris O'Farrell
Cora Gabonton
Denele Crozier
Elizabeth Stroud
Fiona Percy
Heather Bolden
Helen Radoslovich
Jan Powning
Janet Ramsey
Jean Collie
Jenny Beauchamp
Jocelyn Hanson
Judith Cleaver
Judith Roberts
Judy Elton
Julie Dawson
Kathy Solomons
Kim Boyer
Lesley Garton
Liz Furler
Lyn Mackenzie
Lynette Pugh
Marilyn Beaumont
Meredith Taylor

Mervyn Cheung

Miriam Taylor

Nancy Peck

Paula Watt

Raquel Aldunate

Rose Sorger

Sandra Nori

Sharon Jackson

Silvia Kinder

Sue Abbey

Thea Mendelsohn

Vicki Pearce

Yvonne Allan

Michael Jones

Morven Andrews

Onella Stagoll

Philomena Horsely

Rennie Gay

Ruth Dewar

Sandi MacKintosh

Sharon Paul

Stefania Siedlecky

Sue Yarrow

Tim Webster

Wendy Silver

Michelle Kosky

Nancy Layton

Patricia Giles

Rachel Green

Ronelle Brossard

Ruth Morgan

Sharon Hetzel

Shirley Patton

Stephanie Mayman

Susan Stratigos

Vicki Hiscock

Yoland Wadsworth

Bibliography

Abbs, Jude (1987) Letter to the Hon. Dr Neal Blewett, Minister for Health, 12 May, Photocopy.

Abbs, Jude (1994) 'Always one voice—an interview with Jude Abbs', *Queensland Women's Health Network News*, May/June, pp. 4–5.

Aboriginal and Islander Health Worker Journal (2001a) 'La Perouse Stress Free Day', *Aboriginal and Islander Health Worker Journal*, 25:5, September/October, p. 14.

Aboriginal and Islander Health Worker Journal (2001b) 'Ngalawa Wingara-Aboriginal Women's Healing Space', *Aboriginal and Islander Health Worker Journal*, 25:5, September/October, p. 35.

Aboriginal and Islander Health Worker Journal (2001c) 'The Aboriginal and Torres Strait Islander Women's Health Forum', *Aboriginal and Islander Health Worker Journal*, 25:5, September/October, p. 11.

Aboriginal and Islander Health Worker Journal (2004) 'From health worker to health worker, an annotated index of Indigenous health information, 1996–2003', *Aboriginal and Islander Health Worker Journal*.

Aboriginal and Islander Health Worker Journal (2009) 'From health worker to health worker, an annotated index of Indigenous health information, 2004–2008', *Aboriginal and Islander Health Worker Journal*.

Aboriginal and Islander Health Worker Journal, web site, <http://www.aihwj.com.au/issues.html>

Aboriginal Health and Medical Research Council, web site, <http://www.ahmrc.org.au/>, accessed 16 August 2011.

Adams, Rene, Hastings, Cath and Mulder, Liz in conjunction with the North West Plains Aboriginal Women's Gathering Working Party (2002) *The North West Plains Aboriginal Women's Gathering Report*, 26–28 April, Moree, NSW.

Aldunate, Raquel and Revelo, Gladys (1987) 'Racism—a community health hazard', *Options for Action in Community Health*, Proceedings of the First National Community Health Conference on Social and Environmental Health, 24–26 September 1986, Australian Community Health Association, Strawberry Hills, NSW.

Alford, Robert (1975) *Health Care Politics*, University of Chicago Press, Chicago and London.

Allen, Judith (1990) 'Does feminism need a theory of "the state"?' in Watson, Sophie (ed.) *Playing the State: Australian feminist interventions*, Allen & Unwin, Sydney.

Alley, Jane, Chapman, Cris, Geddes, Virginia and Wilson, Kathy (1980) 'Behind closed doors, refuges: close or concede?', *Scarlet Woman*, 10, pp. 3–7.

Alvares, Esther (1992) 'A women's refuge for Bourke: a community initiative', in McKillop, Sandra (ed.) *Aboriginal Justice Issues*, Australian Institute of Criminology Conference Proceedings, 23–25 June, Brisbane, <http://www.aic.gov.au/publications/previous%20series/proceedings/1-27/21.aspx>

Ambanpola, Lilanthi (2005) *Achieving gender and cultural competence by Australia's medical workforce*, Final report, <http://www.awcaus.org.au/resources/documents/Gender%20Culture%20Competence%20Overview%20June%202005.pdf>, accessed 16 August 2011.

Andrews, Susan (2000) 'Alternative' birthing and professional power: national policy and local outcomes, August, Sub-thesis, Master of Letters in the Faculty of Arts, Centre for Women's Studies, The Australian National University, Canberra.

Annandale, Ellen (2009) 'Editorial', *Social Science and Medicine, Virtual Special Issue, Gender and Health*, <http://www.elsevier.com/wps/find/S06_351.cws_home/SSM_vi_gender>, accessed 16 August 2011.

Ansell, Chris and Gash, Alison (2007) 'Collaborative governance in theory and practice', *Journal of Public Administration Research and Theory*, November, pp. 1–29.

A Policy for Women's Health, New Zealand, <http://www.massey.ac.nz/~kbirks/gender/whp.htm>, accessed 12 June 2009.

ARDT Consultants (2007) *Coordinating NSW Government action against domestic and family violence*, Final report, Prepared for the Human Service and Criminal Justice CEOs Cluster, 8 November.

Armstrong, Fiona (2010) 'Good climate for proper reforms', *The Australian*, 8 May.

Armstrong, Pat, Amaratunga, Carol, Bernier, Jocelyne, Grant, Karen, Pederson, Ann and Willson, Kate (2002) *Exposing Privatisation*, Garamond Press, Aurora, Ontario.

Auer, Jocelyn (2003) Women's health centres in SA—a history, Address given to Statewide Women's Health Forum, 25 October 2003, <http://www.whs. sa.gov.au/pub/Jocelyen_Auer_speech.pdf>, accessed 16 August 2011.

Auer, Jocelyn, Boaden, Linda, Kopczynski, Mary, Nicholson, Sally-Anne, Shuttleworth, Clare and Twohig, Julia (1987) 'Consult or collapse', *Options for Action in Community Health*, Proceedings of the First National Community Health Conference on Social and Environmental Health, 24–26 September 1986, Adelaide University Union, Australian Community Health Association, Strawberry Hills, NSW.

Australian Capital Territory (ACT) (2005) *Responding to Sexual Assault: The challenge of change*, Office of the Director of Public Prosecutions and Australian Federal Police, Canberra.

Australian Centre for the Study of Sexual Assault (ACSSA), web site, <http:// www.aifs.gov.au/acssa/>

Australian Council of Trade Unions (ACTU) (2009) 'Equal pay and better jobs to women', *Campaigns*, <http://www.actu.org.au/Campaigns/EqualPay/ default.aspx>, and 'Paid parental leave', <http://www.actu.org.au/ Campaigns/PaidParentalLeave/default.aspx>, accessed 16 August 2011.

Australian College of Midwives (2009) Submission to the Senate Inquiry Health Legislation Amendment (Midwives and Nurse Practitioners) Bill 2009 and two other Bills, <http://www.aph.gov.au/senate/committee/clac_ctte/ health_leg_midwives_nurse_practitioners_09/submissions/sub18.pdf>, accessed 16 August 2011.

Australian College of Midwives, Victorian Branch (1999) *Reforming midwifery: a discussion paper on the introduction of Bachelor of Midwifery programs into Victoria*, Australian College of Midwives, Carlton, Vic.

Australian Domestic and Family Violence Clearinghouse (2006) 'Tasmania's *Safe at Home*: a whole of government response to domestic violence', *Newsletter*, 26 (Spring), pp. 3–8.

Australian Domestic and Family Violence Clearinghouse (2007) *Family Violence Intervention Program (ACT)*, <http://www.adfvc.unsw.edu.au/ gpworddocs/102.rtf>

Australian Health Ministers Advisory Council (AHMAC) (2008) *Primary Maternity Services in Australia: A framework for implementation*, <v.au/ cms_documents/Primary%20Maternity%20Services%20in%20Australia. pdf>, accessed 16 August 2011.

Australian Indigenous Doctors' Association (2008) Submission to the Maternity Services Review Board, 31 October, <http://www.aida.org.au/pdf/submissions/Submission_9.pdf>, accessed 16 August 2011.

Australian Institute for Women's Research and Policy (1997) *Circle across Australia, women and reconciliation*, Report on Consultation with Women's Organisations from the Australian Institute of Women's Research and Policy to the Council for Aboriginal Reconciliation, Griffith University.

Australian Institute of Health and Welfare (AIHW) (1997) 'Health expenditure', *Health Expenditure Bulletin*, Cat. HWE 13, Australian Institute of Health and Welfare, Canberra.

Australian Institute of Health and Welfare (AIHW) (2005a) Domestic violence is a major factor in homelessness among women and children, Media release, 28 September, Australian Institute of Health and Welfare, Canberra.

Australian Institute of Health and Welfare (AIHW) (2005b) *Female SAAP clients and children escaping family and domestic violence, 2003–2004*, Bulletin 30, Cat. AUS 64, Australian Institute of Health and Welfare, Canberra.

Australian Institute of Health and Welfare (AIHW) (2006) *Medical Labour Force, 2006*, National Health Labour Force Series No. 41, Cat. HWL 42, Australian Institute of Health and Welfare, Canberra.

Australian Institute of Health and Welfare (AIHW) (2009) *Health and Community Services Labour Force, 2006*, National Health Labour Series Force No. 42, Cat. HWL 43, Australian Institute of Health and Welfare, Canberra.

Australian Institute of Health and Welfare (AIHW) (2010a) *Australian Hospital Statistics, 2008–09*, Health Services Series 34, Australian Institute of Health and Welfare, Canberra.

Australian Institute of Health and Welfare (AIHW) (2010b) Cardiovascular disease a major threat to Australian women, Media release, 1 June, Australian Institute of Health and Welfare, Canberra, <http://www.aihw.gov.au/mediacentre/2010/mr20100601.cfm>, accessed 16 August 2011.

Australian Institute of Health and Welfare (AIHW) (2010c) *Health Expenditure Australia, 2008–09*, Health and Welfare Expenditure Series 42, Australian Institute of Health and Welfare, Canberra.

Australian Institute of Health and Welfare (AIHW) (2010d) *Women and Heart Disease*, Cat. CVD 49, Australian Institute of Health and Welfare, Canberra.

Australian Institute of Health and Welfare (AIHW) (2011) *Public Health Expenditure in Australia, 2008–09*, Health and Welfare Expenditure Series 43, Cat. HWE 52, Australian Institute of Health and Welfare, Canberra.

Australian Medical Association (AMA) (2008) Submission to the National Maternity Services Review, <http://www.health.gov.au/internet/main/publishing.nsf/Content/maternityservicesreview-submissions>, accessed 16 August 2011.

Australian Nursing Federation (ANF) (2009) Submission to the Health Legislation Amendment (Midwives and Nurse Practitioners) Bill 2009 and two related Bills, <http://www.anf.org.au/pdf/submissions/2009/Sub_Health_Legislation_AmendmentDec09.pdf>, accessed 16 August 2011.

Australian Physiotherapy Association, web site, <http://www.physiotherapy.asn.au/>

Australian Women's Health Network (AWHN) (1988) *Newsletter*, 5 August.

Australian Women's Health Network (AWHN) (2001) *Conference Proceedings, 2001*, Fourth Australian Women's Health Conference, 19–21 February, Adelaide Convention Centre.

Bakalar, Nicholas (2010) 'Study sees a slant in articles on drugs', *The New York Times*, 12 April.

Baker, Jenny (1998) 'One Aboriginal woman's perspective', in Rogers-Clark, Cath and Smith, Angie (ed.), *Women's Health*, McClelland and Petty, Sydney.

Baldry, Eileen (1992) The development of the health consumer movement and its effect on value changes and health policy, PhD thesis, University of New South Wales, Kensington, NSW.

Baldwin-Jones, M. (1989) Women's business, Paper presented to the Human Rights Conference, September, Melbourne.

Barclay, Lesley (2010) 'Legally binding midwives to doctors is not collaboration', *Women and Birth*, 23, pp. 1–2.

Barrett Meyering, Isabelle (2009) 'Time for action: responses from the sector', *Australian Domestic and Family Violence Clearinghouse Newsletter*, 38 (Spring), pp. 4–5.

Barrett Meyering, Isobelle (2010) 'Domestic homicide reviews: recent developments across Australia', *Australian Domestic and Family Violence Clearinghouse Newsletter*, 39 (Summer), pp. 9–11.

Bartlett, Ben and Boffer, John (2001) 'Aboriginal community controlled comprehensive primary health care: the Central Australian Aboriginal Congress', *Australian Journal of Primary Health*, 7:3, pp. 74–82.

Baum, F. E. (2007) *The New Public Health*, Oxford University Press, South Melbourne.

Baum, Fran and Keleher, Helen (2002) 'Public health', *Medical Journal of Australia*, 176:1, p. 36.

Beaumont, Marilyn (1998) 'Development of a five-year Victorian Women's Health Plan', *Australian Journal of Primary Health—Interchange*, 4:3, pp. 6–7.

Behrendt, Larissa (2002) 'Lessons from the mediation session: ensuring that sentencing alternatives focus on Indigenous self-determination', in Strang, Heather and Braithwaite, John (eds), *Restorative Justice and Family Violence*, Cambridge University Press, Oakley, Vic.

Bell, Stephanie (2001) Indigenous women's health—what can make a difference?, Presentation to the Tenth Advanced Course in Obstetrics, Women's Reproductive Health and Care of the Newborn, Joint Consultative Committee on Obstetrics, NSW, 20 July, <http://www.caac.org.au/pr/downloads/conference_indigenous_womens_health_obstetrics_copy1.pdf>, accessed 16 August 2011.

Bell, Stephanie (2010) *Amsant Annual Report, 2009–2010*, p. 4.

Bennett, Scott, Newman, Gerard and Kopras, Andrew (2005) *Commonwealth election 2004*, Research Brief, Department of Parliamentary Services, Parliament House, Canberra.

Blagg, Harry (2002) 'Restorative justice and Aboriginal family violence: opening as a base for healing', in Strang, Heather and Braithwaite, John (eds), *Restorative Justice and Family Violence*, Cambridge University Press, Oakley, Vic.

Blagg, Harry and Valuri, Gieulietta (2003) *An Overview of Night Patrol Services in Australia*, Commonwealth Attorney-General's Department, Canberra.

Boffa, John, Bell, Andrew, Davies, Tanya, Patterson, John and Cooper, David (2007) 'The Aboriginal Medical Services Alliance NT: engaging with intervention to improve primary health care', *Medical Journal of Australia*, 187:11/12, pp. 617–18.

Bönte, Markus, von dem Knesebeck, Olaf, Siegrist, Johannes, Marceau, Lisa, Link, Carol, Arber, S., Adams, Ann and McKinlay, John B. (2008) 'Women and men with coronary heart disease in three countries: are they treated differently?', *Women's Health Issues*, 18:3, pp. 191–8.

Boston Women's Health Collective (1976) *Our Bodies, Ourselves: A book by and for women*, [Second edn], Simon & Schuster, New York.

Boston Women's Health Collective (2006) *The Politics of Women's Health, Can We Trust the Evidence in Evidence Based Medicine?*, <http://www.ourbodiesourselves.org/book/menoexcerpt.asp?id=51>, accessed 16 August 2011.

Bowman, Fran and Keleher, Helen (2002) 'Public health', *Medical Journal of Australia*, 176:1 (7 January), p. 36.

Boxall, Anne-Marie and Flitcroft, Kathy (2007) 'From little things, big things grow: a local approach to system-wide maternity services reform in the absence of definitive evidence', *Australia and New Zealand Health Policy*, 4:18.

Braaf, Rochelle (2008) 'Victoria's integrated response to family violence', *Australian Domestic and Family Violence Clearinghouse Newsletter*, 33 (Winter).

Brady, Maggie (2004) *Indigenous Australians and Alcohol Policy*, UNSW Press, Sydney.

Braun, Virginia (2003) 'Revisiting the orifice: a reappraisal of "a funny thing happened on the way to the orifice: women in gynaecology textbooks', *Feminism and Psychology*, 13:5, pp. 5–10.

BreaCan (2009) *BreaCan Year in Review 08/09*, October, Red Rover Proprietary Limited Printers, South Melbourne.

Breast Cancer Network of Australia, web site, <http://www.bcna.org.au/>

Briscoe, Gordon (1974) 'The Aboriginal Medical Service in Sydney', in Hetzel, Basil S., Dobbin, Malcolm, Lippmann, Lorna and Eggleston, Elizabeth (eds), *Better Health for Aborigines?*, Report of a National Seminar at Monash, University of Queensland Press, St Lucia, pp. 166–70.

Broom, Dorothy (1990) *Research priorities in women's health*, January, Typescript, Report to the Policy Development Division, Commonwealth Department of Community Services and Health, Canberra.

Broom, Dorothy (1991) *Damned If We Do, Contradictions in Women's Health Care*, Allen & Unwin, North Sydney.

Broom, Dorothy (1992) 'Adding insult to injury: the discrimination case against women's health centres', *Refractory Girl*, April, pp. 62–5.

Broom, Dorothy (ed.) (1994) *Double Bind*, Allen & Unwin, St Leonards, NSW.

Broom, Dorothy (1996) *There should be more! Women's use of community health centres*, Final report of a research project funded by the Commonwealth Department of Human Services and Health, Canberra.

Broom, Dorothy (1997) 'The best medicine: women using community health centres', *Australian and New Zealand Journal of Public Health*, 21:3, pp. 275–80.

Broom, Dorothy (1998a) Facing facts, facing futures: challenges to women's health, Paper presented to the Victorian Women's Health Conference, 9–10 June.

Broom, Dorothy (1998b) 'By women for women: the continuing appeal of women's health centres', *Work and Health*, 28:1, pp. 5–22.

Broom, Dorothy (1998c) Re: planning and practice framework draft and national strategies coordination paper, 27 July, Typescript, For AHMAC Subcommittee on Women and Health.

Broom, Dorothy (2001) 'Australian women's health: from margins to mainstream?', in World Health Organisation (WHO), *Women and Health*, Proceedings of WHO Kobe Centre Second International Meeting, 4–6 April, Canberra.

Brown, Chris, Campbell, Chris and Ranald, Pat (1986) It even hurts to shake hands, January, Typescript, Adelaide Women's Community Health Centre.

Browne, M. Elspeth (1979) *Empty Cradle: Fertility control in Australia*, UNSW Press, Sydney.

Bulbeck, Chilla (1997) *Living Feminism*, Cambridge University Press, Melbourne.

Bullimore, Kim (2008) 'Victoria's abortion law reform', *Direct Action*, 5 (October).

Burgmann, Meredith (1984) 'Black sisterhood: the situation of urban Aboriginal women and their relationship to the white women's movement', in Simms, Marion (ed.), *Australian Women and the Political System*, Longman Cheshire, Sydney.

Burrow, Sharon (2008) Exploring key issues affecting women in the workplace, Speech delivered at the Twentieth Women, Management and Employment

Relations Conference, 24 July, Macquarie University, Sydney, <http://www.
actu.asn.au/Images/Dynamic/attachments/6066/Advance%20Australia%20
Fair%20speech.doc>, accessed 16 August 2011.

Bursian, Olga (1995) 'Economic liberalism and the community services industry:
a case study', *Just Policy*, 3 (June), pp. 3–10.

Caddick, Alison and Small, Rhonda (1982) 'W.I.C.H.', *Scarlet Woman*, 15, pp.
9–12.

Caine, Barbara, Gatens, Moira, Grahame, Emma, Larbalestier, Jan, Watson,
Sophie and Webby, Elizabeth (1998) *Australian Feminism. A companion*,
Oxford University Press, Melbourne.

Cameron, R. and Velthuys, J. (2005) The future of women's health depends on
feminism…, Paper given to the Fifth AWHN National Conference on Women's
Health, 20–22 April, Carlton Crest Hotel, Melbourne.

Canadian Institutes of Health Research (2000) *Sex, Gender and Women's Health*,
<http://www.bccewh.bc.ca/publications-resources/documents/cihrreport.
pdf>, accessed 16 August 2011.

Canberra Women's Refuge Collective (1976) *First Annual Report*, June 1974 –
June 1976, Typescript.

Canberra Women's Refuge Collective (1977) *Second Report*, Typescript.

Carmody, Moira (1990) Keeping rates on the political agenda, in *National
Women's Conference 1990: Proceedings*, Write People, Canberra, pp. 303–8.

Carmody, Moira (2009) 'Conceptualising the prevention of sexual assault and
the role of education', *ACSSA Issues*, 10, Australian Centre for the Study of
Sexual Assault.

Carmody, Moira and Carrington, Kerry (2000) 'Preventing sexual assault?', *The
Australian and New Zealand Journal of Criminology*, 33:3, pp. 341–61.

Carmody, Moira and Willis, Karen (2006) *Developing Ethical Sexual Lives: Young
people, sex and sexual assault prevention*, University of Western Sydney and
NSW Rape Crisis Centre, Sydney.

Carrington, Kerry and Phillips, Janet (2006) *Domestic violence in Australia—an
overview of the issues*, E Brief, Parliamentary Library, Parliament of Australia,
Canberra, <http://www.aph.gov.au/library/intguide/sp/Dom_violence.
htm>, accessed 16 August 2011.

Carter, Betty, Hussen, Gillean and Abbott, Lana (1987) 'Aboriginal women and childbirth—the struggle for the Congress Alukura', *Refractory Girl*, 30, pp. 14–17.

Carter, Elizabeth, Lumley, Judith, Wilson, Gai and Bell, Stephanie (2004) '"Alukura...for my daughters and their daughters and their daughters". A review of Congress Alukura', *Australian and New Zealand Journal of Public Health*, 28:3, pp. 229–34.

Cazalet, Daphne and Lane, Mary (2000) 'Women, community artswork and violence', *Women against Violence: An Australian Feminist Journal*, 9 (December), pp. 61–73.

Central Australian Aboriginal Congress (CAAC) (2004–05, 2006–07) *Annual Report*, <http://www.caac.org.au/downloads/caac_annual_report_2004.pdf>, accessed 16 August 2011.

Chappell, Louise (2001) 'Federalism and social policy: the case of domestic violence', *Australian Journal of Public Administration*, 60:1 (March), pp. 59–69.

Chenoweth, Leslie (1993) 'Invisible act: violence against women with disabilities', *Australian Disability Review*, 2:93, pp. 22–8.

Chenoweth, Leslie (1997) 'Violence and women with disabilities: silence and paradox', in Cook, Sandy and Bessant, Judith (eds), *Women's Encounters: Australian experiences*, Sage, Thousand Oaks, Calif.

Clarence, Christine and MacDonald, Jane (1998) 'Lajamanu—women working together', *Aboriginal and Islander Health Worker Journal*, 22:4 (July/August), pp. 2–3.

Clark, Haley, Duncanson, Kirsty and Quadara, Antonia (2009) 'Prevention frameworks', *Aware* [ACSSA newsletter], 22, pp. 7–12.

Clarke, Colleen, Harnett, Paul, Atkinson, Judy and Shochet, Ian (1999) 'Enhancing resilience in Indigenous people: the integration of individual family and community interventions', *Aboriginal and Islander Health Worker Journal*, 23:4 (July/August), pp. 6–10.

Cohen, May and Sinding, Chris (1996) *Changing concepts of women's health—advocating for change*, Women's Health Forum: Canadian and American Commissioned Papers, Minister of Supply and Services, Ottawa, <http://www.cwhn.ca/en/node/23058>

Coker, Ann (2005) 'Opportunities for prevention: addressing IPV in the health care setting', *Family Violence Prevention and Health Practice*, 1 (January).

Commonwealth Department of Health (1978) *Women's Health in a Changing Society*, Proceedings of a Conference on All Aspects of Women's Health, Sponsored by the Commonwealth Department of Health and the National Advisory Committee for International Women's Year, 1, 25–29 August, University of Queensland, Australian Government Publishing Service, Canberra.

Commonwealth Department of Health and Ageing (n.d.), *Midwife Reform Legislation*, Fact sheet, <http://www.health.gov.au/internet/main/publishing.nsf/Content/maternityservicesreview-MidwifeReformLegislationFactsheet>, accessed 16 August 2011.

Commonwealth of Australia (n.d.), Department of the Attorney-General, web site, <http://www.ema.gov.au/www/agd/agd.nsf/Page/Indigenouslawandnativetitle_Indigenouslawprograms_IndigenousLawPrograms>, accessed 20 February 2010.

Commonwealth of Australia (1963) Minute Paper, <http://vrroom.naa.gov.au/print/?ID=19442>, accessed 16 August 2011.

Commonwealth of Australia (1986a) *Looking forward to better health*, Report of the Better Health Commission, 1–3, Australian Government Publishing Service, Canberra.

Commonwealth of Australia (1986b) *Second report*, Medicare Benefits Review Committee, Australian Government Publishing Service, Canberra.

Commonwealth of Australia (1989) *National Women's Health Policy*, Australian Government Publishing Service, Canberra.

Commonwealth of Australia (1991) *National Agenda for Women*, August, Implementation report, Office of the Status of Women, Department of Prime Minister and Cabinet, Australian Government Publishing Service, Canberra.

Commonwealth of Australia (1992) *National Non-English Speaking Background Women's Health Strategy*, Centre for Women's Health Studies, Cumberland College of Health Sciences, University of Sydney, Australian Government Publishing Service, Canberra.

Commonwealth of Australia (1993) *National Women's Health Program. Evaluation and future directions*, Australian Government Publishing Service, Canberra.

Commonwealth of Australia (1994) *A National Aboriginal Health Strategy: Evaluation report 1994*, Office of Aboriginal and Torres Strait Islander Health, Canberra, <http://www.health.gov.au/internet/main/publishing. nsf/Content/health-oatsih-pubs-NAHSeval>

Commonwealth of Australia (1996) *Women's Safety Australia 1996*, ABS Catalogue No. 4128.0, Australian Bureau of Statistics, Canberra.

Commonwealth of Australia (1997) *Report of the National Evaluation of the Second Phase of the National Women's Health Program*, October, Bandt Gatter and Associates and Purdon Associates Proprietary Limited, Canberra.

Commonwealth of Australia (2004a) *National Framework for Sexual Assault Prevention*, Office of the Status of Women, Report prepared by Urbis Keys Young.

Commonwealth of Australia (2004b) *The Cost of Domestic Violence to the Australian Economy*, Access Economics, <http://www.accesseconomics. com.au/publicationsreports/showreport.php?id=23&searchfor=2004&searc hby>

Commonwealth of Australia (2008a) *Australia: the healthiest country by 2020*, Discussion Paper, National Preventive Health Task Force, Canberra, <http:// www.preventativehealth.org.au/internet/preventativehealth/publishing. nsf/Content/nphs-roadmap/$File/nphs-roadmap-1.pdf>, accessed 16 August 2011.

Commonwealth of Australia (2008b) *Rates of Domestic Violence as a Measure of the Effectiveness of the Northern Territory Emergency Response*, Northern Territory Emergency Response Review, <http://www.nterreview.gov.au/ subs/nter_review_report/154_alice_springs_women/154_Alice_Springs_ Women_3.htm>, accessed 16 August 2010.

Commonwealth of Australia (2009a) *Time for Action: The National Council's plans for Australia to reduce violence against women and their children, 2009–2021*, March, Background Paper.

Commonwealth of Australia (2009b) *A Snapshot to Time for Action: The National Council's plans for Australia to reduce violence against women and their children, 2009–2021*, March.

Commonwealth of Australia (2009c) *A healthier future for all Australians*, June, Final Report of the National Health and Hospitals Reform Commission, Canberra.

Commonwealth of Australia (2009d) *Australia: the healthiest country by 2020*, 30 June, Report of the National Preventive Health Task Force, <http://www.preventativehealth.org.au/internet/preventativehealth/publishing.nsf/Content/AEC223A781D64FF0CA2575FD00075DD0/$File/nphs-overview.pdf>

Commonwealth of Australia (2009e) *Domestic Violence Laws in Australia*, Department of Families, Housing, Community Services and Indigenous Affairs, Canberra.

Commonwealth of Australia (2009f) *Extended Medicare Safety Net review report*, A report by the Centre for Health Economics Research and Evaluation, Prepared for the Australian Government Department of Health and Ageing.

Commonwealth of Australia (2009g) *Improving maternity services in Australia*, Report of the Maternity Services Review, Canberra.

Commonwealth of Australia (2009h) *Shut Out: The experience of people with disabilities and their families in Australia*, Canberra.

Commonwealth of Australia (2010a) *Report*, February, Community Affairs Legislation Committee, <http://www.aph.gov.au/senate/committee/clac_ctte/health_leg_midwives_nurse_practitioners_09_nov09/report/report.pdf>

Commonwealth of Australia (2010b) *National Women's Health Policy 2010*, Canberra.

Commonwealth of Australia (2011a) *Evaluation of the Child Health Check Initiative and Expanding Health Service Delivery Initiative*, 31 March, Final report.

Commonwealth of Australia (2011b) *National Disability Strategy*, Council of Australian Governments, web site, <http://www.coag.gov.au/coag_meeting_outcomes/2011-02-13/docs/national_disability_strategy_2010-2020.rtf>

Commonwealth of Australia (2011c) *National Maternity Services Plan*, Australian Health Ministers Conference, <http://midwives.rentsoft.biz/lib/National%20Maternity%20Services%20Plan%20Feb%202011.pdf>

Commonwealth of Australia (2011d) *National Plan to Reduce Violence against Women and Their Children*, <http://www.fahcsia.gov.au/sa/women/progserv/violence/nationalplan/Documents/national_plan.pdf>

Community Development in Health (1988) *Resource Directory*, Community Development in Health Project, <http://www.latrobe.edu.au/publichealth/cdih/cdih_downloads/Resources%20Collection%20Separate%20Chapters/Section%205%20Resource_Directory.pdf>

Connell, R. W. (1987) *Gender and Power*, Stanford University Press, Stanford, Calif.

Conrad, Peter (2004) *The Sociology of Health and Illness. Critical perspectives*, [Seventh edn], Worth, New York.

Cook, Bree, David, Fiona and Grant, Anna (2001) *Sexual violence in Australia*, Research and Policy Paper Series 36, Australian Institute of Criminology, Canberra, <http://www.aic.gov.au/documents/4/3/6/%7B43630977-E669-46BD-ADCC-6B0766447C31%7DRPP36.pdf>

Cooper, Margaret and Temby, Dianne (1995) 'In the hands of the receivers', in Davies J. et al. (eds), *Changing Society for Women's Health*, Proceedings of the Third National Women's Health Conference, 17–19 November, The Australian National University, Canberra, pp. 182–7.

Cooper, Nola (2003) The background herstory of feminist women's health centres (NSW), Address to Women's Health NSW launch of The Nature of Women's Health Past, Present and Future Training Program, 6 March, <http://www.liverpoolwomenshealth.org.au/women/herstory.html>

Cooper, Nola and Spencer, Merry (1978) 'Why women's health centres?, in Commonwealth of Australia, *Women's Health in a Changing Society. Proceedings of a conference on all aspects of women's health*, Australian Government Publishing Service, Canberra.

Cornwall, John (1989) *Just for the Record*, Wakefield Press, Kent Town, SA.

Council of Australian Governments (COAG) (2011) Heads of Agreement—National Health Reform, 13 February, <http://www.coag.gov.au/coag_meeting_outcomes/2011-02-13/docs/communique_attachmentA-heads_of_agreement-national_health_reform_signatures.pdf>

Cox, John W. (2009) 'Timing of transfer for pregnant women from Queensland Cape York communities to Cairns for birthing', *Medical Journal of Australia*, 191:10, pp. 580–1.

Crawford, Phyl and Elliott, Kathleen V. (1994) 'A national survey of services for women with alcohol and other drug-related problems', in Broom, Dorothy (ed.), *Double Bind: Women affected by alcohol and other drugs*, Allen & Unwin, St Leonards, NSW.

Cueto, Marcos (2004) 'The origins of primary health care and selective primary health care', *American Journal of Public Health*, 94:11 (November), pp. 1864–74.

Curthoys, Ann (1984) 'The women's movement and social justice', in Broom, Dorothy H. (ed.), *Unfinished Business*, Allen & Unwin, Sydney.

Davies, A. F. (1964) *Australian Democracy*, [Second edn], Longmans, Melbourne.

Davis, Jill, Andrews, Susan, Broom, Dorothy H., Gray, Gwen and Renwick, Manoa (eds) (1996) *Changing Society for Women's Health*, Proceedings of the Third National Women's Health Conference, 17–19 November, Australian Government Publishing Service, Canberra.

Day, Alice (1977) 'Women at Work', in *Report on the Second National Conference on Women's Health, Newcastle, 22–29 May*, National Conference on Women's Health, Working Women's Centre, Newcastle, [not paginated].

de Beauvoir, Simone (1972) *The Second Sex*, Penguin, Middlesex, UK.

de Jonge, A., van der Goes, B., Ravelli, A., Amelink-Verburg, M., Mol, B., Nijhuis, J., Gravenhorst, J. and Buitendijk, S. (2009) 'Perinatal mortality and morbidity in a nationwide cohort of 529 688 low-risk planned home and hospital births', British Journal Obstetrics and Gynaecology, 116, pp. 1–8.

Dean, Jonathan (2009) 'Who's afraid of third wave feminism?', *International Feminist Journal of Politics*, 11:3, pp. 334–52.

Deller, C., Fatin, N. and Stewart, L. (1979) 'Sexual Assault Referral Centre, Perth: the first thirty months', *Australian Family Physician*, 8 (July), pp. 771–5.

Department of Health and Community Services (2005) *The Health and Well-Being of Northern Territory Women: From the desert to the sea 2005*, Darwin.

Department of Human Services, Victoria, web site, <http://www.dhs.vic.gov.au/home>

Department of Justice (2009) *Review of the Integrated Response to Family Violence: final report*, June, SuccessWorks, Tasmania.

DES Action Australia, web site, <http://www.desaction.org.au/>

Dimech, Mary (1982) 'On racism', *Scarlet Woman*, 14, pp. 14–19.

Domestic Violence Resource Centre Victoria (DVRCV) (2008) 'Federal Government's reforms to family law', *Update on Events and Issues*, <http://www.dvirc.org.au/UpdateHub/FamilyLawReform.htm>

Domestic Violence Resource Centre Victoria (DVRCV) (2009) *Update on Events and Issues*, <http://www.DVIRC.org.au/Update Hub/UpdateIndex.htm>

Donner, Lissa and Pederson, Ann (2004) *Women and primary health care reform: a discussion paper*, Paper prepared for the National Workshop on Women and Primary Health Care, 5–7 February, Winnipeg, Manitoba.

Donovan, Jan (1987) 'Proudly announcing the birth of the Australian Women's Health Network', *Wisenet. Journal of the Women in Science Enquiry Network*, 13 (December), pp. 8–9.

Dowse, Sara (1984) 'The bureaucrat as usurer', in Broom, Dorothy (ed.), *Unfinished Business*, Allen & Unwin, North Sydney.

Dowse, Sara (1988) 'The women's movement fandango with the state: the movement's role in public policy since 1972', in Baldock, Cora and Cass, Bettina (eds), *Social Welfare and the State in Australia*, Allen & Unwin, Sydney.

Dowse, Sara (2009) 'A different kind of politics', *Inside Story*, 19 December, <http://inside.org.au/>

Doyal, Leslie (1983) 'Women, health and sexual division of labour: a case study of the women's health movement in Britain', *Critical Social Policy*, 7 (Summer), pp. 21–33.

Doyal, Leslie (1995) *What Makes Women Sick*, Macmillan, Basingstoke, UK.

Doyle, Bridie (1996) 'Mainstreaming and the question of men', *Women against Violence: AnAustralian Feminist Journal*, 1 (November), pp. 43–6.

Duncanson, Kirsty (2009) 'On theorising the un-naming of men's violence against women. Interview with Adrian Howe', *Aware* [ACSSA Newsletter], 23, pp. 28–31.

Dwyer, Judith (1992a) 'Planning for the future', in *Women and Health Conference Proceedings, University of Adelaide, 22–24 July*.

Dwyer, Judith (1992b) 'Women's health in Australia', in Baum, Fran, Fry, Denise and Lenny, Ian (eds), *Community Health, Policy and Practice in Australia*, Pluto Press, Leichhardt, NSW.

Earle, Jenny, Herron, Alex, Secomb, Linell and Stubbs, Julie (1990) 'The National Domestic Violence Education Program', *Refractory Girl*, 36, pp. 2–6.

Eating Disorders Foundation of Victoria, web site, <http://www.eatingdisorders.org.au/media/key-statistics.html>

Edwards, Alison (1998) 'The Northern Territory domestic violence strategy—all paper, no infrastructure', *Women against Violence: An Australian Feminist Journal*, 4, pp. 46–8.

Edwards, Jean (1984) 'Liverpool Women's Health Centre', *New Doctor*, 33, pp. 22–3.

Ehrenreich, Barbara and English, Deirdre (1973) *Witches, Midwives and Nurses: A history of women healers*, [Second edn], The Feminist Press, Old Westbury, NY.

Eisenstein, Hester (1990) 'Femocrats, official feminism and the uses of power', in Watson, Sophie (ed.) *Playing the State*, Allen & Unwin, North Sydney.

Eisenstein, Hester (1996) *Inside Agitators, Australian Femocrats and the State*, Allen & Unwin, St Leonards, NSW.

Elder, Catriona (2007) *Being Australian: Narratives of Australian identity*, Allen & Unwin, Crows Nest, NSW.

Elizabeth Hoffman House, web site, <http://www.kiams.net/hoffman/about.htm>, accessed 29 September 2009.

Elks, Sarah (2009) 'Premier Bligh rejects bid for Queensland abortion reform', *The Australian*, 29 December, <http://www.theaustralian.com.au/news/nation/premier-bligh-rejects-bid-for-queensland-abortion-reform/story-e6frg6nf-1225814240564>

Ellwood, David (2008) Submission to the National Maternity Services Review, 30 October, <http://www.health.gov.au/internet/main/publishing.nsf/Content/maternityservicesreview-268/$FILE/268_D.Ellwood_scanned.pdf>

Elston, M. A. (1981) 'Medicine as "old husband's tales": the impact of feminism', in Spender, Dale (ed.), *Men's Studies Modified: The impact on the academic disciplines*, Pergamon, New York.

Evans, Robert G. (1993) 'Health care reform: the issue from hell', *Policy Options*, 14:6 (July–August), pp. 35–41.

Evans, Robert G. (1998) *Health for all or wealth for some? Conflicting goals in health care reform*, Health Policy Research Unit Discussion Paper Series, Centre for Health Services and Policy Research, University of British Columbia, Vancouver.

Evans, Susan, Krogh, Chris and Carmody, Moira (2009) 'Time to get cracking: the challenge of developing best practice in Australian sexual assault prevention education', *Australian Centre for the Study of Sexual Assault*, 11.

Farr, Vera (1987) 'Women in health bureaucracy—part one, Western Australia', *National Women's Health Centres Newsletter*, 2, pp. 4–6.

Ferguson, Kathy (1984) *The Feminist Case against Bureaucracy*, Temple University Press, Philadelphia.

Fitzpatrick, Judith M. (1995) 'Obstetric health services in far north Queensland: is choice an option?', *Australian Journal of Public Health*, 19:6, pp. 580–8.

Flick, Barbara (1990) 'Colonisation and decolonisation: an Aboriginal experience', in Watson, Sophie (ed.), *Playing the State*, Allen & Unwin, Sydney.

Foley, Gary (1984) *Aboriginal Community Health Services Workshop: Aboriginal health policy*, Proceedings of the South Australian Community Health Conference, 14–15 September, Angle Park, SA, pp. 111–15.

Fraser, Peg (2008) 'Migrant women and feminism', in *Online Encyclopaedia of Melbourne*, July, <http://www.emelbourne.net.au/about.html>, accessed 20 October 2009.

Fredericks, Bronwyn (2009) '"There is nothing that identifies me to that place": Indigenous women's perceptions of health spaces and places', *Cultural Studies Review*, 15:2, pp. 46–61.

Fredericks, Bronwyn (2010) 'Reempowering ourselves: Australian Aboriginal women', *Signs: Journal of Women in Culture and Society*, 35:3, pp. 546–9.

Fredericks, Karen (1993) 'Women fight back against rape', *Green Left Weekly*, 103.

Freudenberg, Nick (1986) 'The women's health movement—lessons for health educators', *Health/PAC Bulletin*, 16:6 (August), p. 30.

Fuchs, Victor (1974) *Who Shall Live*, Basic Books, New York.

Gaff-Smith, Mavis (2003) *Midwives of the Black Soil Plains*, Triple D Books, Wagga Wagga, NSW.

Gander, Catherine and Champion, Taryn (2009) 'The challenges of integrating domestic violence in a homeless policy framework', *Parity*, 22:10, pp. 25–6.

Ganti, A. K. (2009) 'Another nail in the coffin for hormone replacement therapy?', *The Lancet*, 347:9697, pp. 1217–18.

Garcia, J., Redshaw, M. and Fitzsimons, B. et al. (1998) *First-Class Delivery: A national survey of women's views of maternity care*, Audit Commission, London.

Geddes, Vig (2007) 'DVIRC turns twenty-one', *DVIRC Quarterly*, 4 (Summer), pp. 2–8.

Geelong Rape Crisis Centre (1995–96) *Annual Report*, July.

Giladi, Avner (2010) 'Liminal craft, exceptional law: preliminary notes on midwives in mediaeval Islamic writings', *International Journal of Middle East Studies*, 42, pp. 185–202.

Goldrick-Jones, Amanda (2002) *Men Who Believe in Feminism*, Praeger, Westport, Conn.

Goodall, Heather and Huggins, Jackie (1992) 'Aboriginal women *are* everywhere', in Saunders, K. and Evans, Raymond (eds), *Gender Relations in Australia*, Harcourt Brace Jovanovich, Sydney, pp. 398–424.

Gordon, Josh (2009) 'Furore over midwife report as doctors go on the attack', *WA Today*, 21 February, <http://www.watoday.com.au/national/furore-over-midwife-report-as-doctors-go-on-the-attack-20090221-8e9t.html>

Gosden, Diane (1998) 'Progeny of feminism: the homebirth movement in Australia', *Journal of Interdisciplinary Gender Studies*, 3:1, pp. 39–57.

Gosden, Diane and Noble, Carolyn (2000) 'Social mobilisation around the act of childbirth: subjectivity and politics', *Annual Review of Health Sciences*, 10, pp. 69–79.

Government of Manitoba (1972) *White Paper on Health Policy*, Department of Health and Social Development, Winnipeg.

Government of the Northern Territory (1992) *Women's Health Policy*, Bound typescript, Darwin.

Government of Ontario (1974) *Report of the Health Planning Task Force* [*Mustard Report*], Ministry of Health, Toronto.

Government of Quebec (1970) *Report of the Commission of Enquiry on Health and Social Services* [*Castonguay Report*], Quebec City.

Government of Queensland (2009) *For Our Sons and Daughters: A Queensland Government strategy to reduce domestic and family violence to 2009–2014*, <http://www.communityservices.qld.gov.au/violenceprevention/documents/program-of-action.pdf>

Government of South Australia (2005) *South Australian Women's Health Policy*, Department of Health, Adelaide, <http://www.whs.sa.gov.au/pub/Women_Health_Policy.pdf>

Government of Victoria (2002) *Community Health Plans 2002*, Department of Human Services, Melbourne, <http://www.health.vic.gov.au/healthpromotion/downloads/int_hp_positiveoutcomes.pdf>

Government of Victoria (2009a) *Primary Care Partnerships*, <http://www.health.vic.gov.au/pcps/downloads/better_health_stronger_communities.pdf>

Government of Victoria (2009b) *Respectful Relationships Education*, November, Department of Education and Early Childhood Development, Melbourne.

Grant, Richard (2004) *Less tax or more public spending: twenty years of opinion polling*, Research Paper 13 2003-4, Information and Research Services, Parliamentary Library, Canberra.

Grahame, Emma and Prichard, Janette Joy (1996) *Australian Feminist Organisations 1970–1985*, Women's Studies Centre, University of Sydney, Sydney.

Gray, Gwen (1984) 'The termination of Medibank', *Politics*, 19:2, pp. 1–17.

Gray, Gwen (1997) 'Influencing mainstream medical care: the case of the National Women's Health Policy and Program, 1989–1997', in Crowder, G. et al. (eds), *Australasian Political Studies 1997: Proceedings of the 1997 APSA Conference*, 1 October, Department of Politics, Flinders University of South Australia, pp. 279–94.

Gray, Gwen (1999) 'Women's health in a restructuring state', in Hancock, Linda (ed.), *Women, Public Policy and the State*, Macmillan, South Yarra, Vic.

Gray, Gwen (2003) 'One high standard of health care for all Australians', in Hocking, Jenny and Lewis, Colleen (eds), *It's Time Again: Whitlam and modern Labor*, Circa, Armadale, Vic.

Gray, Gwen (2006) 'Women, federalism and women friendly policies', *Australian Journal of Public Administration*, 65:1, pp. 25–45.

Gray, Gwendolyn (1991) *Federalism and Health Policy*: The development of health systems in Canada and Australia, University of Toronto Press, Toronto.

Gray, Gwendolyn (2004) *The Politics of Medicare*, UNSW Press, Sydney.

Gray, Gwendolyn (2008) 'Institutional, incremental and enduring: women's health action in Canada and Australia', in Grey, Sandra and Sawer, Marian (eds), *Women's Movements, Flourishing or in Abeyance*, Routledge, Abingdon, UK.

Gray, Gwendolyn (2009) Putting health into primary care? Canadian reform initiatives, 2000–08, Unpublished paper.

Gray, Gwendolyn (2010) 'Federalism, feminism and multilevel governance, the elusive search for theory?', in Sawer, Marian, Vickers, Jill and Haussman, Melissa (eds), *Federalism, Feminism and Multilevel Governance*, Ashgate, Aldershot, UK.

Hague, Diane and Milson, Anne (1982) 'ABORTION, the ACTU Congress, 1981', *Refractory Girl*, 23, pp. 15–16.

Hahn, Barry (2002) 'Primary care partnerships: Victoria's answer to primary care reform', *Health Issues*, 72, pp. 16–19.

Hammarstrom, Anne (1999) 'Why feminism in public health?', *Scandinavian Journal of Public Health*, 27, pp. 241–4.

Hancock, Linda (1998) 'How will women's health fare in the latest round of market state reforms?', *Health Issues*, 55 (June), pp. 26–9.

Hancock, W. K. (1961) *Australia*, The Jacaranda Press, Brisbane.

Hart, Julian Tudor (1971) 'The inverse care law', *The Lancet*, Saturday, 27 February, pp. 405–12.

Hartwig, Angela (2009) 'Executive officer report: women's refuge remuneration survey', *Women's Council e News*, Women's Council for Domestic and Family Violence Services, WA.

Haussman, Melissa, Sawer, Marian and Vickers, Jill (eds) (2010) *Federalism, Feminism and Multilevel Governance*, Ashgate, Aldershot, UK.

Healey, Lucy (2009) 'Building the evidence: a report on the status of policy and practice in responding to violence against women with disabilities in Victoria', *Australian Domestic and Family Violence Clearinghouse Newsletter*, 35 (Summer).

Health and Welfare Canada (1972) *Report of the Community Health Centre Project* [*Hastings Report*], Ottawa.

Health Canada (1999) *Health Canada's Women's Health Strategy*, Health Canada, Ottawa.

Heath, Mary (2005) 'The law and sexual offences against adults in Australia', *ACSSA Issues No. 4* (June), Australian Centre for the Study of Sexual Assault, Australian Institute of Family Studies, <http://www.aifs.gov.au/acssa/pubs/issue/i4.html>

Herrnson, P. (1994) 'American political parties: growth and change', in Peele, G. et al. (eds), *Developments in American Politics 2*, [Second edn], Macmillan, London.

Hewitt, Leslie and Worth, Carolyn (n.d.) *Victims Like Us: The development of the Victorian Centres against Sexual Assault*, <http://www.casa.org.au/index. php?page_id=21>

Hicks, Neville (1978) *This Sin and Scandal*, Australian National University Press, Canberra.

Hodges, Jane (1997) 'Women and mental health', *Women against Violence: An Australian Feminist Journal*, 2 (June), pp. 22–30.

Holthouse, Hector (1973) *S'pose I die: The story of Evelyn Maunsell*, Angus & Robertson, London.

Homebirth Access Sydney (2008) Submission to the Maternity Services Review from Homebirth Access Sydney, Based on the *Improving maternity services in Australia* Discussion Paper, <http://www.health.gov.au/internet/main/ publishing.nsf/Content/maternityservicesreview-353>

Horsley, Philomena (1994) 'Women's health services, for and by women. What is the future?', *In Touch, Public Health Association of Australia Newsletter Series*, 11:1 (February), pp. 10, 12.

Howe, Adrian (1984) 'ANZAC DAY—who owns the means of resistance?', *Scarlet Woman*, 19, pp. 22–5.

Howe, Adrian (2009) 'On theorising the un-naming of men's violence against women', *Aware* [ACSSA newsletter], 23, pp. 28–31.

Howe, Keren (1999) 'Violence against women with disabilities', *Women against Violence: AnAustralian Feminist Journal*, 7 (December), pp. 13–17.

Hudson, Bridie (2010) More than rates, roads and rubbish...the road to women's health in local government, Paper given to the Sixth AWHN National Women's Health Conference, 18–21 May, Hobart.

Huggins, Jackie and Blake, Thom (1992) 'Protection or persecution', in Saunders, K. and Evans, Raymond (eds), *Gender Relations in Australia*, Harcourt Brace Jovanovich, Sydney, pp. 42–58.

Hull, Bon (1986) 'Why another women's health centre went to the wall', *The Age*, 1 August, p. 14.

Hunder, Natala (1999) *Supporting Children and Young People Affected by Family Violence*, Geelong Rape Crisis Centre, Department of Human Services, Melbourne.

Hunt, Lynne (1994) 'The women's health movement: one solution', in Waddell, Charles and Peterson, Alan (eds), *Just Health*, Churchill Livingstone, Melbourne.

Immigrant Women's Domestic Violence Service, web site, <http://www.iwdvs.org.au/>, accessed 18 October 2009.

Immigrant Women's Health Service, web site, <http://www.immigrantwomenshealth.org.au/>

Irving, Baiba (1979) 'Women, work and health', *Refractory Girl*, 18/19, pp. 29–32.

Isis, web site, <http://www.isis.org.au/about-us>

Johns, Julie (2009) 'Western collaborative approach', *Research Matters, Newsletter of the South Australian Community Health Research Network*, 18:1, p. 7.

Johnstone, Kim and Bachowski, Rita (2000) *Victorian Women's Health Program—What is it? Past, present and future*, Proceedings of the Women's Health Victoria Forum, 16 November, Typescript.

Jolly, Rhonda, Magarey, Kirsty and Pyburne, Paula (2009) 'Health Legislation Amendment (Midwives and Nurse Practitioners) Bill 2009', 11 August, *Bills Digest*, 11, Department of Parliamentary Services, Parliamentary Library, Canberra, <http://www.aph.gov.au/library/pubs/bd/2009-10/10bd011.pdf>

Jones, M. A. (1990) *The Australian Welfare State*, [Third edn], Allen & Unwin, North Sydney.

Jung, Kyungja (2003) 'The politics of "speaking out": NESB women and the discourse of sexual assault in Australia', *Asian Journal of Women's Studies*, 4:3, pp. 109–45.

Kalantzis, Mary (1990) 'Ethnicity meets gender meets class in Australia', in Sophie Watson (ed.), *Playing the State*, Allen & Unwin, North Sydney.

Kaplan, Gisela (1996) *The Meagre Harvest*, Allen & Unwin, St Leonards, NSW.

Kawachi, Ichiro, Kennedy, Bruce, Gupta, Vanita and Prothrow-Stith, Deborah (1999) 'Women's status and the health of women and men: a view from the States', *Social Science and Medicine*, 48:1, pp. 21–32.

Keel, Monique (2004) *Family violence and sexual assault in Indigenous communities: 'walking the talk'*, ACSSA Briefing No. 4, Australian Institute of Family Studies.

Keel, Monique (2005a) 'Prevention of sexual assault', *Aware* [ACSSA Newsletter], 8 (June), pp. 16–24.

Keel, Monique (2005b) 'State and Territory sexual assault policy', *Aware* [ACSSA Newsletter], 8 (June), pp. 4–9.

Keleher, Helen (2001) 'Why primary health care offers a more comprehensive approach to tackling health inequities than primary care', *Australian Journal of Primary Health*, 7:2, pp. 57–61.

Kelleher, Joan (2009) 'Indigenous issues', *Aware* [ACSSA Newsletter], 20, pp. 13–14.

Kennedy, Jessica, Easteal, Patricia and Taylor, Caroline (2009) 'Rape mythology and the criminal justice system', *Aware* [ACSSA Newsletter], 23.

Kenway, Jane (1992) 'Feminist theories of the state: to be or not to be', in Muetzelfeldt, Michael (ed.), *Society, State and Politics*, Pluto Press, Leichhardt, NSW.

Keville, Terri D. (1994) 'The invisible woman: gender bias in medical research', *Women's Rights Law Reporter*, 15:3 (Spring), pp. 123–42.

Kinder, Sylvia (1980) *Herstory of Adelaide, Women's Liberation, 1969–74*, Salisbury Education Centre, Adelaide.

Kerby-Eaton, E. and Davies, J. (eds) (1986) *Women's Health in a Changing Society*, Proceedings of the Second National Conference on All Aspects of Women's Health, McGill Campus of the SA College of Advanced Education, Adelaide.

Kitzinger, Sheila (2005) *The Politics of Birth*, Elsevier, Amsterdam.

Kong, Grace (1992) 'Aboriginal women', in Smith, Angie (ed.), *Women's Health in Australia*, [Second edn], University of New England, Armidale, NSW.

Koutroulis, Glenda (1990) 'The orifice revisited: women in gynaecological texts', *Community Health Studies*, 14, pp. 73–84.

Krug, Etienne, Mercy, J. A., Dahlberg, L. L. and Zwi, A. B. (2002) *World Report on Violence and Health*, World Health Organisation, Geneva.

Laing, Leslie (2000) *Progress, trends and challenges in Australian responses to domestic violence*, Australian Domestic and Family Violence Clearinghouse Issues Paper 1, <http://www.adfvc.unsw.edu.au/PDF%20files/issuespaper1.pdf>

Lake, Marilyn (1999) *Getting Equal*, Allen & Unwin, St Leonards, NSW.

Lalonde, Marc (1974) *A New Perspective on the Health of Canadians*, Information Canada, Ottawa.

Lane, Karen (in press 2011) 'When is collaboration not collaboration? When it is militarised', *Women and Birth*.

Larbalestier, Jan (1998) 'Identity and difference', in Caine, Barbara (ed.), *Australian Feminism. A companion*, Oxford University Press, Melbourne, pp. 148–58.

Lawson, Henry (1975) *While the Billy Boils: 87 stories from the prose works of Henry Lawson*, Rigby, Adelaide.

Lee, Christina, Dobson, Annette, Brown, Wendy, Bryson, Lois, Byles, Julie, Warner-Smith, Penny and Young, Anne (2005) 'Cohort profile: the Australian Longitudinal Study on Women's Health', *International Journal of Epidemiology*, 34:5, pp. 987–91.

Leichhardt Women's Community Health Centre (LWCHC), web site, <http://www.lwchc.org.au/site/index.php>

Lester, Jane (1992) 'Aboriginal women and family violence', in *Women and Health Conference Proceedings, University of Adelaide, 22–24 July*, pp. 38-40.

Leo, Christopher and Enns, Jeremy (2009) 'Multilevel governance and ideological rigidity: the failure of deep federalism', *Canadian Journal of Political Science*, 42:1, pp. 93–116.

Lewis, Jenny (2009) 'The why and how of partnerships: policy and governance foundations', *Australian Journal of Primary Health*, 15:3, pp. 225–31.

Lilley, Kathleen C. and Stewart, Donald E. (2009) 'The Australian preventive health agenda: what will this mean for workforce development?', *Australia and New Zealand Health Policy*, 6:14.

Lipnack, Jessica (1980) 'The rise of the women's health movement in the USA', *New Age Journal*, March, pp. 122–4.

Litsios, Socrates (2004) 'The Christian Medical Commission and the development of the World Health Organisation's primary care approach', *American Journal of Public Health*, 94:11 (November), pp. 1884–93.

Liverpool Women's Health Centre (n.d.) *A Potted Herstory of Liverpool Women's Health Centre*, <http://www.liverpoolwomen'shealth.or.au/aboutUs/herstory.html>

Loxton, Deborah, Schofield, Margo, Hussain, Rafat and Mishra, Gita (2006) 'History of domestic violence and physical health in midlife', *Women against Violence: An Australian Feminist Journal*, 14:8 (August), pp. 715–31.

Lynch, Lesley (1984) 'Bureaucratic feminisms: bossism and beige suits', *Refractory Girl*, May, p. 38.

Lynn, Robyn and Perkins, Sue (2000) 'A women's community garden: a small step towards a future of peace?', *Women against Violence: An Australian Feminist Journal*, 9 (December), pp. 74–83.

McCarron Benson, Julie (1991) *WEL Women: Recollections of some of the first WEL-ACT women*, Queanbeyan Publishing, Queanbeyan, NSW.

McCormack, Anna (1992) 'Abortion in Queensland', *Refractory Girl*, 43, pp. 40–1.

McFerran, Ludo (1990) 'Interpretation of a frontline state: Australian women's refuges and the state', in Watson, Sophie (ed.), *Playing the State*, Allen & Unwin, Sydney.

McFerran, Ludo (2007) *Taking back the castle: how Australia is making the home safer for women and children*, Australian Domestic and Family Violence Clearinghouse Issues Paper 14, University of New South Wales, Sydney.

McFerran, Ludo (2009) 'The road home: an opportunity to address women, domestic and family violence and homelessness?', *Australian Domestic and Family Violence Clearinghouse Newsletter*, 36 (Autumn).

McGlade, Hannah (2010) 'Time for action: responses from the sector', *Australian Domestic and Family Violence Clearinghouse Newsletter*, 39 (Summer), pp. 4–5.

MacKenzie, Jen (2009) 'Women's health and safety, from practice wisdom to evidence based practice', *Research Matters, Newsletter of the South Australian Community Health Research Unit*, 18:1, p. 6.

McKenzie, Lyn (1979) 'Melbourne Women's Health Collective—problems with funding', in *Lost Sleep over Government Funding. Five case studies*, Victorian Council of Social Services, Collingwood, Vic.

McKeown, Deirdre and Lundie, Rob (2009) *Conscience votes during the Howard Government, 1996–2007*, Research Paper No. 20, 2008–2009, Parliamentary Library, Canberra, <http://www.aph.gov.au/library/Pubs/RP/2008-09/09rp20.htm>

McKeown, T. (1976a) *The Rise of Modern Population*, Edward Arnold, London.

McKeown, T. (1976b) *The Role of Medicine: Dream, mirage or nemesis*, Nuffield Provincial Hospitals Trust, London.

McKeown, T., Record, R. and Turner, R. (1975) 'An interpretation of the decline of mortality in England and Wales during the twentieth century', *Population Studies*, 29, pp. 391–422.

McKinlay, John and McKinlay, Sonja (2004) 'Medical measures and the decline of mortality', in Conrad, Peter (ed.), *The Sociology of Health and Illness*, [Seventh edn], Worth, New York.

McNair, Ruth (2003) 'Outing lesbian health in medical education', *Women and Health*, 37:4, pp. 89–103.

McNair, Ruth (2009) Submission in response to the *New National Women's Health Policy Consultation Discussion Paper 2009*, November, <http://www.awhn.org.au/>

Maddison, Sarah (2001) Uneasy bedfellows: what role now for social movements in the policy process?', Paper given to the National Social Policy Conference, 4–6 July, University of New South Wales, Sydney.

Magnolia Place Team (2007) *Magnolia Place History*, <http://www.lws.org.au/history.htm>

Maltzahn, Kathleen (2009) 'So far, so good, but more can be done to end sex slavery', *The Age*, 18 June.

Marcus, Gaby (2008) *Northern Territory mandatory reporting of domestic and family violence by health professionals*, Australian Domestic and Family Violence Clearinghouse Discussion Paper, <http://www.austdvclearinghouse.unsw.edu.au/RTF%20Files/ADFVC%20submission%20to%20NT%20proposal%20on%20mandatory%20reporting%20of%20DV.rtf>

Marieskind, Helen and Ehrenreich, Barbara (1975) 'Towards socialist medicine: the women's health movement', *Social Policy*, September/October, pp. 34–42.

Martin, Felicity (2000) 'Activism in action, the women's incest survivors network', *Women against Violence: AnAustralian Feminist Journal*, 9 (December), pp. 41–51.

Mason, Carolyn (1994) 'Women's policy in Queensland', *Social Alternatives*, 12:4, pp. 13–16.

Mastroianni, Anna, Faden, Ruth and Federman, Daniel (1994) 'Women and health research: a report from the Institute of Medicine', *Kennedy Institute of Ethics Journal*, 4:1, pp. 55–62.

Maternity Coalition (2008) Submission to the National Maternity Services Review, October, <http://www.health.gov.au/internet/main/publishing.nsf/Content/maternityservicesreview-354>

Maternity Coalition, web site, <http://www.maternitycoalition.org.au/nmap/THE%20FINAL%20NMAP%20Sepember%2024th%202002.pdf>

Matthews, Jill Julius (1984) *Good and Mad Women: The historical construction of femininity in 20th-century Australia*, Allen & Unwin, Sydney.

Matthews, Trevor (1976) 'Interest group access to the Australian Government bureaucracy', in *Royal Commission on Australian Government Administration. Volume 2*, Australian Government Publishing Service, Canberra, Appendix 2.D, pp. 332–64.

Medew, Julia (2011) 'Doctors criticise leukaemia drug study', *Sydney Morning Herald*, 21 January, <http://www.smh.com.au/lifestyle/wellbeing/doctors-criticise-leukaemia-drug-study-20110120-19y3q.html>

Meekosha, Helen (1990) 'Is feminism able bodied?', *Refractory Girl*, 36, pp. 34–42.

Meekosha, Helen (2001) 'In/different health: rethinking gender, disability and health', *Politics, Action Renewal*, Conference Proceedings, Fourth Australian Women's Health Conference, 19–21 February, Adelaide Convention Centre, pp. 357–63.

Melbourne University Consciousness-Raising Group (1974) 'Consciousness raising', in National Women's Conference on Feminism and Socialism, *Papers from the National Conference on Feminism and Socialism*, October, Melbourne, p. 46.

Memmott, Paul, Chambers, Catherine, Go-Sam, Carroll and Thompson, Linda (2006) *Good practice in Indigenous family violence prevention—designing and evaluating successful programs*, Australian Domestic and Family Violence Clearinghouse Issues Paper 11, June, University of New South Wales, Sydney.

Menzies School of Health Research (2008) Submission to the Department of Health and Ageing Maternity Services Review, 31 October, <http://www.health.gov.au/internet/main/publishing.nsf/Content/maternityservicesreview-420/$FILE/420_Menzies%20School%20of%20Health%20Research.pdf>

Metherell, Mark (2010) 'Canberra in mental health talks', *The Age*, 22 June.

Meyer, David S. (2004) 'Protest and political opportunities', *Annual Review of Sociology*, 30, pp. 125–45.

Migrant Women's Support & Accommodation Service (MWSAS), web site, <http://www.mwsas.com.au/>

Milio, Nancy (1984) 'The political anatomy of community health policy in Australia, 1972–1982', *Politics*, 19:2 (November), pp. 18–33.

Millett, Kate (1977) *Sexual Politics*, Virago, London.

Mookai Rosie Bi-Bayan, web site, <http://mookairosie.org.au/new/index.php?option=com_content&view=article&id=23&Itemid=80>, accessed 30 October 2009.

Morgain, Lyn (1994) 'Women's Addiction Recovery Service: a community development model', in Broom, Dorothy (ed.), *Double Bind: Women affected by alcohol and other drugs*, Allen & Unwin, St Leonards, NSW.

Morrison, Zoe (2009) 'Recognising sexual assault', *Parity*, 22:10, pp. 30–1.

Mouzos, Jenny and Makkai, Toni (2004) *Women's Experiences of Male Violence*, Research and Public Policy Series 56, Australian Institute of Criminology, Canberra.

Moynahan, Ray (2003) 'The making of a disease: female sexual dysfunction', *British Medical Journal*, 326:7379, pp. 45–7.

Mugford, Jane (1989) *Domestic Violence*, Australian Institute of Criminology, Canberra, <http://www.aic.gov.au/publications/previous%20series/vt/1-9/vt02.aspx>

Mulrony, Jane (2003a) *Australian prevention programs for young people*, Australian Domestic and Family Violence Clearinghouse Topic Paper, <http://www.adfvc.unsw.edu.au/PDF%20files/prevention_progs_young.pdf>

Mulrony, Jane (2003b) *Trends in inter agency work*, Australian Domestic and Family Violence Clearinghouse Topic Paper, <http://www.adfvc.unsw.edu.au/RTF%20Files/trends_interagency_final.rtf>

Multicultural Centre for Women's Health (MCWH), web site, <http://www.mcwh.com.au/>

Murdolo, Adele (1996) 'Warmth and unity with all women?', *Feminist Review*, 52 (Spring), pp. 69–86.

Murphy, Kate (2006) 'Feminism', in Alexander, Alison (ed.), *The Companion to Tasmanian History*, Centre for Tasmanian Historical Studies, Hobart.

Murray, Suellen (1999) 'Breaking the silence: Nardine Women's Refuge and the politicisation of domestic violence in Western Australia during the 1980s', *Women against Violence: An Australian Feminist Journal*, 7 (December), pp. 4–10.

Murray, Suellen (2002) *More Than Refuge*, University of Western Australia Press, Crawley.

Murray, Suellen and Powell, Anastasia (2008) Sexual assault and adults with a disability, Issues Paper No. 9, Australian Centre for the Study of Sexual Assault, <http://aifs.gov.au/acssa/pubs/issue/i9.html>

Murray, Suellen and Powell, Anastasia (2009) 'What's the problem?: Australian public policy constructions of domestic and family violence', *Women against Violence: An Australian Feminist Journal*, 15, pp. 532–52.

Myers, Helen and Lavender (1997) *An overview of lesbians and health issues*, A COAL Research Paper, Coalition of Activist Lesbians, Typescript.

National Aboriginal Community Controlled Health Organisation (NACCHO), web site, <http://www.naccho.org.au/>

National Health and Medical Research Council (NHMRC) (2000–08) *Disease and Health Issues Based Datasets*, Expenditure Summary, NHMRC Research Funding, <http://www.nhmrc.gov.au/grants/dataset/files/list_of_datasets>

National Health and Medical Research Council (NHMRC) (2000–10) *National Health and Medical Research Council Research Funding, 2000–2010: Disease and health issues based data sets—expenditure summary*, <http://www.nhmrc.gov.au/grants/research-funding-statistics-and-data/summary-funding-data>

National Health and Medical Research Council (NHMRC) (2007) *National Statement on Ethical Conduct in Human Research*, <http://www.nhmrc.gov.au/guidelines/publications/e72>

National Queensland Domestic Violence Resource Service (NQDVRS) (2009) *Christmas Newsletter*, <http://www.nqdvrs.org.au/Newsletters/ Christmas%202009%20v5%202000%20pdf>

National Research Centre for OHS Regulation, web site, <http://ohs.anu.edu. au/>

National Rural Women's Coalition (2008) *Health Infrastructure and Access to Services in Rural and Remote Australia, Particularly focusing on maternity services and their contribution to sustainable rural communities*, <http:// www.nrwc.com.au/>

National Women's Health Centres Newsletter (1987a) *National Women's Health Centres Newsletter*, 1 (July).

National Women's Health Centres Newsletter (1987b) *National Women's Health Centres Newsletter*, 2 (October).

National Women's Health Centres Newsletter (1988) *National Women's Health Centres Newsletter*, 3.

Neame, Alexandra (2003) 'Sexual offences interim report', *Aware* [ACSSA Newsletter], 1 (September), pp. 6–11.

Networknews (1999) 'Women with disabilities win national violence prevention award', *Networknews*, 2:3 (November), p. 4.

Newman, J., Acklin, F., Trindall, A., Arbon, V., Brock, K., Bermingham, M. and Thompson, C. (1999) 'Story-telling: Australian Indigenous women's means of health promotion', *Aboriginal and Islander Health Worker Journal*, 23:4 (July/August), pp. 18–22.

Newman, Lareen, Reiger, Kerreen and Campo, Monica (2011) 'Maternity Coalition, Australia's national maternity consumer advocacy organisation', in O'Reilly, A. (ed.), *The 21st-Century Motherhood Movement: Mothers speak out on why we need to change the world and what to do about it*, Demeter Press, Toronto.

Ngaanyatjarra Pitjantjatjara Yankunytjatjara Women's Council, web site, <http://www.npywc.org.au/>

NGO Submission to the UN Committee on the Elimination of Racial Discrimination (2010) *Freedom Respect Equality Dignity: Action*, Australia, <http://www. rightsaustralia.org.au/images/stories/docs/ngo%20report%20on%20 australia%20to%20hrc%20-%20final.pdf>

Nichols, Betty and Hurley, June (1999) 'The Aboriginal Maternity Service Tamworth', *Aboriginal and Islander Health Worker Journal*, 23:4 (July/ August), pp. 24–8.

Norling, Elaine Odgers and Woodhouse, David (1998) 'Whose labour is it, anyway?', *Sydney Morning Herald*, 13 November, p. 19.

Nottingham, Janie (2008) Submission to the National Health and Hospitals Reform Commission, <http://www.health.gov.au/internet/nhhrc/ publishing.nsf/Content/258/$FILE/258%20-%20SUBMISSION%20-%20 Janie%20Nottingham.pdf>

NSW Department of Health (2000) *Gender Equity in Health*, State Health Publication, Sydney, <http://www.health.nsw.gov.au/pubs/2000/pdf/ gender_equity.pdf>

NSW Department of Health (2010) *Women's Health Plan, 2009–11*, Department of Health, Sydney, <http://www.health.nsw.gov.au/policies/pd/2010/ PD2010_004.html>

NSW Department of Premier and Cabinet (2008) *New South Wales domestic and family violence strategic framework*, December, Discussion Paper, Office for Women, Sydney.

NSW Rape Crisis Centre, web site, <http://www.nswrapecrisis.com.au/>, accessed November 2009.

NSW Women's Advisory Council to the Premier (1987) *A Decade of Change: Women in New South Wales 1976–86*, NSW Government Printer, Sydney.

Nutbeam, Don (2009) 'Defining and measuring health literacy: what can we learn from literacy studies?', *International Journal of Public Health*, 54, pp. 303–5, <http://www.springerlink.com/content/2107484567681523/fulltext. pdf>

Oberin, Julie (2009) Homelessness and violence against women in Australia. Will 'the plan' work?, Speech to the National Homelessness Summit, September, <http://wesnet.org.au/files/J.Oberin.Homelessness%20and%20 Violence%20against%20Women%20in%20Australia.Sept_.09.pdf>

Oliver, Karly and Hawkins, Trent (2008) 'Abortion reform passed in Victoria', *Green Left Weekly*, 770 (15 October).

Organisation for Economic Cooperation and Development (OECD) (2003) *Health care systems: lessons from the reform experience*, Departmental Working Paper No. 374, December, Organisation for Economic Cooperation and Development, Paris.

Organisation for Economic Cooperation and Development (OECD) (2011) *Health Data: Health care activities, surgical procedures by ICD-9-CM, caesarean section, procedures per 1000 live births*, Organisation for Economic Cooperation and Development, Paris.

Orr, Liz (1994) 'The women's refuge movement in Victoria', in Weeks, Wendy (ed.), *Women Working Together*, Longman Cheshire, Melbourne.

Otto, Dianne and Haley, Eileen (1975) 'Health shelter: a history of Adelaide Women's Shelter', *Refractory Girl*, Winter, pp. 11–16.

Outhwaite, Sue (1989) 'Gender and patriarchy', in Smith, Rodney and Watson, Lex (eds), *Politics in Australia*, Allen & Unwin, North Sydney.

Parkinson, Annie (2009) 'Time for action: responses from the sector', *Australian Domestic and Family Violence Clearinghouse Newsletter*, 38 (Spring), p. 5.

Parmer, George and Short, Stephanie (1989) *Health Care & Public Policy: An Australian analysis*, Macmillan, South Melbourne.

Partners in Prevention Victoria, web site, <http://www.dvrcv.org.au/pip/>

Pateras, Vassilka Vicki (1997) 'Accommodating diversity: a NESB focussed women's refuge model', *Women against Violence: An Australian Feminist Journal*, 2 (June), pp. 4–13.

Pear, Robert (2000) 'Research neglects women, studies find', *The New York Times*, 30 April, pp. 1, 16.

Pearce, Sophia (2002) 'Achieving positive health outcomes for Aboriginal women—Aboriginal women's gatherings', *Aboriginal and Islander Health Worker Journal*, 26:3 (May/June), p. 9.

Pearse, Warwick and Refshauge, Chloe (1987) 'Workers' health and safety in Australia: an overview', *International Journal of Health Services*, 17:4, pp. 635–50.

Perera, Suvendrini (1985) 'How long does it take to get it right? Migrant women and the women's movement', *Refractory Girl*, 28, pp. 13–15.

Perkins, Neville (1975) 'Central Australian Aboriginal Congress', in *Report of a Seminar on Aborigines in Australian Society*, 16–19 November, Richardson Hall, Monash University, Clayton, Vic.

Perkins, Sue and Lynn, Robyn (2000) 'A women's community garden', *Women against Violence: An Australian Feminist Journal*, 9 (December), pp. 74–83.

Peters, Alison (2009) NCOSS Submission to the NSW Framework on Domestic and Family Violence Consultation, National Council of Social Services, <http://www.ncoss.org.au/resources/090324-NSW-DV-and-FV-Strategic-Framework-Discussion-Paper-respnse-Mar09.pdf>

Phillips, Ruth (2006) 'Undoing an activist response: feminism and the Australian government's domestic violence policy', *Critical Social Policy*, 26:1, pp. 192–219.

Plibersek, Tanya (2009) Young people educated on respectful relationships, Media release, 2 March.

Pollard, Ruth (2009) 'All domestic violence deaths to be reviewed by State Coroner', *Sydney Morning Herald*, 25 November, pp. 8–9.

Pringle, Rosemary (1973) 'Octavius Beale and the ideology of the birthrate', *Refractory Girl*, 3 (Winter), pp. 19–27.

Pringle, Rosemary and Game, Ann (1983) *Gender at Work*, Allen & Unwin, Sydney.

Pringle, Rosemary and Watson, Sophie (1992) 'Women's interests and the post-structuralist state', in Barrett, Michele and Phillips, Ann (eds), *Destabilising Theory: Contemporary feminist debates*, Polity, Cambridge.

Public Health Association of Australia (2008) Submission from the Public Health Association of Australia to the Senate Select Committee on Men's Health, <http://www.phaa.net.au/documents/SenateSelectMensHealthSubmissionPHAAFeb2009.pdf>

Queensland Women's Health Network (QWHN) (1995) *Annual Report*, Typescript.

Queensland Women's Health Network (QWHN) (2003) *Annual Report*, <http://www.qwhn.asn.au/>

Queensland Women's Health Network (QWHN) (2009) *Queensland Women's Health Network News*, December.

Queensland Working Women's Service (2007–08) *Annual Report*, <http://www.qwws.org.au/information-sheets/view-category>

Radoslovich, Helen (1994) *A Piece of the Cake: A celebration and herstory of metropolitan women's health centres in South Australia*, Combined Women's Health Centre of South Australia, Adelaide.

Ramsay, Janet (2004) The making of domestic violence policy by the Australian Commonwealth Government and the Government of the State of New South Wales between 1970 and 1985, PhD E thesis, University of Sydney, Sydney, <http://ses.library.usyd.edu.au/bitstream/2123/724/9/adt-NU20060205.17311202chapter1.pdf>

Randall, Melanie (1988) 'Feminism and the state: questions for theory and practice', *RFR/DRF*, 17:3, pp. 10–16.

Redman, Sally, Turner, Jane and Davis, Cindy (2003) 'Improving supportive care for women with breast cancer in Australia: the challenge of modifying health systems', *Psycho-Oncology*, 12, pp. 521–31.

RedOrbit News (2009) 'Women with stroke treated worse than men', *Health News*, <http://www.redorbit.com/news/health/1643897/women_with_stroke_treated_worse_than_men/>

Reiger, Kerreen (1999a) 'Birthing in the post-modern moment: struggles over defining maternity care needs', *Australian Feminist Studies*, 14:30, pp. 387–404.

Reiger, Kerreen (1999b) '"Sort of part of the women's movement, but different": mother's organisations and Australian feminism', *Women's Studies International Forum*, 22:6, pp. 585–95.

Reiger, Kerreen (2000) 'The politics of midwifery in Australia: tensions, debates and opportunities', *Health Sociology Review*, 10:1, pp. 53–64.

Reiger, Kerreen (2001) *Our Bodies and Our Babies: The forgotten women's movement*, Melbourne University Press, Carlton South, Vic.

Reiger, Kerreen (2006) 'A neoliberal quickstep: contradictions in Australian maternity policy', *Health Sociology Review*, 15:4 (October), pp. 330–40.

Riverland Domestic Violence Action Group, web site, <http://www.rdvag.com.au/>

Roberts, Jan and Stewart, Bev (1999) *We're Not Ladies, We're Women! A herstory of the Wagga Wagga Women's Health Centre*, Wagga Wagga Women's Health Centre, Wagga Wagga, NSW.

Robertson, Geraldine (compiler) (n.d.), 'Women working together: suffrage and onwards', *Womensweb*, <http://home.vicnet.net.au/~women/Introduction.html>, accessed 16 August 2011.

Rodwin, Victor and Croce-Galis, Melanie (2004) 'Population health in Utah and Nevada: an update on Victor Fuchs' tale of two States', in Conrad, Peter (ed.), *The Sociology of Health and Illness*, [Seventh edn], Worth, New York.

Rosenberg, Harriet and Allard, Daniel (2007) 'Evidence for caution: women and statin use', *Women and Health Protection*, <http://www.whp-apsf.ca/pdf/statinsEvidenceCaution.pdf>

Rosenman, Elena (2003) *Talking Like a Toora Woman*, Toora Women Incorporated, Campbell, ACT.

Rosewarne, Clive, Vaarzon-Morel, Petronella, Bell, Stephanie, Carter, Elizabeth, Liddle, Margaret and Liddle, Johnny (2007) 'The historical context of developing an Aboriginal community-controlled health service: a social history of the first ten years of the Central Australian Aboriginal Congress', *Health and History*, 9:2, pp. 114–43.

Ross, Liz (1987) 'Sisters are doing it for themselves...and us', *Hecate*, 13:1, pp. 83–99.

Royal Australasian College of Physicians (n.d.) *College Roll*, <http://www.racp.org.nz/page/library/college-roll/college-roll-detail&id=115>

Royal Australasian College of Physicians, web site, <http://www.racp.edu.au/>

Russell, Lesley (2009) 'Commonwealth Indigenous budget bulletin', *Macroeconomics*, June, <http://www.macroeconomics.com.au/files/Commonwealth%20Indigenous%20Budget%20Bulletin%20-%20June%202009.pdf>

Russell, Lesley (2010) Innovations in care—where is mental health in the health reform agenda?, Paper presented to the Policy Innovations Seminar Series, 20 May, Menzies Centre for Health Policy, University of Sydney, Sydney, <http://www.aihw.gov.au/mediacentre/2010/mr20100601.cfm>

Ruzek, Sheryl (1978) *The Women's Health Movement*, Praeger, New York.

Ryan, Lyndal, Ripper, Margie and Buttfield, Barbara (1994) *We Women Decide: Women's experiences of seeking abortion in Queensland, South Australia and Tasmania, 1985–92*, Women's Studies Unit, Flinders University, Bedford Park, SA.

Saggers, Sherry and Gray, Dennis (1991) *Aboriginal Health & Society*, Allen & Unwin, St Leonards, NSW.

Saltman, Richard, Rico, Ana and Boerma, Wienke (eds) (2006) *Primary Care in the Driver's Seat?*, European Observatory on Health Systems and Policies Series, Open University Press, Maidenhead and Berkshire, UK.

Sandall, Philippa (1974) 'The Leichhardt story', in *From the Gilded Cage*, WEL Said, Dulwich Hill, NSW, pp. 88–9.

Sawer, Marian (1989) 'Women: the long march through the institutions', in Head, Brian and Patience, Allan (eds), *From Fraser to Hawke*, Longman Cheshire, Melbourne.

Sawer, Marian (1990) *Sisters in Suits*, Allen & Unwin, North Sydney.

Sawer, Marian (1994) 'Reclaiming the state: liberalism and social liberalism', *Australian Journal of Politics and History. Special Issue*, pp. 159–72.

Sawer, Marian (2003) *The Ethical State? Social liberalism in Australia*, Melbourne University Press, Carlton, Vic.

Sawer, Marian (2008a) 'Disappearing tricks', *Dialogue*, 27:3, pp. 4–9.

Sawer, Marian (2008b) *Making Women Count*, UNSW Press, Sydney.

Sawer, Marian (2010) 'The case for Liberal women', *Australian Review of Public Affairs*, February, <http://www.australianreview.net/digest/2010/02/sawer.html>

Sawer, Marian (2011) Entering too late? Women in parliamentary politics in New South Wales, Paper presented to the Sixth ECPR General Conference, 25–27 August, University of Iceland, Reykjavik.

Sawer, Marian and Simms, Marian (1984) *A Woman's Place*, Allen & Unwin, Sydney.

Sax, Sidney (1980) 'Community health developments in Australia', *Public Health Reviews*, 1X:3–4, pp. 269–99.

Sax, Sidney (1984) *A Strife of Interests*, Allen & Unwin, Sydney.

Scarlet Alliance, web site, <http://www.scarletalliance.org.au/who/history/>

Schattschneider, Elmer Eric (1960) *The Semi Sovereign People*: *A realist's view of democracy in America*, Holt, Reinhardt & Wilson, New York.

Schoen, Cathy, Osborn, Robin, Squires, David, Doty, Michelle, Pierson, Roz and Applebaum, Sandra (2010) 'How health insurance design affects access to care and costs, by income, in 11 countries', *Health Affairs*, 29:12, pp. 2323–34.

Schofield, Toni (1996) 'An update of the national NESB women's health strategy', in Davis, Jill, Andrews, Susan, Broom, Dorothy, Gray, Gwen and Renwick, Manoa (eds), *Changing Society for Women's Health*, Proceedings of the Third National Women's Health Conference, Australian Government Publishing Service, Canberra.

Schofield, Toni (1998) 'Health', in Caine, Barbara (ed.) *Australian Feminism. A companion*, Oxford University Press, Melbourne, pp. 123–32.

Scotton, R. B. (1978) 'Health services and the public sector', in Scotton, R. B. and Ferber, H. (eds), *Public Expenditures and Social Policy in Australia. Volume 1*, Longman Cheshire, Melbourne.

Scully, Diana and Bart, Pauline (1973) 'A funny thing happened on the way to the orifice: women in gynaecology textbooks', *AJS*, 78:4, pp. 1045–9.

Senate Community Affairs Legislation Committee (2010), *Health Legislation Amendment (Midwives and Nurse Practitioners) Bill 2009 and two related Bills*, 1 February, Parliament of Australia, Canberra, <http://www.aph.gov.au/senate/committee/clac_ctte/health_leg_midwives_nurse_practitioners_09_nov09/report/index.htm>

Sera's Women's Shelter, North Queensland Domestic Violence Resource Service and the North Queensland Combined Women's Services (2006) *Dragonfly Whispers*.

Shaw, Lea and Tilden, Jan (1990) *Creating Health for Women: A community health promotion handbook*, Women's Health Development Program, Brisbane Women's Community Health Centre.Shea, Brian (1970) 'The organisation of health and medical care services in Australia—the state's point of view', in *The Delivery of Health Services in Australia*, American College of Hospital Administrators, Chicago, pp. 37–63.

Shoebridge, A. and Shoebridge, K. (2010) Snapshot Australia: women in paid work, Paper presented to the Third National Congress on Women, Health and Work, 2–5 June, Stockholm, Sweden.

Shuttleworth, Clare (1992) 'Thorn in the side: women's health movement in SA', *Women and Health Conference Proceedings*, 22–24 July, University of Adelaide.

Siedlecky, Stefania (1977) 'Reactions to the Leichhardt Women's Health Centre', *New Doctor*, 5, pp. 29–32.

Siedlecky, Stefania and Wyndham, Diana (1990) *Populate or Perish*, Allen & Unwin, Sydney.

Simmons, Amy (2009) 'Sexual assault "woven through Australia's landscape"', [Interview with Carolyn Worth], *News Online*, <http://fightforjustice. blogspot.com/2009/03/sexual-assault-woven-through-australias.html>

Simpson, Denise (2003) 'Change processes within a feminist organisation', *Australian Domestic and Family Violence ClearinghouseNewsletter*, 13 (January), pp. 6–9.

Singer, Natasha (2009) 'Medical papers by ghostwriters pushed therapy', *The New York Times*, 5 August, p. A1, <http://www.nytimes.com/2009/08/05/ health/research/05ghost.html>

Singer, Natasha and Wilson, Duff (2009) 'A push to root out industry-financed ghostwriting from medical journals', *The New York Times*, 17 September, p. B1, <http://www.nytimes.com/2009/08/05/health/research/05ghost. html?ref=business>

Skues, Jennifer and Kirby, Robert (1996) 'Women, work and health', *Australian Journal of Primary Care—Interchange*, 2:4, pp. 54–61.

Smith, Alison (1985) 'Women's refuges: the only resort?', in Parry, Don and Botsman, Peter (eds), *Public/Private*, UNSW Press, Kensington, NSW.

Smith, Angie (ed.) (1992) *Women's Health in Australia*, [Second edn], University of New England, Armidale, NSW.

Smith, Mamie (1979), 'Women seek refuge', *The Herald*, 14 September, p. 26.

Smith, Meg (1984) 'The struggle for women's health centres in New South Wales', *Refractory Girl*, May, pp. 3–6.

Smith, Mick (n.d.) *Looking Back: Support groups for people with mood disorders*, <http://www.mhcc.org.au/documents/DrMegSmith.pdf>

Snyder, Emmi (1977) 'Making changes: 2nd National Women's Health Conference', *Refractory Girl*, September, pp. 15–17.

Sorensen, Georg (2004) *The Transformation of the State*, Palgrave Macmillan, Basingstoke, UK, and New York.

South Western Centre Against Sexual Assault (CASA) (2003–04) 'Wananga kooneem pa-cease fear', *Women against Violence*: *AnAustralian Feminist Journal*, 15, pp. 49–50.

Spinney, Angela (n.d. [ca. 2008–09]) *Challenges of Working With/Supporting Children in the Refuge Environment: The Safe from the Start Project*,

Reproduced by the National Homelessness Information Clearinghouse, <http://www.homelessnessinfo.net.au/dmdocuments/the_safe_from_the_start_project_-_national_homelessness_information_clearinghouse.rtf>

Stein, Michael and Turkewitsch, Lisa (2008) The concept of multi-level governance in studies of federalism, Paper given to the International Political Science Association International Conference: New Theories and Regional Perspectives, Concordia University, Montreal, <http://montreal2008.ipsa.org/site/images/PAPERS/section3/RC%2028-%20Stein%20Turkewitsch%203.4.pdf>

Stephen, Kylie (n.d.) 'Changes to Western Australia's abortion law in 1998', *Pro-Plus Choice Forum*, <http://www.prochoiceforum.org.uk/about.php>

Stevens, Joyce (1985) *A History of International Women's Day in Words and Images*, IWD Press, <http://www.isis.aust.com/iwd/stevens/postscript.htm>

Stevens, Joyce (1995) *Healing Women: A history of Leichhardt Women's Community Health Centre*, First 10 Years History Project.

Stratigos, Susan (n.d.) *Review of the Prevention of Violence against Women Program*, Typescript.

Stroud, Elizabeth (1989) 'Women's health on the move…again', *Australian Women's Health Network Newsletter*, January–March, p. 3.

Stuart, Lynette (1995) Alukura—an Aboriginal Women's Community-Controlled Health and Birthing Centre, Paper given to the third National Rural Health Conference, 3–5 February, Mt Beauty, Vic.

Summers, Anne (1986) 'Mandarins or missionaries: women in the federal bureaucracy', in Grieve, Norma and Burns, Alisa (eds), *Australian Women*, Oxford University Press, Melbourne.

Summers, Anne (1999) *Ducks on the Pond*, Penguin Books, Ringwood, Vic.

Summers, John (2006) 'The federal system', in Parkin, Andrew, Summers, John and Woodward, Dennis (eds), *Government, Politics, Power and Policy in Australia*, [Eighth edn], Pearson, Frenchs Forest, NSW, pp. 135–59.

Support Services in Australia, Office for Women and WESNET, Canberra, <http://wesnet.org.au/files/0511EAOOW_report.pdf>

Szoke, Helen (1988) 'Federal health budget: rhetoric but no dollars', *Health Issues*, 16 (December).

Taft, Angela (1999) 'The Osland "family" doctor', *Women against Violence: An Australian Feminist Journal*, 6 (July), pp. 64–6.

Taft, Angela, Watson, Lyn and Lee, Christina (2003) 'Health and experience of violence amongst young Australian women', *The Australian Longitudinal Study on Women's Health*, <www.newcastle.edu.a new/centre/wha>

Tarrow, Sydney (1996) *Power in Movement: Social movements, collective action and politics*, Cambridge University Press, Cambridge.

Tassie, Jane (1997) 'Home-based workers at risk: outworkers and occupational health and safety', *Safety Science*, 25:1–3, pp. 179–86.

Taylor, Jean (2003) Untitled story on Women's Web, Women's Stories—Women's Actions, Victorian Honour Roll of Women, Biographies, <http://home.vicnet.net.au/~womenweb/sources/Later%20Stories/Jean%20Taylor.htm>

Taylor, Malcolm (1979) *Health Insurance and Canadian Public Policy*, McGill-Queens University Press, Montreal.

The Australian Women's Register, Working Women's Centre at Melbourne (1975–84), <http://www.womenaustralia.info/biogs/AWE0012b.htm>

The Commonwealth Fund (2010) *In the Literature: Highlights from Commonwealth Fund supported studies in professional journals*, <http://www.commonwealthfund.org/Content/Publications/In-the-Literature/2010/Nov/How-Health-Insurance-Design-Access-Care-Costs.aspx>

Thomas, Carol and Selfe, Joanne (1992) 'Aboriginal women and the law', in McKillop, Sandra (ed.), *Aboriginal Justice Issues*, Australian Institute of Criminology Conference Proceedings, 23–25 June, Brisbane, <http://www.aic.gov.au/publications/previous%20series/proceedings/1-27/21.aspx>

Thornton, Margaret (1984) 'The legitimation of sexual harassment', *Scarlet Woman*, 18, pp. 2–5.

Tilley, Christine (2000) 'The contributions of the Australian Government in meeting the health needs of Queensland women with physical disabilities', *Sexuality and Disability*, 18:1, pp. 61–71.

Torpey, Janet, Linm, Cassio and Glass, Richard (2003) 'Men and women *are* different', *Journal of the American Medical Association*, 289:4, p. 510.

Townsend, Lynn (1994) *Establishment of Women's Emergency Services Network, WESNET (Inc.)*, Report to the WESNET Steering Committee.

Ussher, Jane (1991) *Women's Madness: Misogyny or mental illness?*, Harvester Wheatsheaf, New York.

Valencia, Carolina (2007) *Migrant and refugee women's health project*, Report 2006/2007, Hobart Women's Health Centre.

van Kesteren, John, Mayhew, Pat and Nieuwbeerta, Paul (2000) *Criminal Victimisation in Seventeen Industrialised Countries: Key findings from the 2000 International Crime Victims Survey*, Ministry of Justice, No. 187, The Hague.

Vernon, Barbara (2011) 'The right to be a midwife', *Health Issues*, Summer, pp. 35–8.

VicHealth (2004) *The Health Costs of Violence: Measuring the burden of disease caused by intimate partner violence*, Department of Human Services, Melbourne, <http://www.vichealth.vic.gov.au/~/media/ResourceCentre/ PublicationsandResources/Mental%20health/IPV%20BOD%20web%20 version.ashx>

VicHealth (2009) *National Survey on Community Attitudes to Violence against Women 2009*, Melbourne.

VicHealth (2010) *National Survey on Community Attitudes to Violence against Women 2009*, <http://www.vichealth.vic.gov.au/en/Publications/Freedom- from-violence/National-Community-Attitudes-towards-Violence-Against- Women-Survey-2009.aspx>

VicHealth (n.d.[a]) *Partnerships*, <http://www.vichealth.vic.gov.au/~/media/ About%20Us/Attachments/Fact20SheetPartnerships1.ashx>, accessed 16 August 2011.

VicHealth (n.d.[b]) *ThePartnerships Analysis Tool*, <http://www.vichealth.vic. gov.au/~/media/About%20Us/Attachments/VHP%20part%20toollow%20 res.ashx>, accessed 16 August 2011.

Wainer, Jo (2006) *Lost: Illegal abortion stories*, Melbourne University Press, Carlton, Vic.

Wanada, web site, <http://wanada.org.au/>

Webb, Christine (ed.) (1986) *Feminist Practice in Women's Health Care*, John Wiley, Chichester, UK.

Weeks, Wendy (1994) *Women Working Together*, Longman Cheshire, Melbourne.

Weeks, Wendy (2002) *Cultural diversity and services against sexual violence*, A Report from the National Association of Services against Sexual Violence, CASA House for the NSASAV, Melbourne.

Weeks, Wendy and Gilmour, Kate (1996) 'How violence against women became an issue on the national policy agenda', in Dalton, Tony, Draper, Mary, Weeks, Wendy and Weisman, John (eds), *Making Social Policy in Australia*, Allen & Unwin, St Leonards, NSW.

Weeks, Wendy and Oberin, Julie (2004) *Women's Refuges, Shelters, Outreach and Support Services in Australia: From Sydney squat to complex services challenging domestic and family violence*, An electronic resource.

Weigers, Therese A. (2009) 'The quality of maternity care services as experienced by women in the Netherlands', *BMC Pregnancy and Childbirth*, 9:18, <http://www.ncbi.nlm.nih.gov/pmc/articles/PMC2689853/>, accessed 16 August 2011.

Weisman, Carol S. (1998) *Women's Health Care*, Johns Hopkins University Press, Baltimore and London.

Weiss, Karen (2009) '"Boys will be boys" and other gendered accounts: an exploration of victims' excuses and justification for unwanted sexual contact and coercion', *Women against Violence: An Australian Feminist Journal*, 15:7, pp. 810–34.

Weldon, S. Laurel (2002) *Protest, Policy and the Problem of Violence against Women*, University of Pittsburgh Press, Pittsburgh.

Whittle, Priscilla and Williams, Libby (2001) Improving access and equity in rural and remote Australia—provision of women's health services by female GPs in remote and rural areas, Paper given to the Sixth National Rural Health Conference, 4–7 March, Canberra, <http://nrha.ruralhealth.org.au/conferences/docs/papers/6_C_4_1.pdf>, accessed 16 August 2011.

Wilkinson, Richard and Pickett, Kate (2009) *The Spirit Level: Why more equal societies almost always do better*, Allen Lane, London.

Willcox, Karen (2006) 'Tasmania's Safe at Home: a whole of government response to domestic violence', *Australian Domestic and Family Violence Clearinghouse Newsletter*, 26 (Spring), pp. 5–8.

Willcox, Karen (2008) 'Multiagency responses to domestic violence—from good ideas to good practice', *Australian Domestic and Family Violence Clearinghouse Newsletter*, 33 (Winter), pp. 4–6.

Willis, Evan (1983) *Medical Dominance*, Allen & Unwin, North Sydney.

Women against Rape Collective (n.d. [ca. 1976]) *Herstory of Women against Rape.*

Women in Industry Contraception & Health (1989) *Annual Report*, Carlton, Victoria.

Women's Electoral Lobby New South Wales (WEL NSW) (2005) *The History and Achievements of WEL NSW*, <http://users.comcen.com.au/~welnsw/pages/WELNSW%20HISTORY.pdf>

Women's Emergency Services Network (WESNET), web site, <http://wesnet.org.au/>

Women's Health Information Resource Collective (1987) *Women's Health Information Resource Collective: More than an annual report*, Carlton, Vic.

Women's Health in the North (2009) *New National Women's Health Policy*, July, Submission to the National Women's Health Policy.

Women's Health in the North, web site, <http://www.whin.org.au/>

Women's Health NSW, web site, <http://www.whnsw.asn.au/>

Women's Health Strategy Unit (WHSU) (2003) *Young Women's Sexual Health Project: Evaluation report*, October, Department of Health and Community Services, Darwin.

Women's Health Unit (2003), *Operating Plan 2003–05*, Women's Health Unit, A division of Population Health, Central Sydney Area Health Service.

Women's Health Victoria (WHV) (2010) Women's health advocates call for Australian clinical guidelines to ensure equal representation of women in medical trials, Media release, 10 June.

Women's Health Victoria, web site, <http://whv.org.au/>

Women's Health West, web site, <http://www.whwest.org.au/>

Women's Liberation Halfway House Collective (1977) *Herstory of the Halfway House, 1974–1976*, Melbourne.

Women's Policy Coordination Unit (1987) *Women's Budget Program Victoria*, Department of the Premier and Cabinet, Melbourne.

Women with Disabilities Australia (WWDA), web site, <http://www.wwda.org.au/>

WorkCover Corporation and the Working Women's Centre (2005) *Gender, workplace injury and return to work: a South Australian perspective*, February, Report.

Working Women's Centre (1980) 'Sexual harassment—an industrial responsibility', *Scarlet Woman*, 12, pp. 27–30.

World Health Organisation (WHO) (2003) *The Solid Facts: The social determinants of health*, [Second edn], International Centre for Health and Society, Copenhagen.

World Health Organisation (WHO) (2008a) *Closing the Gap in a Generation: Health equity through action on the social determinants of health*, Commission on the Social Determinants of Health, Geneva.

World Health Organisation (WHO) (2008b) *Now More Than Ever. Primary Health Care: The World Health Report*, World Health Organisation, Geneva.

World Health Organisation (WHO) (2009) *Women and Health: Today's evidence, tomorrow's agenda*, World Health Organisation, Geneva.

Wyndham, Diana (1983) 'He was her medical man, but he done her wrong', *New Doctor* 29/*Social Alternatives* 3:4, pp. 28–31.

Yarrow Place, web site, <http://www.yarrowplace.sa.gov.au>

Yeatman, Anna (1994) 'Women and the state', in Pritchard Hughes, Kate (ed.), *Contemporary Australian Feminism*, Longman Cheshire, Melbourne.

Index

Morand, Maxine, 207

Multicultural Centre for Women's Health, 61, 80, 158, 207, 306

Multicultural Women's Health Centre, 101, 333

Nappaljari Jones, Jilpia, 99

National Aboriginal Community Controlled Health Organisation, 8

National Aboriginal Health Strategy, 248, 253,

National Agenda for Women, 13, 142, 184, 229, 246, 254, 255

National Association of Services against Sexual Assault, 151, 241

National Committee on Violence against Women, 255, 234

National Council to Reduce Violence against Women and their Children, 67, 76, 232, 253, 257, 258, 259, 309, 312, 313, 315, 339, 340

National Disability Strategy, 265

National Domestic Violence Education Campaign, 255, 334

National Health and Hospitals Reform Commission, 309, 316, 319, 320, 321, 340

National Health and Medical Research Council, 34, 185, 268

National Midwives Association, 182

National Network against Trafficking in Women, 138

National Party, 95, 285, 292

National Plan to Reduce Violence against Women and their Children, 258, 309, 313, 340

National Preventive Health Task Force, 172, 322, 339, 340

Nationals, The, 4

National Women's Health Policy, 14–16, 38, 66, 89, 110, 119, 140, 143, 145, 146, 149, 170, 184, 187, 215, 217, 218, 222, 223,

226, 228–230, 245, 248, 249, 253–255, 262, 263, 269, 270, 273, 279, 280, 288–291, 293–295, 298, 300, 311, 314

National Women's Health Program, 80, 90, 105, 108–110, 119, 144, 146, 190, 227, 230, 231, 250, 252, 253, 266, 267, 273, 284, 291, 309

NESB Women's Health Strategy, 254

Nettle, Kerry, 285, 286

New Zealand, 257, 280, 294, 295, 296, 302, 317, 319

Newby, Liza, 38, 140, 226, 246, 247, 334

Ngaanyatjarra Pitjantjatjara Yankunytjatjara Women's Council, 90, 100, 331

non-Labor, 245, 292, 293, 299

NSW Rape Crisis Centre, 240

NSW Women's Health Policy Review Committee, 104

occupational health and safety, 14, 62, 165–170

OECD, 3, 17, 19, 39, 156, 190, 193, 195, 200, 279, 282, 295, 317, 319

Office of Aboriginal and Torres Strait Islander Health, 149

Office of the Status of Women, 142, 148, 247, 255, 257, 289, 334

Older Women's Network, 137

O'Loughlin, Carmel, 230

Operation Pegasus, 134

Osborne, Paul, 204–205

Our Bodies, Ourselves, 29, 82, 328

out-of-pocket expenses, 63, 189, 296

Parish, Jo, 229

Parliamentary Group on Population and Development, 286

Partnerships against Domestic Violence, 78, 256, 257, 260

partnerships, 155–157, 159, 172–4, 219, 234, 256, 265